CONTEMPORARY ENDOCRINOLOGY

Series Editor:
P. Michael Conn, PhD
Oregon Health & Science University
Beaverton, OR

For other titles published in this series, go to
www.springer.com/series/7680

MARCELLO D. BRONSTEIN
Editor

Cushing's Syndrome

Pathophysiology, Diagnosis and Treatment

First Edition

Catalina Norman, MD

Humana Press

Editor
Marcello D. Bronstein
Division of Endocrinology and Metabolism
Hospital das Clínicas
University of Sao Paulo Medical School
Sao Paulo
Brazil
mdbronstein@uol.com.br

ISBN 978-1-60327-448-7 e-ISBN 978-1-60327-449-4
DOI 10.1007/978-1-60327-449-4
Springer New York Dordrecht Heidelberg London

Library of Congress Control Number: 2010937016

Printed on acid-free paper

Humana Press is part of Springer Science+Business Media (www.springer.com)

Preface

I usually say to my residents that when I was a resident myself, I was much more confident at diagnosing and treating Cushing's syndrome than I am today! This statement aims at pointing out that the deeper you go in dealing with clinical, laboratorial, and image aspects of the differential diagnosis of the many etiologies of the syndrome, as well as the various treatment modalities, the more you will encounter cases that are exceptions to the rules, leading to diagnosis and treatment pitfalls. However, notwithstanding that, only insights provided by experts will help physicians dealing with Cushing's syndrome to provide better care to their patients, avoiding the above-mentioned pitfalls.

This medical text, which Humana Press kindly invited me to edit, was initially intended to be a handbook on Cushing's syndrome, giving insights on the various aspects of its diagnosis and treatment to trainee endocrinologists, internists, pediatricians, neurosurgeons, and urologists. Pursuing that task, I invited basic and clinical researchers with great experience in their respective areas, and I was gratified by their agreement to cooperate with the book. However, their chapters were so comprehensive and profound that I ended up with a true textbook on Cushing's syndrome, from the bench to bedside, encompassing molecular, physiological, clinical, and therapeutic aspects of all the many causes of hypercortisolism. As many chapters overlapped on some issues, duplication was inevitable. Nevertheless, I tried to keep the originality of each manuscript as much as possible, also aiming to stress important data for the reader by repeating the arguments under different perspectives.

I am indebted to Humana Press for the opportunity to edit a book with so distinguished a team of collaborators, and extremely grateful to all the colleagues who gave their outstanding knowledge and their time to enrich this work.

Sao Paulo, SP **Marcello D. Bronstein**

Contents

Contributors

DIMA ABDELMANNAN, MD • *Division of Clinical and Molecular Endocrinology, Department of Medicine, Case Western Reserve, University School of Medicine and VA Health Services Research & Development, Center for Quality Improvement Research, Louis Stokes Cleveland VAMC, Cleveland, OH, USA*

FARHAD AFSHAR, MD • *Department of Endocrinology, Barts and the London School of Medicine and Dentistry, John Vane Science Centre, Charterhouse Square, London, UK*

NORA ALBIGER, PhD • *Division of Endocrinology, School of Medicine, University of Padua, via Ospedale 105, 35128 Padua, Italy*

KRYSTALLENIA I. ALEXANDRAKI, MD/PhD/MSC/MSC • *Department of Endocrinology, St. Bartholomew's Hospital, London, UK*

MADSON Q. ALMEIDA, MD • *Unidade de Endocrinologia do Desenvolvimento e Laboratório de Hormônios e Genética Molecular LIM-42, Hospital das Clínicas da Faculdade de Medicina da Universidade de São Paulo, São Paulo, Brasil*

DAVID C. ARON, MD/MS • *Division of Clinical and Molecular Endocrinology, Department of Medicine, Case Western Reserve University, School of Medicine and VA Health Services Research & Development, Center for Quality Improvement Research, Louis Stokes Cleveland VAMC, Cleveland, OH, USA*

GUILLAUME ASSIE • *Service des Maladies Endocriniennes et Métaboliques, Centre de Référence des Maladies Rares de la Surrénale, INSERM U-567, Institut Cochin, Hôpital Cochin, Faculté de Médecine Paris Descartes, Université Paris 5, Paris, France*

ANAT BEN-SHLOMO, MD • *Cedars-Sinai Medical Center, Pituitary center Los Angeles, CA, USA*

XAVIER BERTAGNA, MD • *Service des Maladies Endocriniennes et Métaboliques, Centre de Référence des Maladies Rares de la Surrénale, INSERM U-567, Institut Cochin, Hôpital Cochin, Faculté de Médecine Paris Descartes, Université Paris 5, Paris, France*

JÉRÔME BERTHERAT • *Service des Maladies Endocriniennes et Métaboliques, Centre de Référence des Maladies Rares de la Surrénale, INSERM U-567, Institut Cochin, Hôpital Cochin, Faculté de Médecine Paris Descartes, Université Paris 5, 27, rue Fg St Jacques 75014, Paris, France*

ISABELLE BOURDEAU, MD • *Division of Endocrinology, Department of Medicine, Centre hospitalier de l'Université de Montréal (CHUM), Montréal, Canada*

MARCELLO D. BRONSTEIN, MD • *Division of Endocrinology and Metabolism, Hospital das Clinicas, University of São Paulo Medical School, São Paulo, Brasil*

OSCAR D. BRUNO, MD • *Consultant Professor of Medicine, Hospital de Clínicas, University of Buenos Aires, Buenos Aires, Argentina*

MARGARET CASTRO, MD • *Professor of Endocrinology, Department of Internal Medicine, University of Sao Paulo at Ribeirao Preto, São Paulo, Brasil*

FRANCESCO CAVAGNINI, MD • *Chair of Endocrinology, Ospedale San Luca, Istituto Auxologico Italiano IRCCS, Università di Milano, Via Spagnoletto 3, Milano 20149, Milan, Italy*

MARTINA DE MARTIN, MD • *Chair of Endocrinology, Ospedale San Luca, Istituto Auxologico Italiano IRCCS, Università di Milano, Milan, Italy*

RENUKA P. DIAS, MD • *Department of Endocrinology, Barts and the London School of Medicine and Dentistry, John Vane Science Centre, Charterhouse Square, London, UK*

SORAHIA DOMENICE, MD • *Laboratório de Hormônios e Genética, Faculdade de Medicina da Universidade de São Paulo, Unidade de Endocrinologia do Desenvolvimento da, Hospital das Clínicas, Molecular LIM/42, São Paulo, Brasil*

IAN F. DUNN, MD • *Clinical Instructor in Surgery, Neurosurgery Department, Brigham & Women's Hospital, Boston, MA 02115, USA*

LUCILA LEICO KAGOHARA ELIAS, MD/PhD • *Associated Professor of Physiology, Department of Physiology, University of São Paulo at Ribeirao Preto, São Paulo, Brasil*

PAULA CONDE LAMPARELLI ELIAS, MD • *Assistant Physician of Endocrinology, Department of Internal Medicine, University of Sao Paulo at Ribeirao Preto, São Paulo, Brasil*

RICHARD A. FEELDERS, MD • *Department of Internal Medicine, Sector of Endocrinology, Erasmus MC, 's Gravendijkwal 230, 3015 CE Rotterdam, The Netherlands*

JAMES W. FINDLING, MD • *Professor of Clinical Medicine, Director of Community Endocrine Services, Department of Medicine, Endocrinology Center, Medical College of Wisconsin, Menomonee Falls, WI, USA*

MARIA CANDIDA BARISSON VILLARES FRAGOSO, MD • *Laboratório de Hormônios e Genética Molecular LIM/42, Unidade de Endocrinologia do Desenvolvimento da Faculdade de Medicina da Universidade de São Paulo, São Paulo, Brasil*

FRANCESCA PECORI GIRALDI, MD • *Chair of Endocrinology, Ospedale San Luca, Istituto Auxologico Italiano, Università di Milano, Milan, Italy*

ASHLEY B. GROSSMAN, MD/BA/BSC/FRCP/FMEDSCI • *Department of Endocrinology, Barts and the London School of Medicine and Dentistry, John Vane Science Centre, Charterhouse Square, London, UK*

LAURENCE GUIGNAT • *Service des Maladies Endocriniennes et Métaboliques, Faculté de Médecine Centre de Référence des Maladies Rares de la Surrénale, INSERM U-567, Institut Cochin, Hôpital Cochin, Paris Descartes, Université Paris 5, Paris, France*

WOUTER W. DE HERDER, MD/PhD • *Department of Internal Medicine, Sector of Endocrinology, Erasmus MC, 's Gravendijkwal 230, 3015 CE Rotterdam, The Netherlands*

ANDREA M. ISIDORI, MD • *Department of Endocrinology, St. Bartholomew's Hospital, London, UK*

JAY JAGANNATHAN, MD • *Department of Neurological Surgery, University of Virginia Health Sciences Center, Charlottesville, VA, USA*

BRADLEY R. JAVORSKY, MD • *Assistant Professor of Medicine, Department of Medicine, Endocrinology Center, Medical College of Wisconsin, Building A, Suite 203, Menomonee Falls, WI 53051, USA*

NIKI KARAVITAKI, MD • *Department of Endocrinology, Oxford Centre for Diabetes, Endocrinology and Metabolism, Churchill Hospital, Oxford, 0X37LJ, UK*

SIBYLLE KOHLER, MD • *Department of Endocrinology, Oxford Centre for Diabetes, Endocrinology and Metabolism, Churchill Hospital, Oxford, 0X37LJ, UK*

ANDRÉ LACROIX, MD • *Professor of Medicine, Division of Endocrinology, Department of Medicine, Centre hospitalier de l'Université de Montréal (CHUM), Montréal, Canada*

STEVEN W.J. LAMBERTS MD/PhD • *Erasmus MC University Medical Center, Department of Internal Medicine, 's-Gravendijkwal 230, 3015 CE Rotterdam, The Netherlands*

ANTOINE LAMPRON, MD • *Division of Endocrinology, Department of Medicine, Centre hospitalier de l'Université de Montréal (CHUM), Montréal, Canada*

ANA CLAUDIA LATRONICO • *Associate Professor of Medicine, Unidade de Endocrinologia do Desenvolvimento e Laboratório de Hormônios e Genética Molecular LIM/42, Hospital das Clínicas, da Faculdade de Medicina da Universidade de São Paulo, Av. Dr. Enéas de carvelho Aguiar, 155, 2 andar Bloco 6, São Paulo, Brasil*

EDWARD R. LAWS, JR, MD • *Department of Neurological Surgery, Brigham & Women's Hospital, Boston, MA, USA*

ANTONIO M. LERÁRIO, MD • *Division of Endocrinology and Metabolism, Hospital das Clinicas, University of São Paulo Medical School, São Paulo, Brasil*

NING-AI LIU, MD • *Cedars-Sinai Medical Center, 8700 Beverly Blvd., Room 2015 Pituitary center, Los Angeles, CA, USA*

FRANCO MANTERO, MD • *Division of Endocrinology, School of Medicine, University of Padua, via Ospedale 105, 35128 Padua, Italy*

TÂNIA LONGO MAZZUCO, MD • *Division of Endocrinology, Department of Medicine, Centre hospitalier de l'Université de Montréal (CHUM), Montréal, Canada*

SHLOMO MELMED, MD • *Cedars-Sinai Medical Center, 8700 Beverly Blvd., Room 2015 Pituitary center, Los Angeles, CA, USA*

BERENICE BILHARINHO MENDONCA, MD • *Unidade de Endocrinologia do Desenvolvimento da Faculdade de Medicina Laboratório de Hormônios e Genética Molecular LIM/42, Hospital das Clínicas, da Universidade de São Paulo, São Paulo, Brasil*

AYRTON CUSTODIO MOREIRA, MD/PhD • *Professor of Endocrinology, Department of Internal Medicine, University of São Paulo at Ribeirao Preto, São Paulo, Brasil*

JOHN NEWELL-PRICE MA/PhD/FRCP • *Reader and Consultant Endocrinologist, Academic Unit of Diabetes and Endocrinology, Royal Hallamshire Hospital, Room 0U142, Floor O, University of Sheffield, Sheffield, UK*

EMILIA M. PINTO, MD • *Unidade de Endocrinologia do Desenvolvimento e Laboratório de Hormônios e Genética Molecular LIM-42, Hospital das Clínicas da Faculdade de Medicina da Universidade de São Paulo, São Paulo, Brasil*

NICHOLAS P. PLOWMAN, MD • *Department of Endocrinology, Barts and the London School of Medicine and Dentistry, John Vane Science Centre, Charterhouse Square, London, UK*

ELISABETH F.C. VAN ROSSUM, MD/PhD • *Erasmus MC University Medical Center, Department of Internal Medicine, 's-Gravendijkwal 230, 3015 CE Rotterdam, The Netherlands*

MARTIN O. SAVAGE, MD • *Department of Endocrinology, Barts and the London School of Medicine and Dentistry, John Vane Science Centre, Charterhouse Square, London, UK*

JASON P. SHEEHAN, MD/PhD • *Assistant Professor of Neurological Surgery and Radiation Oncology, Department of Neurological Surgery, University of Virginia Health Sciences Center, Charlottesville, VA, USA*

HELEN L. STORR, MD • *Department of Endocrinology, Barts and the London School of Medicine and Dentistry, John Vane Science Centre, Charterhouse Square, London, UK*

CONSTANTINE STRATAKIS, MD/D(MED)SCI • *Section on Endocrinology, Genetics (SEGEN), Program on Developmental Endocrinology & Genetics (PDEGEN), National Institute of Child Health and Human Development (NICHD), National Institutes of Health, Bethesda, MD, USA*

GEOFFREY B. THOMPSON, MD • *Division of Gastroenterologic and General Surgery, Mayo Clinic, Rochester, MN, USA*

PETER J. TRAINER, MD/FRCP • *Professor, Department of Endocrinology, The Christie NHS Foundation Trust, Wilmslow Road, Manchester, UK*

JOHN A.H. WASS, MD • *Department of Endocrinology, Oxford Centre for Diabetes, Endocrinology and Metabolism, Churchill Hospital, Oxford, OX3 7LJ, UK*

WILLIAM F. YOUNG, JR., MD/MSC • *Divisions of Endocrinology, Diabetes, Metabolism, Nutrition and Internal Medicine, Mayo Clinic, Rochester, MN, USA*

1 Physiology and Pathophysiology of the HPA Axis

Margaret Castro, Lucila Leico Elias, Paula Conde Lamparelli Elias, and Ayrton Custodio Moreira

Contents

Summary

The corticotrophin releasing hormone (CRH), the main hypothalamic regulator of adrenocorticotropic hormone (ACTH) secretion, is mainly synthesized in the parvocellular, but also in the magnocellular neurons, of the paraventricular nucleus (PVN). CRH neurons of the PVN receive adrenergic afferent from nucleus tractus solitarius, *locus coeruleus*, and ventro-lateral medulla. CRH is secreted into the hypophyseal portal blood and binds to high affinity membrane type I CRH receptors (CRH-R1) in the anterior pituitary corticotrophs to stimulate pro-opiomelanocortin (POMC) gene transcription through a process that includes the activation of adenylyl cyclase. The CRH stimulates POMC gene transcription in vivo and in vitro and also in response to stress and adrenalectomy. ACTH, synthesized within the anterior pituitary as part of a large POMC 241-amino-acid precursor, is the principal hormone stimulating adrenal glucocorticoid biosynthesis and secretion. Angiotensin II, activin, inhibin, and cytokines (TNF-β and leptin) synergize with or inhibit the effects of ACTH on the adrenal cortex. The hypothalamic pituitary adrenal (HPA) axis is also regulated by biological rhythms resulting from a complex interaction of genetic output of the endogenous circadian pacemaker and environmental synchronizers. ACTH is secreted in a pulsatile pattern with a circadian rhythm so that levels are the highest on waking and decline throughout the day, reaching the nadir values in the evening.

From: *Contemporary Endocrinology: Cushing's Syndrome: Pathophysiology, Diagnosis and Treatment*
Edited by: M.D. Bronstein (ed.), DOI 10.1007/978-1-60327-449-4_1,

Other regulator of the HPA axis is the stress system, which has main components the CRH and locus coeruleus-norepinephrine autonomic systems and their peripheral effectors. Basal and stress induced activity of the HPA axis is constrained by glucocorticoid negative feedback. Glucocorticoids and catecholamines affect major immune functions such as antigen presentation, leukocyte proliferation and traffic, secretion of cytokines and antibodies, and selection of the T helper (Th) 1 versus Th2 responses. The proinflammatory cytokines, notably interleukin-1, interleukin-6, tumor necrosis factor β, and leukemia inhibitory factor also increase ACTH secretion either directly or by augmenting the effect of CRF. Glucocorticoids exert an immunoregulatory feedback by several mechanisms, involving the blockade of lymphocyte activation, the production and action of IL-2, IL-1, γ-interferon, TNF, and prostaglandins. Another important aspect of the regulation of the HPA axis is the negative feedback control exerted by glucocorticoid, which inhibits the basal expression of CRH and AVP mRNA synthesis and secretion in the hypothalamus and also inhibits POMC gene transcription in the anterior pituitary. Glucocorticoid exerts its effects by activation of cytosolic receptors that belong to the nuclear receptor superfamily, the corticosteroid type I, or mineralocorticoid, and corticosteroid type II, or glucocorticoid, receptors. Several molecular mechanisms underlying glucocorticoid actions have been elucidated, most of which involve transcriptional regulation of gene expression. One of the most important factors regulating the access of endogenous glucocorticoid to its receptor is local metabolism of the steroids within the target cells by 11β-hydroxysteroid dehydrogenase (11β-HSD) enzymes, a phenomenon sometimes termed prereceptor metabolism. Cortisol/corticosterone are responsible for the salt and water homeostasis and blood pressure control and influence carbohydrate, protein, lipid, and bone metabolism. They are also important regulators of immune and inflammatory processes and are required for numerous processes associated with host defense. On the other hand, prolonged or high dose glucocorticoid therapy as well as an excess of endogenous production of glucocorticoids exert a large spectrum of deleterious actions in the whole body. Our understanding on the HPA axis biology has given significant insight into the critical role of glucocorticoids in the maintenance of homeostasis and, when dysregulated, in the pathogenesis of diseases.

Key Words: Hypothalamic-pituitary-adrenal-axis, stress response, cortisol circadian rhythm, glucocorticoid feedback, pathophysiology

NEUROENDOCRINE CONTROL OF THE HYPOTHALAMO-PITUITARY-ADRENAL AXIS

The corticotrophin releasing hormone (CRH) is the main hypothalamic regulator of the ACTH secretion *(1–3)*. CRH belongs to a family of related peptides which includes, besides CRH, sauvagine, urotensin, and the urocortin. These peptides, which possess 20–45% homology in their amino acid sequence, show in some species a role in the osmoregulation, behavior, appetite, inflammation, and cardiovascular adaptations to stress *(4, 5)*. CRH synthesis occurs mainly in the parvocellular neurons of the PVN. Immunolocalization of CRH was also observed in magnocellular neurons of the PVN, in the preoptical area and dorsal medial nucleus of the hypothalamus *(6)*. CRH neurons of the PVN receive adrenergic efferent from nucleus tractus solitarius, *locus ceruleus* and ventro-lateral medulla. In the hypothalamus, CRH co-localizes with vasopressin (AVP), cholecystokinin, encephalin, vasoactive peptides, neurotensin, and angiotensin II *(7)*. The physiological meaning of the CRH co-localization with other neuropeptides has not been completely established, but these peptides seem to act synergically to modulate CRH effects on ACTH secretion from corticotrophs. The expression of CRH in the hypothalamus is under influence of diverse factors such as catecholamines, serotonin, acetylcholine, cytokines (IL-1 and IL-6), gamma aminobutyric acid, and glucocorticoids (Fig. 1) *(8, 9)*.

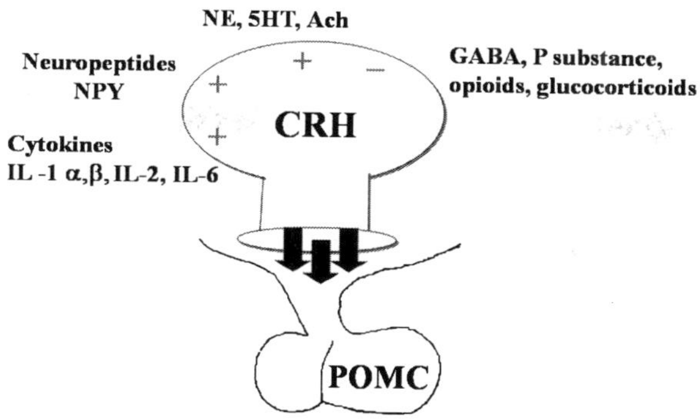

Fig. 1. Regulation of corticotrophin releasing hormone (CRH) synthesis and secretion in the parvocellular neuron of the hypothalamic paraventricular nucleus. CRH secretion is influenced by diverse factors such as catecholamines (NE), serotonin (5HT), acetylcholine (Ach), cytokines (IL-1 and IL-6), gamma aminobutyric acid (GABA), neuropeptide Y (NPY), P substance, opioids, and glucocorticoids.

CRH is also synthesized in extra-hypothalamic areas, such as cerebral cortex, limbic system, *locus coeruleus*, cerebellum, and brain stem, as well as in peripheral tissues, such as gastrointestinal tract, adrenal medulla, testis, and immune cells *(10–12)*In placenta, there is an increased secretion during pregnancy resulting in a threefold increase in circulating CRH levels. It is likely that circulating CRH reflects its synthesis in peripheral tissues *(13)*.

The CRH is secreted into the hypophyseal portal blood, where it binds to high affinity membrane type I CRH receptors (CRH-R1) in the anterior pituitary corticotrophs *(14)* to stimulate pro-opiomelanocortin (POMC) gene transcription through a process that includes the activation of adenylyl cyclase (Fig. 2) *(15, 16)*. The CRH stimulates POMC gene transcription in vivo and in vitro *(17)*, and it is also the main mediator of POMC gene transcription in response to stress and adrenalectomy *(18)*. Plasma ACTH levels present a biphasic pattern of response postsynthetic ovine corticotropin-releasing factor (oCRH) stimulus. It is characterized by a rapid increase after 15min followed by a gradual decline until 90min, then presenting a second peak 2–3h after the stimulus *(19)*. The peak ACTH response to CRH does not differ throughout the day, but it is affected by endogenous function of the hypothalamus-pituitary-adrenal (HPA) axis and its responsiveness is reduced in subjects treated with corticosteroids but increased in subjects with Cushing's disease. In the circulation, CRH is bound to CRH-binding protein and determines the availability of free CRH to its target tissues *(15–17)*. Increased levels of CRH as well as increased levels of CRH-binding protein levels are observed during pregnancy and due to this balance, cortisol secretion is not markedly elevated in pregnancy *(20)*.

ACTH is the principal hormone stimulating adrenal glucocorticoid biosynthesis and secretion. ACTH has 39 amino acids but is synthesized within the anterior pituitary as part of a large POMC 241-amino-acid precursor. Two different cell lines express POMC, the melanotroph cells in the intermediate lobe (vestigial in human) and the corticotroph cells in the anterior lobe of pituitary *(21)*. The ACTH synthesis requires a coordinate action of multiple transcription factors (TFs), which act in specific regions of each gene. The *pituitary cell-restricted T box factor* (Tpit) is exclusively expressed in corticotrophs and melanotrophs. Tpit was identified as an specific factor for corticotroph differentiation and fundamental to pituitary POMC expression *(22)*. The POMC expression is under regulation of many different factors, such as CRH, glucocorticoids, and leukemia inhibitor factor (LIF). LIF stimulates the promoter region of the *POMC* gene acting on STAT 1 and STAT 3 (*signal transducer and activator of transcription*) *(23)*. The activation of *POMC* gene expression by CRH can also be modulated by the nurr1/nur77, a member of the subfamily of nuclear receptors *(24)*.

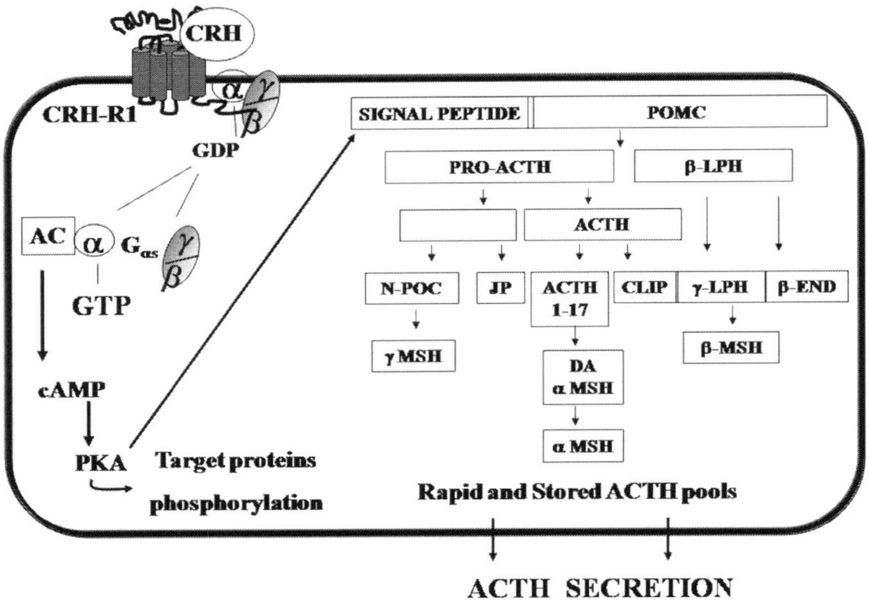

Fig. 2. Intracellular regulation of ACTH secretion. CRH binds to high affinity membrane type I CRH receptors (CRH-R1) in the anterior pituitary corticotrophs to stimulate pro-opiomelanocortin (POMC) gene transcription through a process that includes the activation of adenylyl cyclase (AC) and protein kinase A (PKA). In the anterior pituitary, POMC is cleaved by pro-hormone convertase (PC)1 to generate β-lipoprotein (β-LPH) and pro-ACTH. The latter is further cleaved to an N-terminal peptide (N-POC), 16-kDa joining peptide (JP), and ACTH. In the intermediate lobe of the pituitary and in the hypothalamus, where both PC1 and PC2 are expressed, the cleavage of POMC results in the secretion of melanocyte stimulate hormone (γ-MSH and α-MSH), corticotrophin-like intermediate lobe peptide (CLIP), β-MSH, and β-endorphin.

The POMC is cleaved in a tissue-specific pattern to generate smaller peptide hormones by prohormone convertase 1 and 2 (PC1 and PC2). In the anterior pituitary, POMC is cleaved by PC1 to generate β-lipoprotein and pro-ACTH, the latter is further cleaved to an N-terminal peptide, 16-kDa joining peptide, and ACTH *(25)*. The functions of the N-terminal peptide and β-lipoprotein are unknown, although they have weak steroidogenic activity and may augment the effect of ACTH on stimulating adrenal growth. The first 24 amino acids of ACTH are common to all species. Synthetic ACTH 1–24 (Synacthen) is commercially available for clinical testing of HPA axis and assessment of adrenal function. In the intermediate lobe of the pituitary and in the hypothalamus, where either PC1 and PC2 are expressed, the cleavage of POMC results in γ-MSH, α-MSH, CLIP (corticorophin-like intermediate lobe peptide), β-MSH, and β-endorphin *(26)*. The increased pigmentation characteristic of Addison's disease is related to increased ACTH binding to the melanocortin-1 receptor in the skin, rather than the result of increased α-MSH secretion (Fig. 2) *(27)*.

Angiotensin II, activin, inhibin, and cytokines (TNF-β and leptin) synergize with or inhibit the effects of ACTH on the adrenal cortex *(28–30)*. Acutely, steroidogenesis is stimulated through a StAR-mediated increase in cholesterol delivery to the CYP11A1 enzyme in the inner mitochondrial membrane *(31)*. Chronically (after 24–26h of exposure), ACTH acts to increase the synthesis of all steroidogenic CYP enzymes and adrenodoxin *(32)*, and such effects are mediated at the transcriptional level. ACTH also increases synthesis of LDL and HDL receptors and possibly also 3-hydroxy-3-methylglutaryl coenzyme A reductase, the rate-limiting step in cholesterol biosynthesis. ACTH increases adrenal weight by inducing both hyperplasia and hypertrophy. Adrenal atrophy is a feature of ACTH deficiency.

CIRCADIAN RHYTHM

The ACTH-corticosteroid rhythm is an endogenous rhythm regulated by the brain-adrenal neurohumoral circuit. The biological rhythms result from a complex interaction of genetic output of the endogenous circadian pacemaker and environmental synchronizers. Several clock genes and their cognate proteins have been described and create molecular cycles that approximate the 24-h environmental cycle *(33)*. The ontogenetic changes in the development of cortisol circadian rhythm may reflect prenatal and postnatal concurrent maturation of the suprachiasmatic nucleus and its specific neuroanatomical pathways (Fig. 3a). The circadian system seems to be functional in late fetal life. The main synchronizing factors of the fetal circadian cycles are received from maternal circadian inputs *(34, 35)*. The major postnatal action of the environment is to synchronize the circadian rhythms by periodic factors, such as light–dark, rest–activity and sleep–wake cycles, food ingestion, and social cues *(35–37)*. In human, the cortisol circadian rhythm emerged at a mean age of 8 postnatal weeks, suggesting that, in most normal infants, the development of HPA axis circadian maturation may occur at a much earlier age than previously described *(37)*. However, the effects of these synchronizers on circadian rhythm are superimposed by inherited characteristics of ACTH/glucocorticoid regulation. ACTH is secreted in a pulsatile pattern with a circadian rhythm so that levels are highest on waking and decline throughout the day, reaching nadir values in the evening (Fig. 3b) *(38)*. ACTH pulse frequency is higher in normal adult men than in women. The circadian ACTH rhythm appears to be mediated mainly by an increased ACTH pulse amplitude between 5 and 9a.m. but also by a reduction in ACTH pulse frequency between 6 and 12p.m. *(39, 40)*. Circadian rhythm can be disrupted by day–night shift working patterns and by long-distance travel across time zones *(41)*. In these conditions, it may take up to two weeks for circadian rhythm to reset to a new day–night cycle. Endogenous causes

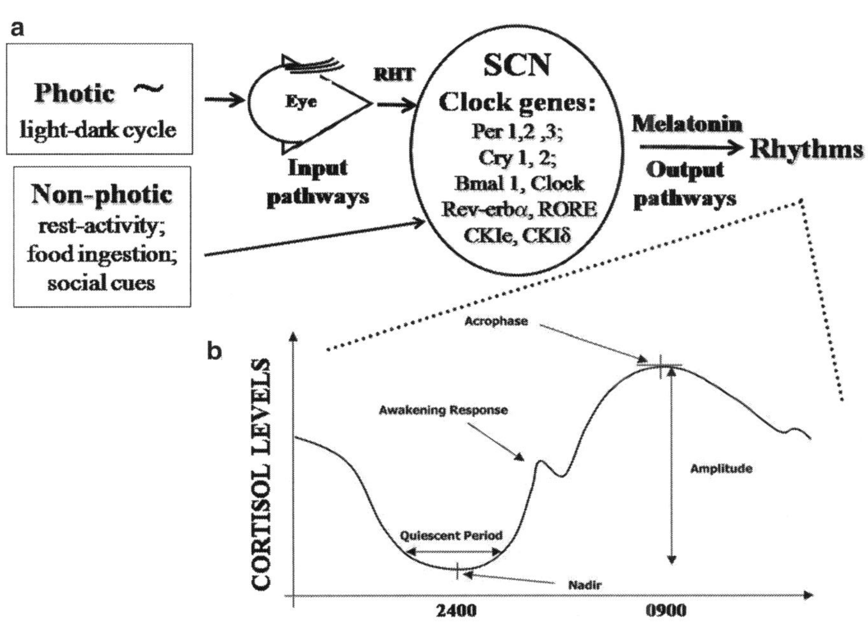

Fig. 3. (**a**) Schematic representation of the environmental input pathways (photic and nonphotic stimulus) to suprachiasmatic nucleus (SCN), where they synchronize clock genes: Period (Per 1,2,3), Cryptochrome (Cry 1,2), Bmal 1, Clock Orphan nuclear receptors (Rev-erbα and RORE), casein kinase I epsilon or delta (CKIe,CKIδ) genes. Interaction between environment and genes results in output pathways to coordinate biological rhythms, including cortisol circadian rhythm (**b**). *RHT* retino-hypothalamic tract.

of Cushing's syndrome result in loss of normal feedback mechanism of the HPA axis and circadian rhythm of cortisol secretion. Therefore, cortisol measurement at midnight has been demonstrated to be a sensitive test for screening Cushing's syndrome in adults and children *(42–45)*.

THE STRESS RESPONSE AND IMMUNE-ENDOCRINE AXIS

The main components of the stress system are CRH and locus ceruleus–norepinephrine autonomic systems and their peripheral effectors, the HPA axis and the autonomic system (Fig. 4). Activation of the HPA axis by stress is an important regulatory mechanism in most mammals to maintain homeostasis after multiple types of challenges. Conversely, basal and stress induced activity of the HPA axis is constrained by glucocorticoid negative feedback *(46, 47)*. In response to stressors, the HPA axis is driven by CRH, the primary ACTH secretagogue and a tonic facilitator during stress, and AVP and oxytocin (OT), weaker secretagogues of ACTH, from the PVN. These neuropeptides induce ACTH release from the anterior pituitary, which in turn stimulates the release of glucocorticoid from the adrenals *(44)*. In the short term, this response allows the animal to cope with the immediate demands imposed by the stressful event. However, longer or more chronic exposures to stress hormones can result in a number of negative effects, particularly in regard to neurobiological function *(48)*. Throughout an individual's lifespan, both the magnitude and duration of the hormonal stress response change dramatically. Neonates show reduced stress reactivity in response to stressors that typically elicit robust stress responses in adults *(49)*. Conversely, aged adults show heightened and more prolonged stress responses compared to younger adults *(50)*.

Several stress paradigms, including fever, surgery, burn injury, hypoglycemia, hypotension, and exercise increase ACTH and cortisol secretion mediated by CRH and AVP stimulation *(51–54)*. Acute psychological stress raises cortisol levels, but secretion rate appears to be normal in patients

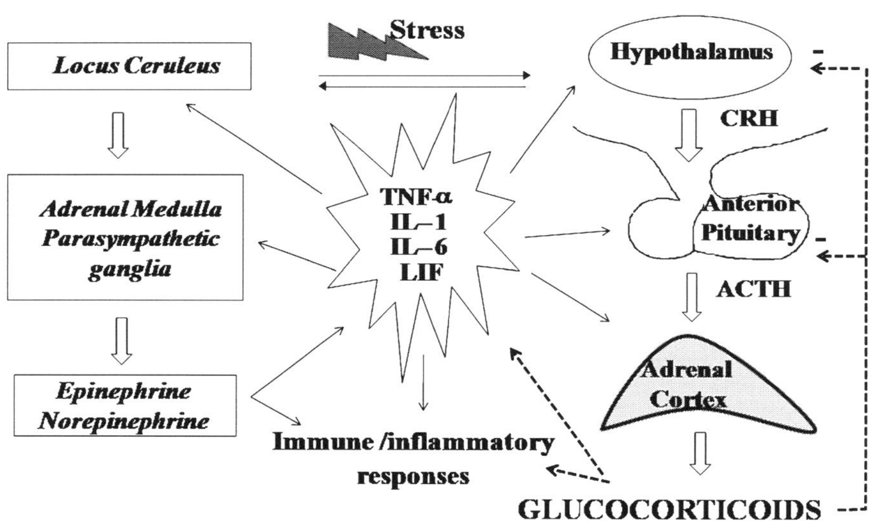

Fig. 4. The main components of the stress system are hypothalamic CRH and locus coeruleus–norepinephrine autonomic systems and their peripheral effectors. Glucocorticoids and catecholamines affect major immune/inflammatory functions. The proinflammatory cytokines, notably interleukin-1 (IL-1), interleukin-6 (IL-6), tumor necrosis factor (TNF-α), and leukemia inhibitory factor (LIF) also increase ACTH secretion either directly or by augmenting CRH secretion. Besides their negative feedback inhibition of HPA axis, glucocorticoids also exert an immunoregulatory feedback.

with chronic anxiety and underlying psychotic illness. However, depression is associated with high circulating cortisol concentrations, and this an important differential diagnosis of Cushing's syndrome *(55–57)*. Experience with stressors can also influence stress reactivity. For instance, in adults, repeated exposure to a stressor leads to habituation of the stress response, such that stress hormone levels are blunted *(58–60)*.

Stress alters the secretion of the hypothalamic factors and the type of stressor determines the role of these secretagogues in the ACTH response. CRH not only activates the HPA axis but also sets in motion a coordinated series of behavioral and physiologic responses, suggesting that the central nervous system may coordinate both behavioral and immunologic adaptation during stressful situations *(61)*. The principal stress hormones glucocorticoids and catecholamines affect major immune functions, such as antigen presentation, leukocyte proliferation and traffic, secretion of cytokines and antibodies, and selection of the T helper (Th) 1 versus Th2 responses *(62)*. The proinflammatory cytokines, notably interleukin-1, interleukin-6, and tumor necrosis factor (TNF) β, also increase ACTH secretion either directly or by augmenting the effect of CRF *(63, 64)*. Leukemia inhibitory factor, a cytokine of the interleukin-6 family, is a further activator of the HPA axis *(65)*. Besides the glucocorticoid negative feedback in the HPA axis, glucocorticoids also exert an immunoregulatory feedback by several mechanisms involving the blockage of lymphocyte activation, the production and action of IL-2, IL-1, γ-interferon, TNF, and prostaglandins (Fig. 4) *(66)*.

NEGATIVE FEEDBACK CONTROL

An important aspect of CRH and ACTH secretion is the negative feedback control exerted by glucocorticoids *(29)*. The basal expression of CRH and AVP mRNA synthesis and secretion in the hypothalamus are under the inhibitory control of glucocorticoids *(9, 67)*. Glucocorticoids inhibit *POMC* gene transcription in the anterior pituitary, directly or indirectly, by rapid (minutes) and delayed (hours) mechanisms *(9, 47)*. The rapid feedback negative mechanism involves the inhibition of stimulated ACTH and CRH secretion and seems to be dependent on nitric oxide release *(68)* and also appears to be mediated by the glucocorticoid induced synthesis and release of endogenous cannabinoids *(69, 70)*. In addition, studies conducted in different species suggest that the rapid effects of glucocorticoids are mediated, or at least dependent on membrane-associated G protein-coupled receptors and activation of downstream signaling cascades. The membrane-initiated actions of glucocorticoids may also provide an additional mechanism for the regulation of gene transcription *(71)*. The delayed feedback negative mechanism involves ACTH release (45–120min after glucocorticoid exposure) and later ACTH synthesis. CRH secretion and synthesis are both affected by intermediate and delayed feedback negative mechanism. The delayed glucocorticoid actions are mediated, mainly, by activation of known cytosolic receptors that belong to the nuclear receptor superfamily, the corticosteroid type I, or mineralocorticoid, and corticosteroid type II, or glucocorticoid, receptors (Fig. 5a) *(71)*. The negative feedback effect is dependent upon the dose, potency, half-life, and duration of administration of glucocorticoid and has important physiologic and diagnostic consequences. Suppression of the HPA axis by pharmacologic corticosteroids may persist for many months after cessation of therapy, and adrenocortical insufficiency should be anticipated. The withdrawal of feedback mechanism in Addison's disease explains ACTH hypersecretion, whereas the autonomous production explains the undetectable ACTH levels in patients with cortisol-secreting adrenal adenoma. The negative feedback control of ACTH secretion in Cushing's disease is reset at higher level than normal. Thus, cortisol levels in Cushing's disease do not suppress with low-dose, but do so following high-dose of dexamethasone *(73)*.

CORTICOSTEROID HORMONE ACTION

In the brain and pituitary, glucocorticoid binds to high affinity type I corticosteroid receptors and also to lower affinity type II receptors *(72)*. Type I receptor is expressed in restricted brain areas, such as limbic system and brain stem. On the other hand, type II receptor is largely expressed in the brain: in the limbic system, cerebral cortex, PVN, as well as in other hypothalamic nuclei. Type I receptor is saturated with low glucocorticoid concentration, while type II receptor requires high concentrations and are saturated during the circadian rhythm peak and also in response to elevated glucocorticoid secretion during stress. Therefore, type I receptor might be involved in the control of basal activity of the HPA axis and type II receptor in the stress HPA response *(46)*. The hippocampus presents both type I and II receptors, and is involved in the circadian rhythm of the HPA axis, activation of stress response, and glucocorticoid negative feedback *(74)*.

Several molecular mechanisms underlying glucocorticoid actions have been elucidated, most of which involve transcriptional regulation of gene expression (Fig. 5b). Glucocorticoid receptor (GR) not

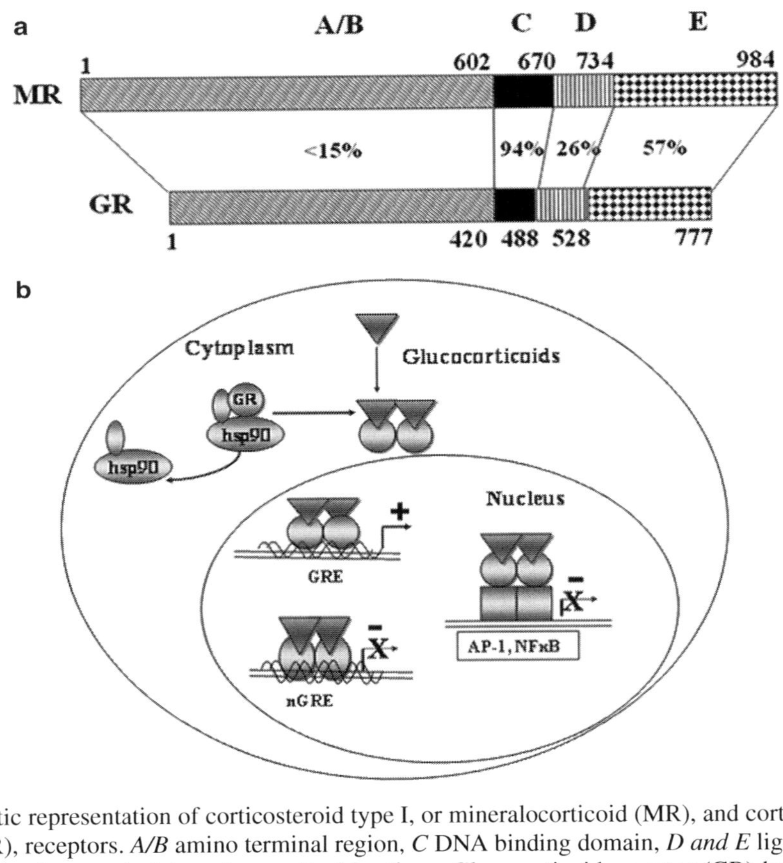

Fig. 5. (**a**) Schematic representation of corticosteroid type I, or mineralocorticoid (MR), and corticosteroid type II, or glucocorticoid (GR), receptors. *A/B* amino terminal region, *C* DNA binding domain, *D and E* ligand binding domain. (**b**) Molecular mechanisms underlying glucocorticoid actions. Glucocorticoid receptor (GR) belongs to the nuclear receptor superfamily. GR not bound to ligand localizes, predominantly, within the cytoplasm but rapidly and efficiently translocates to the nucleus following hormone binding. Binding of glucocorticoids induces conformational changes in the receptor, dissociation from chaperone proteins, such as heat shock protein 90 (hsp90), dimerization of the receptor, nuclear import, and DNA binding. Glucocorticoid signaling not only comprises the binding of the GR to its GRE or binding to nGREs, but it also involves indirect regulation of the glucocorticoid-responsive genes by regulating or interacting with other transcription factors, such as activating protein 1 (AP-1) and nuclear factor kB (NF-*k*B), interfering with their upstream transduction pathways.

bound to ligand localizes, predominantly, within the cytoplasm but rapidly and efficiently translocates to the nucleus following hormone binding. Binding of glucocorticoids induces conformational changes in the receptor, dissociation from chaperone proteins, dimerization of the receptor, nuclear import, and DNA binding *(75)*. Therefore, it has become increasingly clear that glucocorticoid signaling not only comprises the binding of the GR to its responsive element *(76)*, and by binding to negative glucocorticoid responsive elements (nGREs), but it also involves indirect regulation of the glucocorticoid-responsive genes by regulating or interacting with other TFs, a process referred as "crosstalk." In the indirect crosstalk, GR interferes with upstream transduction pathways of other TFs. In the direct crosstalk, GR and TFs modulate each other's activity when bound to the promoters of their target genes *(77–81)*. Activated GR also selectively recruits cofactors in a coordinated fashion. Co-activators and corepressors are cofactors that increase or decrease the total activity of most steroid receptor complexes. The prevailing model is that the nature of the ligand binding to receptors acts as a molecular switch, with agonist steroids causing both the dissociation of corepressors from ligand-free or antagonist-bound receptors and the association of co-activators *(82–84)*. Many of the GR-related co-activators contain intrinsic histone acetyltransferase and methyltransferase activity, which alter chromatin structure and facilitate access of transcription machinery components to DNA *(85, 86)*. The full understanding of the mechanisms of glucocorticoid action will provide the therapeutic relevant discrimination of genomic mechanisms into transactivation and transrepression leading to the development of optimized glucocorticoids and selective glucocorticoid receptor agonists that will improve clinical medicine *(87)*.

Glucocorticoids are essential for life but are also increasingly implicated in the pathogenesis of disease and produce many unwanted effects when given therapeutically. Approximately, 95% of cortisol/corticosterone in the circulation is bound to a carrier protein (corticosteroid-binding globulin, CBG). In principle, only the free steroid has ready access to target cells. However, in some cases (e.g., in inflamed tissues) local serine proteases facilitate delivery by liberating free steroid from its binding globulin, while in others (e.g., pituitary gland) locally expressed CBG may limit access by absorbing free steroid *(88)*. Affinity for synthetic corticosteroids is negligible, except prednisolone, which has an affinity for CBG about 50% of that of cortisol. Circulating CBG concentrations levels are increased by estrogens and in some patients with chronic active hepatitis but reduced by glucocorticoids and in patients with cirrhosis, nephrosis, and hyperthyroidism *(89)*. Inherited abnormalities in CBG synthesis are rare and include elevated CBG, partial and complete deficiency of CBG, or CBG variants with reduced affinity for cortisol *(90–92)*. Ability of glucocorticoids in the systemic circulation to reach target cells is also affected by transporter proteins, which belong to the ATP-binding cassette family. These proteins are expressed in a tissue-specific manner and, like CBG, show substrate specificity, providing a mechanism for tissue- and steroid-specific delivery of glucocorticoids to target cells, a phenomenon that may contribute to the subtle differences in pharmacological profile of various corticosteroids and to development of glucocorticoid resistance *(93)*. The circulating half-life of cortisol varies between 70 and 120min *(94, 95)*. The free cortisol excreted through the kidneys is termed urinary free cortisol and represents only 1% of the total cortisol secretion rate.

The most important factor regulating the access of endogenous glucocorticoid to its receptor is local metabolism of the steroids within the target cells themselves by 11β-hydroxysteroid dehydrogenase (11β-HSD) enzymes, a phenomenon sometimes termed as prereceptor metabolism. 11β-HSD type 1 and 2 catalyze the interconversion of cortisol and the inactive metabolite cortisone in humans (or corticosterone and 11-deoxycorticosterone in rodents). Stewart et al. described the first case of adult 11β-HSD2 deficiency as a condition of apparent mineralocorticoid excess characterized by hypertension, hypokalemia, suppression of the renin–angiotensin system, and impaired conversion of cortisol to cortisone *(96)*. Subsequent studies revealed that MR-expressing tissues, which are normally highly sensitive to aldosterone (kidney, parotid sweat glands, and colon), show high levels of 11β-HSD activity. On the other hand, other tissues in which MRs are abundant (e.g., brain, heart) show little if any 11β-HSD activity, suggesting that cortisol (or corticosterone) is the primary MR ligand at these sites *(97)*. These landmark studies opened a new chapter in the biology of glucocorticoids and it is now apparent that "prereceptor" interconversion of active and inactive glucocorticoids plays a key role in determining not only the specificity of the MR but also the degree of GR activation in a number of tissues *(96, 97)*. Evidence that 11β-HSD1 blockade promotes insulin secretion led to the view that 11β-HSD1 may be an important factor in the development of insulin resistance, obesity, and other metabolic disturbances *(98–100)*. Consequently, drugs that block 11β-HSD1 selectively are now an important target for the pharmaceutical industry *(101)*. There is also a growing interest in the role of 11β-HSD1 in the brain, particularly in the hypothalamus, hippocampus, cortex, and cerebellum, where the enzyme is expressed in abundance. Of particular note is a recent study that demonstrated improved cognitive function in elderly subjects treated with an inhibitor of 11β-HSD1 and evidence from a genetic study that demonstrated an association between haplotypes of the 11β-HSD1 gene and susceptibility to Alzheimer's disease *(102)*.

HYPERCORTISOLISM AND PATHOPHYSIOLOGICAL FUNCTIONS

Cortisol/corticosterone are responsible for the salt and water homeostasis and blood pressure control and influence carbohydrate, protein, and lipid metabolism. They are also important regulators of immune and inflammatory processes and are required for numerous processes associated with host defense. On the other hand, prolonged or high dose glucocorticoid therapy as well as an excess of endogenous production of glucocorticoids exerts a large spectrum of deleterious actions in the whole body. These include a significant redistribution of fat; protein wasting associated with muscle weakness; hyperglycemia and insulin resistant diabetes mellitus; hypertension, elevated cholesterol, altered serum lipids, salt and water retention; immunodeficiency, poor wound healing and loss of connective tissue leading to easy bruising; impaired growth and development; osteoporosis; menstrual irregularities, infertility and other endocrine-related changes; depression and, sometimes, impaired cognitive function.

Cushing's syndrome is associated in 79–97% of the cases with typical central (visceral) redistribution of adipose tissue together with a characteristic "moon face" and "buffalo hump" *(103–105)*. The mechanism of the typical fat redistribution in hypercortisolism is not completely understood. One of the reasons is probably the site-specific regulation of enzymes of intracellular lipolysis (hormone-sensitive lipase) and intravascular lipolysis (lipoprotein lipase) *(106)*. Catecholamines are hormones that also play an important role in the regulation of lipolysis. Studies have showed significantly increased lipolysis in subcutaneous adipose tissue and increased local concentrations of catecholamines and their metabolites in subcutaneous tissue of patients with Cushing's syndrome *(107)*. Besides lipolysis, glucocorticoids also promote gluconeogenesis in the liver, the degradation of proteins to free amino acids in muscle and muscle atrophy *(102, 108, 109)*. The principal role of 11β-HSD1 is to amplify the local concentration of active glucocorticoids in tissues, in which the steroids have a key regulatory role, for example, the liver. A number of studies, including phenotypic analysis of 11β-HSD1-null mice, have emerged supporting this hypothesis. These mice have elevated corticosterone levels due to impaired glucocorticoid feedback but are resistant to the hyperglycemia induced by stress or overfeeding. In addition, they show increased levels of high-density lipoprotein cholesterol, lowered low-density lipoprotein cholesterol, and reduced triglycerides. The metabolic responses appear to be driven by key changes, which, by preventing amplification of the local corticosterone concentration, reduce gluconeogenesis and β-oxidation of lipids in the liver and possibly also attenuate glucocorticoid-dependent functions in visceral adipose tissue. When these animals are placed on a high fat diet, 11β-HSD1-null mice gain less weight than their wild type counterparts and tend to deposit fat in subcutaneous rather than the visceral sites associated with metabolic disease *(101, 102)*. On the other hand, a transgenic mice overexpressing 11β-HSD1 selectively in adipose tissue, similar to that found in adipose tissue from obese humans, had increased adipose levels of corticosterone and developed visceral obesity that was exaggerated by a high-fat diet. These mice also exhibited pronounced insulin-resistant diabetes, hyperlipidemia, and, surprisingly, hyperphagia despite hyperleptinemia. Increased adipocyte 11β-HSD1 activity may be a common molecular etiology for visceral obesity and the metabolic syndrome *(108)*.

Chronic hypercortisolism has also been associated with higher GR binding sites and GR mRNA expression and decreased affinity in intraabdominal than subcutaneous adipose tissue samples. In addition, the beta isoform GR mRNA expression was also increased compared with controls. Therefore, Cushing's syndrome is accompanied by a reversible decrease in GR affinity, possibly related to an increased GR beta expression, which may be a compensatory mechanism to GC excess *(109–111)*.

Hypercortisolism causes general obesity and growth retardation in children *(112)*. Glucocorticoids slow longitudinal growth by reducing the proliferation of chondrocytes and inducing apoptosis of these cells. Inhibition of insulin-like growth factor I signaling is one mechanism underlying decreased chondrocyte proliferation *(113)*.

Glucocorticoid excess leads to an increase of blood pressure by the interplay of several pathophysiological mechanisms regulating plasma volume, peripheral cardiovascular resistance, and cardiac output *(114)*. In the kidney, cortisol acts on distal nephron to cause sodium retention and potassium loss (mediated by the MR), ensuing an increase in blood volume *(115)*. Dexamethasone treated rats demonstrated increased mean arterial pressure, urine flow rate, and urinary excretion of both sodium and urea. These alterations in body water observed with glucocorticoid excess may be a result, in part, of impaired urinary concentrating capacity, downregulation of urea transporters UT-A1 and UT-A3, and increased urea excretion *(116)*.

In addition to 11β-HSD2 inhibition, the factors that contribute to increase in plasma volume include co-secretion of mineralocorticoids (deoxycorticosterone, corticosterone); a redistribution of sodium to extracellular compartment; a greater cardiac output mediated by epinephrine induced by increased phenylethanolamine-*N*-methyltransferase activity; and activation of ouabain-sensitive Na–K dependent ATPase *(117)*. A second mechanism involves an increased systemic vascular resistance resulted from potentiation of vasopressor responses to angiotensin II, catecholamines, AVP, and erythropoietin *(118)*. The enhanced response to angiotensin II is due to the induction of angiotensin II receptors by glucocorticoids. In addition, an increased systemic vascular resistance occurs due to the inhibition of vasodilatory systems such as nitric oxide, kinin/kallikrein, prostacyclin, inhibition of peripheral catabolism of catecholamine, in particular of norepinephrine, by the direct action of glucocorticoids on cardiovascular receptors, increased calcium uptake and calcium channel antagonist binding in vascular smooth muscle cells, and decreased atrial natriuretic peptide (ANP)-mediated cyclic guanosine monophosphate formation, leading to diminished ANP-dependent vasodilatation *(119–121)*.

Although glucocorticoids do not affect the number or affinity of *a*1-adrenergic receptors, they potentiate downstream α1-adrenergic signaling *(122, 123)*. Localized changes in vasoreactivity may contribute to the beneficial effects of combined treatment with glucocorticoids and β2-agonists in patients with asthma. This illustrates one of the potential advantages of inhaled glucocorticoids developed to target lung tissue, and thus decrease the adverse effects of systemic delivery *(124)*.

Glucocorticoids clearly act on diverse targets through multiple mechanisms to control inflammation. In the peripheral blood, glucocorticoids reduce T- and B-lymphocyte counts acutely by redistributing lymphocytes from the intravascular compartment to spleen, lymph nodes, and bone marrow. Eosinophil counts also fall rapidly while neutrophil counts increase after glucocorticoid administration *(125, 126)*. The immunologic actions of glucocorticoids involve direct actions on both T- and B-lymphocytes that include inhibition of immunoglobulin synthesis and stimulation of lymphocyte apoptosis *(127)*, as well as inhibition of monocyte differentiation into macrophages, macrophage phagocytosis, and cytotoxic activity. Glucocorticoids reduce the local inflammatory response by preventing the action of histamine and plasminogen activators. Glucocorticoids block several inflammatory pathways including inhibition of prostaglandin production through three independent mechanisms: the induction and activation of annexin I (also called lipocortin-1), the induction of Mitogen-activated protein kinase (MAPK) phosphatase 1, and the repression of transcription of cyclooxygenase 2 *(128–132)*. Mice lacking annexin I have elevated levels of cPLA2α, an exaggerated inflammatory response, and partial resistance to the antiinflammatory action of glucocorticoids *(133)*. Cytokines, bacterial and viral infections, and ultraviolet radiation activate Mitogen-activated protein (MAPK) cascades by the activation of Jun N-terminal kinase, which in turn phosphorylates the TF c-Jun. This factor binds to DNA sequences called activator protein 1 response elements and induces the transcription of inflammatory and immune genes by protein–protein interactions, a major antiinflammatory mechanism *(134)*. The cortisol–GR complex also physically interacts with NF-*k*B to block its transcriptional activity. In its inactive state, NF-*k*B is sequestered in the cytoplasm by an inhibitory protein named I*k*B. TNF-*a*, interleukin-1, microbial pathogens, viral infections, and other inflammatory signals trigger signaling cascades that activate I*k*B kinases. Phosphorylation of I*k*B leads to its ubiquitination and degradation by the proteasome, unmasking a nuclear localization signal on NF-*k*B. In the nucleus, NF-*k*B binds DNA sequences called NF-*k*B elements and stimulates the transcription of cytokines, chemokines, cell adhesion molecules, complement factors, and receptors for these molecules *(135, 136)*. NF-*k*B also induces the transcription of cyclooxygenase 2, an enzyme essential for prostaglandin production. Thus, glucocorticoid-induced antagonism of NF-*k*B and repression of cyclooxygenase 2 is the third mechanism for the inhibition of prostaglandin synthesis after the induction of the antagonists of cPLA2α, annexin I, and Mitogen-activated protein (MAPK) phosphatase 1 *(131)*. Glucocorticoids and the GR also modulate the activity of other TFs *(135)*. Recent work suggests that glucocorticoids can have rapid effects on inflammation that are not mediated by changes in gene expression. This called nongenomic mechanism involves the activation of phosphatidylinositol 3-kinase leading to phosphorylation of Akt, which in turn phosphorylates and activates endothelial nitric oxide synthetase, resulting in the production of nitric oxide *(137, 138)*. More research is needed to clarify the role of nontranscriptional mechanisms in the inhibition of vasodilation, vascular permeability, and migration of leukocytes across endothelium *(131)*. Another mechanism of the glucocorticoid-induced inhibition of inflammation involves decreased stability of mRNA of genes for inflammatory proteins such as vascular endothelial growth factor and cyclooxygenase 2 *(139, 140)*. Based on these actions, infections are common in patients with Cushing's syndrome because the normal inflammatory response is suppressed. Reactivation of tuberculosis and opportunistic fungal infections of the skin and nails have been reported *(141, 142)*. Wound infections are common and contribute to poor wound healing *(143)*. In addition, a recent study suggested a complex interaction between Cushing's syndrome and inflammation. In particular, the raised levels of IL-8 and osteoprotegerin despite glucocorticoid excess may represent an inflammatory and pro-atherogenic phenotype *(144)*. Indeed, in patients with Cushing's syndrome, serum osteoprotegerin levels are increased and appear to be associated with coronary risk *(145)*.

Glucocorticoids cause catabolic changes in muscle, skin, and connective tissue by inhibiting epidermal cell division and DNA synthesis and reducing collagen synthesis and production *(146–148)*. Hypercortisolism results in skin thinning and purple striae, easy bruisability. Thin and fragile skin that bruises easily are signs of discriminatory value to the early diagnosis of Cushing's syndrome *(149)*. Acne may occur over the face, chest, and back. The typical red-purple striae, common in younger patients, greater than 1cm in diameter are most frequently found on the abdomen, upper thighs, breasts, and arms. Increased skin pigmentation can be associated to ACTH-dependent hypercortisolism because of overstimulation of melanocyte receptors by ACTH. Acanthosis nigricans occurs in 30% of patients with Cushing's syndrome and it is related to insulin resistance due to the metabolic effects of hypercortisolism. Glucocorticoids cause catabolic changes in muscle due to the inhibition of protein synthesis, degradation of proteins to free amino acids and decreased amino acid uptake by the muscle, leading to muscle weakness and atrophy *(150, 151)*. The myopathy of Cushing's syndrome involves the proximal muscles of the lower limb and the shoulder.

Osteoporotic fractures may be the presenting symptom of an otherwise silent glucocorticoid excess and can precede the diagnosis of hypercortisolism by up to two years. The glucocorticoid excess mainly affects trabecular bone, leading to vertebral fractures in up to 70% of patients *(152)*. Glucocorticoids have complex effects on bone exerting both positive and negative effects on cell growth and are proapoptotic which lead to osteoporosis and an increased risk of fractures *(153, 154)*. Osteoporosis is mediated in part by the binding of GRs to nGREs that inhibit transcription of osteocalcin as well as IGF-I in osteoblasts; osteocalcin is an important extracellular matrix protein that promotes bone mineralization *(155)*. Glucocorticoids exacerbate osteoporosis by inducing apoptosis of osteoblasts and increasing the activity of osteoclasts. Some of these effects are directly mediated by GRs in bone cells, whereas indirect effects are mediated by interactions with other endocrine signals *(156)*. In addition to blocking cytokine signaling, glucocorticoids inhibit the synthesis of matrix metalloproteinases and collagen, which are important factors in wound repair *(157–159)*. Glucocorticoids also induce a negative calcium balance by inhibiting vitamin D actions on intestinal calcium absorption and increasing renal calcium excretion *(160–162)*. As a consequence, parathyroid hormone secretion is usually increased resulting in increased osteoclastic activity. Moreover, glucocorticoids increase the expression of receptor activator of NF-*k*B ligand (RANK-L) and decrease the expression of its soluble decoy receptor, osteoprotegerin, in stromal and osteoblastic cells; glucocorticoids also enhance the expression of colony stimulating factor-1, which in the presence of RANK-L induces osteoclastogenesis. Studies on resorption markers in patients with Cushing's syndrome are contradictory showing normal, high, or even reduced levels *(163, 165)*.

Glucocorticoids suppress centrally the thyroid and gonadal axis, probably through a direct action on thyroid-stimulating hormone, luteinizing hormone, and follicle-stimulating hormone release. In addition, peripherally, hypercortisolism inhibits 5α-deiodinase contributing to hypothyroidism. Hypogonadism is reversible upon correction of hypercortisolism. Menstrual irregularity in females and loss of libido in both sexes are common and hirsutism is frequently found in female patients *(166–168)*. GH secretion is reduced, possibly mediated by increased somatostatinergic tone.

Brain is an important target tissue for glucocorticoids *(101, 169)*. Increased HPA activity is common in major depression, anorexia nervosa, obsessive-compulsive disorders, and panic states, whereas HPA function is generally reduced in posttraumatic stress and seasonal affective disorders *(170–173)*. These changes have been attributed, in part, to failure of the negative feedback effects of cortisol in the brain and pituitary gland. Human studies report cognitive impairment consistent with hippocampal neuronal death in depression, bipolar disorder, Cushing's disease, and in those individuals receiving exogenous corticosteroids *(174, 175)*. In addition, there is a high incidence of apparent diffuse loss of brain volume in patients who have Cushing's syndrome. These aspects may underlie the interest in glucocorticoids and cognitive function, memory, and neurodegenerative diseases, such as Alzheimer's disease *(176–178)*. Recent studies indicate at least partial reversibility and rapid improvement in the psychiatric state following correction of hypercortisolism by medical or surgical therapy *(179)*. Our understanding on the glucocorticoids biology has increased exponentially. The findings have given significant insight into the critical role of glucocorticoids in the maintenance of homeostasis and, when dysregulated, in the pathogenesis of diseases.

REFERENCES

1. Bruhn TO, Sutton RE, Rivier CL, Vale WW. Corticotropin-releasing factor regulates proopiomelanocortin messenger ribonucleic acid levels in vivo. Neuroendocrinology 1984;39:170–175.
2. Rivier C, Rivier J, Vale W. Inhibition of adrenocorticotropic hormone secretion in the rat by immunoneutralization of corticotropin-releasing factor. Science 1982;218:377–379.
3. Vale W, Spiess J, Rivier C, Rivier J. Characterization of a 41-residue ovine hypothalamic peptide that stimulates secretion of corticotropin and beta-endorphin. Science 1981;213:1394–1397.
4. Coste SC, Quintos RF, Stenzel-Poore MP. Corticotropin-releasing hormone-related peptides and receptors: emergent regulators of cardiovascular adaptations to stress. Trends Cardiovasc Med 2002;12:176–182.
5. Venihaki M, Majzoub J. Lessons from CRH knockout mice. Neuropeptides 2002;36:96–102.
6. Plotsky PM. Pathways to the secretion of adrenocorticotropin: a view from the portal. J Neuroendocrinol 1991;3:1–9.
7. Swanson LW, Sawchenko PE, Rivier J, Vale WW. Organization of ovine corticotropin-releasing factor immunoreactive cells and fibers in the rat brain: an immunohistochemical study. Neuroendocrinology 1983;36:165–186.
8. McKinley MJ, Gerstberger R, Mathai ML, Oldfield BJ, Schmid H. The lamina terminalis and its role in fluid and electrolyte homeostasis. J Clin Neurosci 1999;6:289–301.
9. Sawchenko PE, Swanson LW, Vale WW. Co-expression of corticotropin-releasing factor and vasopressin immunoreactivity in parvocellular neurosecretory neurons of the adrenalectomized rat. Proc Natl Acad Sci USA 1984;81:1883–1887.
10. Grino M, Chrousos GP, Margioris AN. The corticotropin releasing hormone gene is expressed in human placenta. Biochem Biophys Res Commun 1987;148:1208–1214.
11. Sasaki A, Sato S, Murakami O, Go M, Inoue M, Shimizu Y, Hanew K, Andoh N, Sato I, Sasano N, et al. Immunoreactive corticotropin-releasing hormone present in human plasma may be derived from both hypothalamic and extrahypothalamic sources. J Clin Endocrinol Metab 1987;65:176–182.
12. Suda T, Tomori N, Tozawa F, Mouri T, Demura H, Shizume K. Distribution and characterization of immunoreactive corticotropin-releasing factor in human tissues. J Clin Endocrinol Metab 1984;59:861–866.
13. Campbell EA, Linton EA, Wolfe CD, Scraggs PR, Jones MT, Lowry PJ. Plasma corticotropin-releasing hormone concentrations during pregnancy and parturition. J Clin Endocrinol Metab 1987;64:1054–1059.
14. Chen R, Lewis KA, Perrin MH, Vale WW. Expression cloning of a human corticotropin-releasing-factor receptor. Proc Natl Acad Sci USA 1993;90:8967–8971.
15. Giguere V, Labrie F, Cote J, Coy DH, Sueiras-Diaz J, Schally AV. Stimulation of cyclic AMP accumulation and corticotropin release by synthetic ovine corticotropin-releasing factor in rat anterior pituitary cells: site of glucocorticoid action. Proc Natl Acad Sci USA 1982;79:3466–3469.
16. Perrin MH, Haas Y, Rivier JE, Vale WW. Corticotropin-releasing factor binding to the anterior pituitary receptor is modulated by divalent cations and guanyl nucleotides. Endocrinology 1986;118:1171–1179.
17. Levin N, Roberts JL. Positive regulation of proopiomelanocortin gene expression in corticotropes and melanotropes. Front Neuroendocrinol 1991;12:1–22.
18. Dallman MF, Makara GB, Roberts JL, Levin N, Blum M. Corticotrope response to removal of releasing factors and corticosteroids in vivo. Endocrinology 1985;117:2190–2197.
19. Orth DN, Jackson RV, DeCherney GS, DeBold CR, Alexander AN, Island DP, Rivier J, Rivier C, Spiess J, Vale W. Effect of synthetic ovine corticotropin-releasing factor. Dose response of plasma adrenocorticotropin and cortisol. J Clin Invest 1983;71:587–595.
20. Linton EA, Wolfe CD, Behan DP, Lowry PJ. A specific carrier substance for human corticotrophin releasing factor in late gestational maternal plasma which could mask the ACTH-releasing activity. Clin Endocrinol (Oxf) 1988;28:315–324.
21. Lundblad JR, Roberts JL. Regulation of proopiomelanocortin gene expression in pituitary. Endocr Rev 1988;9: 135–158.
22. Pulichino AM, Vallette-Kasic S, Tsai JP, Couture C, Gauthier Y, Drouin J. Tpit determines alternate fates during pituitary cell differentiation. Genes Dev 2003;17:738–747.

23. Mynard V, Guignat L, Devin-Leclerc J, Bertagna X, Catelli MG. Different mechanisms for leukemia inhibitory factor-dependent activation of two proopiomelanocortin promoter regions. Endocrinology 2002;143:3916–3924.
24. Murphy EP, Conneely OM. Neuroendocrine regulation of the hypothalamic pituitary adrenal axis by the nurr1/nur77 subfamily of nuclear receptors. Mol Endocrinol 1997;11:39–47.
25. Smith AI, Funder JW. Proopiomelanocortin processing in the pituitary, central nervous system, and peripheral tissues. Endocr Rev 1988;9:159–179.
26. Seidah NG, Benjannet S, Hamelin J, Mamarbachi AM, Basak A, Marcinkiewicz J, Mbikay M, Chretien M, Marcinkiewicz M. The subtilisin/kexin family of precursor convertases. Emphasis on PC1, PC2/7B2, POMC and the novel enzyme SKI-1. Ann NY Acad Sci 1999;885:57–74.
27. Suzuki I, Cone RD, Im S, Nordlund J, Abdel-Malek ZA. Binding of melanotropic hormones to the melanocortin receptor MC1R on human melanocytes stimulates proliferation and melanogenesis. Endocrinology 1996;137:1627–1633.
28. Bornstein SR, Rutkowski H, Vrezas I. Cytokines and steroidogenesis. Mol Cell Endocrinol 2004;215:135–141.
29. Ehrhart-Bornstein M, Hinson JP, Bornstein SR, Scherbaum WA, Vinson GP. Intraadrenal interactions in the regulation of adrenocortical steroidogenesis. Endocr Rev 1998;19:101–143.
30. Krug AW, Vleugels K, Schinner S, Lamounier-Zepter V, Ziegler CG, Bornstein SR. Ehrhart-Bornstein M. Human adipocytes induce an ERK1/2 MAP kinases-mediated upregulation of steroidogenic acute regulatory protein (StAR) and an angiotensin II-sensitization in human adrenocortical cells. Int J Obes (Lond) 2007;31:1605–1616.
31. Lin D, Sugawara T, Strauss JF, 3rd, Clark BJ, Stocco, DM, Saenger P, Rogol A, Miller WL. Role of steroidogenic acute regulatory protein in adrenal and gonadal steroidogenesis. Science 1995;267:1828–1831.
32. Simpson ER, Waterman MR. Regulation of the synthesis of steroidogenic enzymes in adrenal cortical cells by ACTH. Annu Rev Physiol 1988;50:427–440.
33. Lowrey PL, Takahashi JS. Mammalian circadian biology: elucidating genome-wide levels of temporal organization. Annu Rev Genomics Hum Genet 2004;5:407–441.
34. Reppert SM, Schwartz WJ. Maternal suprachiasmatic nuclei are necessary for maternal coordination of the developing circadian system. J Neurosci 1986;6:2724–2729.
35. Seron-Ferre M, Ducsay CA, Valenzuela GJ. Circadian rhythms during pregnancy. Endocr Rev 1993;14:594–609.
36. Duffy JF, Wright KP, Jr. Entrainment of the human circadian system by light. J Biol Rhythms 2005;20:326–338.
37. Santiago LB, Jorge SM, Moreira AC. Longitudinal evaluation of the development of salivary cortisol circadian rhythm in infancy. Clin Endocrinol (Oxf) 1996;44:157–161.
38. Mistlberger RE, Skene DJ. Nonphotic entrainment in humans? J Biol Rhythms 2005;20:339–352.
39. Krieger DT, Allen W, Rizzo F, Krieger HP. Characterization of the normal temporal pattern of plasma corticosteroid levels. J Clin Endocrinol Metab 1971;32:266–284.
40. Veldhuis JD, Iranmanesh A, Johnson ML, Lizarralde G. Amplitude, but not frequency, modulation of adrenocorticotropin secretory bursts gives rise to the nyctohemeral rhythm of the corticotropic axis in man. J Clin Endocrinol Metab 1999;71:452–463.
41. Desir D, Van Cauter E, Fang VS, Martino E, Jadot C, Spire JP, Noel P, Refetoff S, Copinschi G, Golstein J. Effects of "jet lag" on hormonal patterns. I. Procedures, variations in total plasma proteins, and disruption of adrenocorticotropin-cortisol periodicity. J Clin Endocrinol Metab 1981;52:628–641.
42. Castro M, Elias PC, Quidute AR, Halah FP, Moreira AC. Out-patient screening for Cushing's syndrome: the sensitivity of the combination of circadian rhythm and overnight dexamethasone suppression salivary cortisol tests. J Clin Endocrinol Metab 1999;84:878–882.
43. Raff H, Raff JL, Findling JW. Late-night salivary cortisol as a screening test for Cushing's syndrome. J Clin Endocrinol Metab 1998;83:2681–2686.
44. Herman JP, Figueiredo H, Mueller NK, Ulrich-Lai Y, Ostrander MM, Choi DC, Cullinan WE. Central mechanisms of stress integration: hierarchical circuitry controlling hypothalamo-pituitary-adrenocortical responsiveness. Front Neuroendocrinol 2003;24:151–180.
45. Martinelli CE, Jr, Sader SL, Oliveira EB, Daneluzzi JC, Moreira AC. Salivary cortisol for screening of Cushing's syndrome in children. Clin Endocrinol (Oxf) 1999;51:67–71.
46. Dallman MF, Akana SF, Cascio CS, Darlington DN, Jacobson L, Levin N. Regulation of ACTH secretion: variations on a theme of B. Recent Prog Horm Res 1987;43:113–173.
47. Keller-Wood ME, Dallman MF. Corticosteroid inhibition of ACTH secretion. Endocr Rev 1984;5:1–24.
48. McEwen BS. Glucocorticoids, depression, and mood disorders: structural remodeling in the brain. Metabolism 2005;54:20–23.
49. Sapolsky RM, Meaney MJ. Maturation of the adrenocortical stress response: neuroendocrine control mechanisms and the stress hyporesponsive period. Brain Res 1986;396:64–76.

50. Sapolsky RM. Glucocorticoids, stress, and their adverse neurological effects: relevance to aging. Exp Gerontol 1999;34: 721–732.
51. Fish HR, Chernow B, O'Brian JT. Endocrine and neurophysiologic responses of the pituitary to insulin-induced hypoglycemia: a review. Metabolism 1986;35:763–780.
52. Luger A, Deuster PA, Kyle SB, Gallucci WT, Montgomery LC, Gold PW, Loriaux DL, Chrousos GP. Acute hypothalamic-pituitary-adrenal responses to the stress of treadmill exercise. Physiologic adaptations to physical training. N Engl J Med 1987; 316:1309–1315.
53. Udelsman R, Norton JA, Jelenich SE, Goldstein DS, Linehan WM, Loriaux DL, Chrousos GP. Responses of the hypothalamic-pituitary-adrenal and renin-angiotensin axes and the sympathetic system during controlled surgical and anesthetic stress. J Clin Endocrinol Metab 1987;64:986–994.
54. Vaughan GM, Becker RA, Allen JP, Goodwin CW, Jr, Pruitt BA, Jr, Mason AD, Jr. Cortisol and corticotrophin in burned patients. J Trauma 1982;22:263–273.
55. Aguilera G. Regulation of pituitary ACTH secretion during chronic stress. Front Neuroendocrinol 1994;15:321–350.
56. Linkowski P, Mendlewicz J, Kerkhofs M, Leclercq R, Golstein J, Brasseur M, Copinschi G, Van Cauter E. 24-hour profiles of adrenocorticotropin, cortisol, and growth hormone in major depressive illness: effect of antidepressant treatment. J Clin Endocrinol Metab 1987;65:141–152.
57. Streeten DH, Anderson GH, Jr, Dalakos TG, Seeley D, Mallov JS, Eusebio R, Sunderlin FS, Badawy SZ, King RB. Normal and abnormal function of the hypothalamic-pituitary-adrenocortical system in man. Endocr Rev 1984;5: 371–394.
58. Harris RB, Gu H, Mitchell TD, Endale L, Russo M, Ryan DH. Increased glucocorticoid response to a novel stress in rats that have been restrained. Physiol Behav 2004;81:557–568.
59. Helmreich DL, Morano MI, Akil H, Watson SJ. Correlation between changes in stress-induced corticosterone secretion and GR mRNA levels stress. 1997;2:101–112.
60. Marti O, Armario A. Influence of regularity of exposure to chronic stress on the pattern of habituation of pituitary-adrenal hormones. Prolactin Glucose Stress 1997;1:179–189.
61. Sternberg EM, Chrousos GP, Wilder RL, Gold PW. The stress response and the regulation of inflammatory disease Ann Intern Med 1992;117:854–866.
62. Elenkov IJ, Chrousos GP. Stress system—organization, physiology and immunoregulation. Neuroimmunomodulation 2006;13:257–267.
63. Chrousos GP. The hypothalamic-pituitary-adrenal axis and immune-mediated inflammation. N Engl J Med 1995;332: 1351–1362.
64. Vamvakopoulos NC, Chrousos GP. Hormonal regulation of human corticotropin-releasing hormone gene expression: implications for the stress response and immune/inflammatory reaction. Endocr Rev 1994;15,:409–420.
65. Ray DW, Ren SG, Melmed S. Leukemia inhibitory factor (LIF) stimulates proopiomelanocortin (POMC) expression in a corticotroph cell line. Role of STAT pathway. J Clin Invest 1996;97:1852–1859.
66. Besedovsky H, del Rey A, Sorkin E, Dinarello CA. Immunoregulatory feedback between interleukin-1 and glucocorticoid hormones. Science 1986;233:652–654.
67. Antoni FA. Hypothalamic control of adrenocorticotropin secretion: advances since the discovery of 41-residue corticotropin-releasing factor. Endocr Rev 1986;7:351–378.
68. Sandi C, Venero C, Guaza, C. Nitric oxide synthesis inhibitors prevent rapid behavioral effects of corticosterone in rats. Neuroendocrinology 1996;63:446–453.
69. Di S, Malcher-Lopes R, Halmos KC, Tasker JG. Nongenomic glucocorticoid inhibition via endocannabinoid release in the hypothalamus: a fast feedback mechanism. J Neurosci 2003;23:4850–4857.
70. Malcher-Lopes R, Di S, Marcheselli VS, Weng FJ, Stuart CT, Bazan NG, Tasker JG. Opposing crosstalk between leptin and glucocorticoids rapidly modulates synaptic excitation via endocannabinoid release. J Neurosci 2006;26: 6643–6650.
71. Tasker JG, Di S, Malcher-Lopes R. Minireview: rapid glucocorticoid signaling via membrane-associated receptors. Endocrinology 2006;147:5549–5556.
72. de Kloet ER, Oitzl MS, Joels M. Functional implications of brain corticosteroid receptor diversity. Cell Mol Neurobiol 1993;13:433–455.
73. Castro M, Elias LL, Elias PC, Moreira AC. A dose-response study of salivary cortisol after dexamethasone suppression test in Cushing's disease and its potential use in the differential diagnosis of Cushing's syndrome. Clin Endocrinol (Oxf) 2003 59:800–805.
74. Jacobson L, Sapolsky R. The role of the hippocampus in feedback regulation of the hypothalamic-pituitary-adrenocortical axis. Endocr Rev 1991;12:118–134.

75. Bamberger CM, Schulte HM, Chrousos GP. Molecular determinants of glucocorticoid receptor function and tissue sensitivity to glucocorticoids. Endocr Rev 1996;17:245–261.
76. Hauner H, Entenmann G, Wabitsch M, Gaillard D, Ailhaud G, Negrel R, Pfeiffer EF. Promoting effect of glucocorticoids on the differentiation of human adipocyte precursor cells cultured in a chemically defined medium. J Clin Invest 1989;84:1663–1670.
77. Autelitano DJ. Glucocorticoid regulation of c-fos, c-jun and transcription factor AP-1 in the AtT-20 corticotrope cell. J Neuroendocrinol 1994;6:627–637.
78. Chambon P. The nuclear receptor superfamily: a personal retrospect on the first two decades. Mol Endocrinol 2005;19: 1418–1428.
79. Evans RM. The nuclear receptor superfamily: a rosetta stone for physiology. Mol Endocrinol 2005;19:1429–1438.
80. Kassel O, Herrlich P. Crosstalk between the glucocorticoid receptor and other transcription factors: molecular aspects. Mol Cell Endocrinol 2007;275:13–29.
81. Therrien M, Drouin J. Pituitary pro-opiomelanocortin gene expression requires synergistic interactions of several regulatory elements. Mol Cell Biol 1991;11:3492–3503.
82. Glass CK, Rosenfeld MG. The coregulator exchange in transcriptional functions of nuclear receptors. Genes Dev 2000; 14:121–141.
83. Hu X, Li Y, Lazar MA. Determinants of CoRNR-dependent repression complex assembly on nuclear hormone receptors. Mol Cell Biol 2001;21:1747–1758.
84. Wang Q, Blackford JA, Jr, Song LN, Huang Y, Cho S, Simons SS, Jr. Equilibrium interactions of corepressors and coactivators with agonist and antagonist complexes of glucocorticoid receptors. Mol Endocrinol 2004;18:1376–1395.
85. Lonard DM, O'Malley BW. Expanding functional diversity of the coactivators. Trends Biochem Sci 2005;30:126–132.
86. Trotter KW, Archer TK. Nuclear receptors and chromatin remodeling machinery. Mol Cell Endocrinol 2007; 265–266:162–167.
87. Stahn C, Lowenberg M, Hommes DW, Buttgereit F. Molecular mechanisms of glucocorticoid action and selective glucocorticoid receptor agonists. Mol Cell Endocrinol 2007;275:71–78.
88. Hammond GL. Molecular properties of corticosteroid binding globulin and the sex-steroid binding proteins. Endocr Rev 1990;11:65–79.
89. Brien TG. Human corticosteroid binding globulin. Clin Endocrinol (Oxf) 1981;14:193–212.
90. Brunner E, Baima J, Vieira TC, Vieira JG, Abucham J. Hereditary corticosteroid-binding globulin deficiency due to a missense mutation (Asp367Asn, CBG Lyon) in a Brazilian kindred. Clin Endocrinol (Oxf) 2003;58:756–762.
91. Roitman A, Bruchis S, Bauman B, Kaufman H, Laron Z. Total deficiency of corticosteroid-binding globulin. Clin Endocrinol (Oxf) 1984;21:541–548.
92. Smith CL, Power SG, Hammond GL. A Leu—His substitution at residue 93 in human corticosteroid binding globulin results in reduced affinity for cortisol. J Steroid Biochem Mol Biol 1992;42:671–676.
93. Meijer OC, Karssen AM, de Kloet ER. Cell- and tissue-specific effects of corticosteroids in relation to glucocorticoid resistance: examples from the brain. J Endocrinol 2003;178:13–18.
94. Mendel CM. The free hormone hypothesis: a physiologically based mathematical model. Endocr Rev 1989;10:232–274.
95. Peterson RE, Wyngaarden JB, Guerra SL, Brodie BB, Bunim JJ. The physiological disposition and metabolic fate of hydrocortisone in man. J Clin Invest 1955;34:1779–1794.
96. Stewart PM, Corrie JE, Shackleton CH, Edwards CR. Syndrome of apparent mineralocorticoid excess. A defect in the cortisol-cortisone shuttle. J Clin Invest 1988;82:340–349.
97. Edwards CR, Benediktsson R, Lindsay RS, Seckl JR. 11 beta-Hydroxysteroid dehydrogenases: key enzymes in determining tissue-specific glucocorticoid effects. Steroids 1996;61:263–269.
98. De Sousa Peixoto RA, Turban S, Battle JH, Chapman KE, Seckl JR, Morton NM. Preadipocyte 11beta-hydroxysteroid dehydrogenase type 1 is a keto-reductase and contributes to diet-induced visceral obesity in vivo. Endocrinology 2008;149:1861–1868.
99. Iwasaki Y, Takayasu S, Nishiyama M, Tsugita M, Taguchi T, Asai M, Yoshida M, Kambayashi M, Hashimoto K. Is the metabolic syndrome an intracellular Cushing state? Effects of multiple humoral factors on the transcriptional activity of the hepatic glucocorticoid-activating enzyme (11beta-hydroxysteroid dehydrogenase type 1) gene. Mol Cell Endocrinol 2008;285:10–18.
100. Schnackenberg CG. 11beta-hydroxysteroid dehydrogenase type 1 inhibitors for metabolic syndrome. Curr Opin Investig Drugs 2008;9:295–300.
101. Buckingham JC. Glucocorticoids: exemplars of multi-tasking. Br J Pharmacol 2006;147(Suppl 1):S258–268.
102. Seckl JR. Prenatal glucocorticoids and long-term programming. Eur J Endocrinol 2004;151(Suppl 3):U49–62.

103. Hiramatsu R, Yoshida K, Sato T A body measurement to evaluate the pattern of fat distribution in central obesity. A screening and monitoring technique for Cushing's syndrome. JAMA 1983;250:3174–3178.
104. Lamberts SW, Birkenhager JC. Body composition in Cushing's disease. J Clin Endocrinol Metab 1976;42:864–868.
105. Yoshida S, Inadera H, Ishikawa Y, Shinomiya M, Shirai K, Saito Y. Endocrine disorders and body fat distribution. Int J Obes 1991;15(Suppl 2):37–40.
106. Bujalska IJ, Walker EA, Tomlinson JW, Hewison M, Stewart PM. 11Beta-hydroxysteroid dehydrogenase type 1 in differentiating omental human preadipocytes: from de-activation to generation of cortisol. Endocr Res 2002;28:449–461.
107. Krsek M, Rosicka M, Nedvidkova J, Kvasnickova H, Hana V, Marek J, Haluzik M, Lai EW, Pacak K. Increased lipolysis of subcutaneous abdominal adipose tissue and altered noradrenergic activity in patients with Cushing's syndrome: an in-vivo microdialysis study. Physiol Res 2006;55:421–428.
108. Masuzaki H, Paterson J, Shinyama H, Morton NM, Mullins JJ, Seckl JR, Flier JS. A transgenic model of visceral obesity and the metabolic syndrome. Science 2001;294:2166–2170.
109. Rebuffe-Scrive M, Bronnegard M, Nilsson A, Eldh J, Gustafsson JA, Bjorntorp P. Steroid hormone receptors in human adipose tissues. J Clin Endocrinol Metab 1990;71:1215–1219.
110. Bronnegard M, Arner P, Hellstrom L, Akner G, Gustafsson JA. Glucocorticoid receptor messenger ribonucleic acid in different regions of human adipose tissue. Endocrinology 1990;127:1689–1696.
111. Hagendorf A, Koper JW, de Jong FH, Brinkmann AO, Lamberts SW, Feelders RA. Expression of the human glucocorticoid receptor splice variants alpha, beta, and P in peripheral blood mononuclear leukocytes in healthy controls and in patients with hyper- and hypocortisolism. J Clin Endocrinol Metab 2005;90:6237–6243.
112. Storr HL, Chan LF, Grossman AB, Savage MO. Paediatric Cushing's syndrome: epidemiology, investigation and therapeutic advances. Trends Endocrinol Metab 2007;18:167–174.
113. van der Eerden BC, Karperien M, Wit JM. Systemic and local regulation of the growth plate. Endocr Rev 2003; 24:782–801.
114. Magiakou MA, Smyrnaki P, Chrousos GP. Hypertension in Cushing's syndrome. Best Pract Res Clin Endocrinol Metab 2006;20:467–482.
115. Stewart PM, Krozowski ZS. 11 beta-Hydroxysteroid dehydrogenase Vitam Horm 1999;57:249–324.
116. Li C, Wang W, Summer SN, Falk S, Schrier RW. Downregulation of UT-A1/UT-A3 is associated with urinary concentrating defect in glucocorticoid-excess state. J Am Soc Nephrol 2008;19:1975–1981.
117. Arnaldi G, Mancini T, Polenta B, Boscaro, M) Cardiovascular risk in Cushing's syndrome. Pituitary 2004;7:253–256.
118. Ullian ME. The role of corticosteriods in the regulation of vascular tone Cardiovasc Res 1999;41:55–64.
119. Grunfeld JP, Eloy L. Glucocorticoids modulate vascular reactivity in the rat. Hypertension 1987;10:608–618.
120. Sala C, Ambrosi B, Morganti A. Blunted vascular and renal effects of exogenous atrial natriuretic peptide in patients with Cushing's disease. J Clin Endocrinol Metab 2001;86:1957–1961.
121. Saruta T, Suzuki H, Handa M, Igarashi Y, Kondo K, Senba S. Multiple factors contribute to the pathogenesis of hypertension in Cushing's syndrome. J Clin Endocrinol Metab 1986;62:275–279.
122. Brieva J, Wanner A. Adrenergic airway vascular smooth muscle responsiveness in healthy and asthmatic subjects. J Appl Physiol 2001;90:665–669.
123. Knox AJ, Mortimer K. Combining inhaled glucocorticoids and long acting beta(2)-adrenoceptor agonists in asthma and COPD. Br J Pharmacol 2008;153:1085–1086.
124. Derendorf H, Meltzer EO. Molecular and clinical pharmacology of intranasal corticosteroids: clinical and therapeutic implications. Allergy 2008;63:1292–1300.
125. Boumpas DT, Chrousos GP, Wilder RL, Cupps TR, Balow JE. Glucocorticoid therapy for immune-mediated diseases: basic and clinical correlates. Ann Intern Med 1993;119:1198–1208.
126. Yu DT, Clements PJ, Paulus HE, Peter JB, Levy J, Barnett EV. Human lymphocyte subpopulations. Effect of corticosteroids. J Clin Invest 1974;53:565–571.
127. Cidlowski JA, King KL, Evans-Storms RB, Montague JW, Bortner CD, Hughes FM, Jr. The biochemistry and molecular biology of glucocorticoid-induced apoptosis in the immune system. Recent Prog Horm Res 1996;51:457–490; discussion 90–91.
128. Antonicelli F, De Coupade C, Russo-Marie F, Le Garrec Y. CREB is involved in mouse annexin A1 regulation by cAMP and glucocorticoids. Eur J Biochem 2001;268:62–69.
129. Kim SW, Rhee HJ, Ko J, Kim YJ, Kim HG, Yang JM, Choi EC, Na DS. Inhibition of cytosolic phospholipase A2 by annexin I. Specific interaction model and mapping of the interaction site. J Biol Chem 2001;276:15712–15719.
130. Mizuno H, Uemura K, Moriyama A, Wada Y, Asai K, Kimura S, Kato T. Glucocorticoid induced the expression of mRNA and the secretion of lipocortin 1 in rat astrocytoma cells. Brain Res 1997;746:256–264.

131. Rhen T, Cidlowski JA. Anti-inflammatory action of glucocorticoids—new mechanisms for old drugs. N Engl J Med 2005;353:1711–1723.
132. Solito E, de Coupade C, Parente L, Flower RJ, Russo-Marie F. IL-6 stimulates annexin 1 expression and translocation and suggests a new biological role as class II acute phase protein. Cytokine 1998;10:514–521.
133. Roviezzo F, Getting SJ, Paul-Clark MJ, Yona S, Gavins FN, Perretti M, Hannon R, Croxtall JD, Buckingham JC, Flower RJ. The annexin-1 knockout mouse: what it tells us about the inflammatory response. J Physiol Pharmacol 2002;53:541–553.
134. De Bosscher K, Vanden Berghe W, Haegeman G. The interplay between the glucocorticoid receptor and nuclear factor-kappaB or activator protein-1: molecular mechanisms for gene repression. Endocr Rev 2003;24:488–522.
135. Barnes PJ, Karin M. Nuclear factor-kappaB: a pivotal transcription factor in chronic inflammatory diseases. N Engl J Med 1997;336:1066–1071.
136. Scheinman RI, Cogswell PC, Lofquist AK, Baldwin AS, Jr. Role of transcriptional activation of I kappa B alpha in mediation of immunosuppression by glucocorticoids. Science 1995;270:283–286.
137. Hafezi-Moghadam A, Simoncini T, Yang Z, Limbourg FP, Plumier JC, Rebsamen MC, Hsieh CM, Chui DS, Thomas KL, Prorock AJ, Laubach VE, Moskowitz MA, French BA, Ley K, Liao JK. Acute cardiovascular protective effects of corticosteroids are mediated by non-transcriptional activation of endothelial nitric oxide synthase. Nat Med 2002;8:473–479.
138. Simoncini T, Mannella P, Fornari L, Caruso A, Varone G, Genazzani AR. Genomic and non-genomic effects of estrogens on endothelial cells. Steroids 2004;69:537–542.
139. Gille J, Reisinger K, Westphal-Varghese B, Kaufmann R. Decreased mRNA stability as a mechanism of glucocorticoid-mediated inhibition of vascular endothelial growth factor gene expression by cultured keratinocytes. J Invest Dermatol 2001;117:1581–1587.
140. Lasa M, Abraham SM, Boucheron C, Saklatvala J, Clark AR. Dexamethasone causes sustained expression of mitogen-activated protein kinase (MAPK) phosphatase 1 and phosphatase-mediated inhibition of MAPK p38. Mol Cell Biol 2002;22:7802–7811.
141. Graham BS, Tucker WS, Jr. Opportunistic infections in endogenous Cushing's syndrome. Ann Intern Med 1984;101: 334–338.
142. Hill AT, Stewart PM, Hughes EA, McLeod DT. Cushing's disease and tuberculosis. Respir Med 1998;92:604–606.
143. Leibovich SJ, Ross R. The role of the macrophage in wound repair. A study with hydrocortisone and antimacrophage serum. Am J Pathol 1975;78:71–100.
144. Kristo C, Ueland T, Godang K, Aukrust P, Bollerslev J. Biochemical markers for cardiovascular risk following treatment in endogenous Cushing's syndrome. J Endocrinol Invest 2008;31:400–405.
145. Dovio A, Allasino B, Palmas E, Ventura M, Pia A, Saba L, Aroasio E, Terzolo M, Angeli A. Increased osteoprotegerin levels in Cushing's syndrome are associated with an adverse cardiovascular risk profile. J Clin Endocrinol Metab 2007;92:1803–1808.
146. Perez P, Page A, Bravo A, Del Rio M, Gimenez-Conti I, Budunova I, Slaga TJ, Jorcano JL. Altered skin development and impaired proliferative and inflammatory responses in transgenic mice overexpressing the glucocorticoid receptor. FASEB J 2001;15:2030–2032.
147. Rokowski RJ, Sheehy J, Cutroneo KR. Glucocorticoid-mediated selective reduction of functioning collagen messenger ribonucleic acid. Arch Biochem Biophys 1981;210:74–81.
148. Sarnstrand B, Brattsand R, Malmstrom A. Effect of glucocorticoids on glycosaminoglycan metabolism in cultured human skin fibroblasts. J Invest Dermatol 1982;79:412–417.
149. Ross EJ, Linch DC. Cushing's syndrome—killing disease: discriminatory value of signs and symptoms aiding early diagnosis. Lancet 1982;2:646–649.
150. Block NE, Buse MG. Effects of hypercortisolemia and diabetes on skeletal muscle insulin receptor function in vitro and in vivo. Am J Physiol 1989;256:E39–48.
151. Wajchenberg BL, Bosco A, Marone MM, Levin S, Rocha M. Lerario AC, Nery M, Goldman J, Liberman B. Estimation of body fat and lean tissue distribution by dual energy X-ray absorptiometry and abdominal body fat evaluation by computed tomography in Cushing's disease. J Clin Endocrinol Metab 1995;80:2791–2794.
152. Chiodini I, Torlontano M, Carnevale V, Trischitta V, Scillitani A. Skeletal involvement in adult patients with endogenous hypercortisolism. J Endocrinol Invest 2008;31:267–276.
153. Mazziotti G, Angeli A, Bilezikian JP, Canalis E, Giustina A. Glucocorticoid-induced osteoporosis: an update. Trends Endocrinol Metab 2006;17:144–149.
154. Schacke H, Docke WD, Asadullah K. Mechanisms involved in the side effects of glucocorticoids. Pharmacol Ther 2002;96:23–43.

155. Dostert A, Heinzel T. Negative glucocorticoid receptor response elements and their role in glucocorticoid action. Curr Pharm Des 2004;10:2807–2816.
156. Canalis E, Delany AM. Mechanisms of glucocorticoid action in bone. Ann NY Acad Sci 2002;966:73–81.
157. Chakraborti S, Mandal M, Das S, Mandal A, Chakraborti T. Regulation of matrix metalloproteinases: an overview. Mol Cell Biochem 2003;253:269–285.
158. Cutroneo KR. How is Type I procollagen synthesis regulated at the gene level during tissue fibrosis. J Cell Biochem 2003;90:1–5.
159. Nuutinen P, Riekki R, Parikka M, Salo T, Autio P, Risteli J, Oikarinen A. Modulation of collagen synthesis and mRNA by continuous and intermittent use of topical hydrocortisone in human skin. Br J Dermatol 2003;148:39–45.
160. Laake H. The action of corticosteroids on the renal reabsorption of calcium. Acta Endocrinol (Copenh) 1960;34: 60–64.
161. Peck WA. The effects of glucocorticoids on bone cell metabolism and function. Adv Exp Med Biol 1984;171: 111–119.
162. Wajchenberg BL, Pereira VG, Kieffer J, Ursic S. Effect of dexamethasone on calcium metabolism and 47Ca kinetics in normal subjects. Acta Endocrinol (Copenh) 1969;61:173–192.
163. Canalis E, Giustina A. Glucocorticoid-induced osteoporosis: summary of a workshop. J Clin Endocrinol Metab 2001; 86:5681–5685.
164. Francucci CM, Pantanetti P, Garrapa GG, Massi F, Arnaldi G, Mantero F. Bone metabolism and mass in women with Cushing's syndrome and adrenal incidentaloma. Clin Endocrinol (Oxf) 2002;57:587–593.
165. Mancini T, Doga M, Mazziotti G, Giustina A. Cushing's syndrome and bone. Pituitary 2004;7:249–252.
166. Chrousos GP, Torpy DJ, Gold PW. Interactions between the hypothalamic-pituitary-adrenal axis and the female reproductive system: clinical implications. Ann Intern Med 1998;129:229–240.
167. Lado-Abeal J, Rodriguez-Arnao J, Newell-Price JD, Perry LA, Grossman AB, Besser GM, Trainer PJ. Menstrual abnormalities in women with Cushing's disease are correlated with hypercortisolemia rather than raised circulating androgen levels. J Clin Endocrinol Metab 1998;83:3083–3088.
168. Luton JP, Thieblot P, Valcke JC, Mahoudeau JA, Bricaire H. Reversible gonadotropin deficiency in male Cushing's disease. J Clin Endocrinol Metab 1977;45:488–495.
169. McEwen BS, De Kloet ER, Rostene W. Adrenal steroid receptors and actions in the nervous system. Physiol Rev 1986;66:1121–1188.
170. Dorn LD, Burgess ES, Dubbert B, Simpson SE, Friedman T, Kling M, Gold PW, Chrousos GP. Psychopathology in patients with endogenous Cushing's syndrome: 'atypical' or melancholic features. Clin Endocrinol (Oxf) 1995;43: 433–442.
171. Dorn LD, Burgess ES, Friedman TC, Dubbert B, Gold PW, Chrousos GP. The longitudinal course of psychopathology in Cushing's syndrome after correction of hypercortisolism. J Clin Endocrinol Metab 1997;82:912–919.
172. Pariante CM, Thomas SA, Lovestone S, Makoff A, Kerwin RW. Do antidepressants regulate how cortisol affects the brain? Psychoneuroendocrinology 2004;29:423–447.
173. Regestein QR, Rose LI, Williams GH. Psychopathology in Cushing's syndrome. Arch Intern Med 1972;130: 114–117.
174. Maheu FS, Mazzone L, Merke DP, Keil MF, Stratakis CA, Pine DS, Ernst M. Altered amygdala and hippocampus function in adolescents with hypercortisolemia: a functional magnetic resonance imaging study of Cushing syndrome. Dev Psychopathol 2008;20:1177–1189.
175. Sapolsky RM, Krey LC, McEwen BS. Prolonged glucocorticoid exposure reduces hippocampal neuron number: implications for aging. J Neurosci 1985;5:1222–1227.
176. Dai J, Buijs R, Swaab D. Glucocorticoid hormone (cortisol) affects axonal transport in human cortex neurons but shows resistance in Alzheimer's disease. Br J Pharmacol 2004;143:606–610.
177. Elgh E, Lindqvist Astot A, Fagerlund M, Eriksson S, Olsson T, Nasman B. Cognitive dysfunction, hippocampal atrophy and glucocorticoid feedback in Alzheimer's disease. Biol Psychiatry 2006;59:155–161.
178. Landfield PW, Blalock EM, Chen KC, Porter NM. A new glucocorticoid hypothesis of brain aging: implications for Alzheimer's disease. Curr Alzheimer Res 2007;4:205–212.
179. Bourdeau I, Bard C, Forget H, Boulanger Y, Cohen H, Lacroix A. Cognitive function and cerebral assessment in patients who have Cushing's syndrome. Endocrinol Metab Clin North Am 2005;34:357–369, ix.

2 Etiologies of Cushing's Syndrome

John Newell-Price

Contents

Summary

Harvey Cushing described the first case of Cushing's syndrome with a severe phenotype in 1912. Since then investigation and management of Cushing's syndrome has remained a significant clinical challenge *(1, 2)*, and patients suspected of this diagnosis warrant referral to major centers. Knowledge of the varying etiologies of Cushing's syndrome is important so that the likelihood of a precise cause may be considered during initial consultation and diagnostic workup.

Key Words: Diagnosis, Cushing's, ACTH-dependent, ACTH-independent, pituitary, adrenal, ectopic, CRH, PPNAD, AIMAH, McCune–Albright, cortisol

DEFINITION OF CUSHING'S SYNDROME

Cushing's syndrome is due to the chronic, excessive, and inappropriate exposure to glucocorticoid: in man this is cortisol in endogenous Cushing's syndrome.

Exogenous Cushing's Syndrome

By far the commonest cause of Cushing's syndrome in the modern era is by using exogenous glucocorticoids, frequently needed to treat inflammatory conditions. The clinical "Cushingoid" phenotype is well recognized and is due to the long-term adverse effects of excess glucocorticoid, and may be indistinguishable from endogenous Cushing's syndrome on clinical grounds alone. With the exception of exogenous hydrocortisone and cortisone acetate, where cortisol will be measured in serum

From: *Contemporary Endocrinology: Cushing's Syndrome: Pathophysiology, Diagnosis and Treatment*
Edited by: M.D. Bronstein (ed.), DOI 10.1007/978-1-60327-449-4_2,

assays, excessive exogenous glucocorticoids cause a Cushing's phenotype but with suppression of the endogenous hypothalamo-pituitary adrenal axis. Since glucocorticoids are prescribed to millions of people worldwide the numbers of patients with glucocorticoid excess are vast. Because of this, and the fact that there may be cross reactivity between some synthetic glucocorticoids and cortisol assays, it is essential that in the diagnostic workup of suspected Cushing's syndrome that clinical history taking includes a search for exogenous sources of glucocorticoid including tablets, creams, rectal and parentral preparations, inhalers, and over-the-counter drugs and remedies *(3)*.

Endogenous Cushing's Syndrome

When presentation is florid the diagnosis is usually straightforward, but in modern practice Cushing's syndrome is frequently and increasingly considered in mild cases in the absence of the classical signs in the context of osteoporosis, diabetes, hypertension, in gynecology and psychiatric clinics, and achieving a diagnosis can be difficult. Appropriate management of Cushing's syndrome is dependent on correctly identifying the cause of excess cortisol. Separating adrenocorticotropin (ACTH)-independent causes (adrenal tumors and hyperplasia) from ACTH-dependent causes (pituitary or ectopic secretion of ACTH, and rare ectopic CRH production) is usually simple. However, many ectopic sources are occult and the differentiation of the source of ACTH secretion may require meticulous and repeated investigation to enable the appropriate surgery to be undertaken.

Other Conditions with Hypercortisolemia Without Cushing's Syndrome

Hypercortisolemia may be found due to activation of the hypothalamo-pituitary adrenal axis, without physical features of Cushing's syndrome, as found in severe chronic illness, for example during a protracted stay on the intensive care unit, during acute illness, surgery, malnutrition, anorexia, and excess cortisol-binding globulin (estrogen therapy being the commonest cause) *(3)*. In some specific conditions, there may be some mild clinical features of Cushing's syndrome, namely, pregnancy, depression, alcohol dependence, morbid obesity, poorly controlled diabetes mellitus, and glucocorticoid resistance. This latter group has often been called pseudo-Cushing's, but this term may be confusing and hinder diagnosis and is better not used. Instead one approach is to consider that there is hypercortisolemia, but to then establish whether this is true autonomous hypercortisolemia – Cushing's syndrome.

ETIOLOGY AND PATHOGENESIS

Endogenous Cushing's syndrome is usually sporadic and divided into ACTH-dependent and ACTH-independent causes (Table 1). Overall, ACTH-dependent causes account for approximately 80% of cases, and of these 80% are due to corticotrope pituitary adenomas (Cushing's disease) with an excess female predominance, and the remaining 20% due to the ectopic ACTH syndrome *(2)*. Cushing's disease, the ectopic ACTH syndrome and adrenal adenomas may also be found in the context of multiple endocrine neoplasia type 1. Ectopic corticotrophin-releasing hormone (CRH) production has been described rarely over the last two decades and accounts for <1% of all cases of ACTH-dependent causes, and may mimic Cushing's disease on biochemical testing, including bilateral inferior petrosal sinus sampling *(4–7)*. The majority of tumors reported to cause ectopic CRH secretion are, however, evident on radiological imaging, facilitating diagnosis.

Table 1
Etiology of Cushing's Syndrome

Cause of Cushing's Syndrome	*F:M*	*%*
ACTH-dependent[a]		
Cushing's disease	3.5:1[b]	70
Ectopic ACTH syndrome	1:1	10
Unknown source of ACTH[c]	5:1	5
ACTH-independent	4:1	10
Adrenal adenoma	1:1	5
Adrenal carcinoma		<2
Other causes (PPNAD, AIMAH, McCune–Albright)		

PPNAD primary pigmented nodular adrenal disease, *AIMAH* ACTH-independent massive adrenal hyperplasia
[a]In women 9:1 ratio of Cushing's disease to ectopic ACTH
[b]Male preponderance in children
[c]Patients may ultimately prove to have Cushing's disease, ectopic CRH <1% of all cases of ACTH-dependent disease

ACTH-Dependent Cushing's Syndrome

Cushing's Disease

The average age of onset of Cushing's disease is 36 years. Severity of presentation varies widely, but a milder clinical phenotype in a patient presenting with Cushing's syndrome, especially if female, is more likely to be due to Cushing's disease than other etiologies. Most cases of Cushing's disease are due to corticotrope microadenomas, a few millimeters in diameter, only being larger than 1 cm (macroadenoma) in 6% of cases *(1, 8)*. In 40% of cases, no tumor is visible on T1-weighted 1.5-tesla MRI scans *(1)*. These tumors express the pro-opiomelanocortin gene (*POMC*) to form at 1,200-nt transcript, the peptide product of which is subsequently cleaved to ACTH (Fig. 1). POMC processing is usually efficient in corticotroph microadenomas, but less so in macroadenomas, which may secrete relatively large amounts of unprocessed POMC. Some pituitary macroadenomas are "silent corticotroph adenomas," and may present with tumor mass effects (e.g., optic chiasm compression) alone: on follow-up initial absence of Cushingoid features may progress to overt clinical Cushing's syndrome. Approximately 90% of tumors express the CRH-1 receptor, as evidenced by the release of ACTH in response to exogenously administered CRH *(9, 10)*. Tumors also express the vasopressin-3 (V3) receptor *(11–14)*, and respond to vasopressin and desmopressin *(15)*.

Tumors causing Cushing's disease are relatively resistant to the effects of glucocorticoids, but *POMC* expression and ACTH secretion are reduced by higher doses of dexamethasone in 80% of cases *(2, 16)*. Glucocorticoids act to reduce POMC expression by binding directly to a negative glucocorticoid response element at -57 bp on the *POMC* promoter *(17)*, and also by antagonizing the effects of the positively acting transcription factor Nur77 *(18)*. Resistance to glucocorticoid repression may also be caused by "miss-expression" of the "bridging protein" *Brg* 1 (which is important for glucocorticoid inhibitory feedback on *POMC* expression) found in corticotrope tumors, and may be one event determining tumorigenesis *(19)*. *Brg* 1 acts to recruit histone decetylases to inhibit expression by condensation of chromatin on the *POMC* promoter. Corticotrope tumors also show overexpression

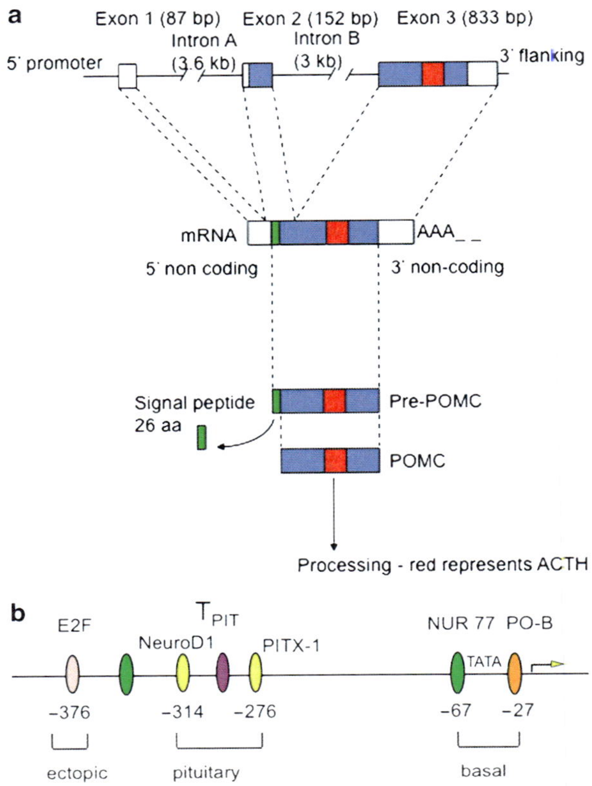

Fig. 1. Structural organization of the human pro-opiomelanocortin gene, its promoter and peptide product. (**a**) Schematic representation of exonic structure, mRNA, peptide product. (**b**) Promoter. Note that upstream region activated in ectopic ACTH syndrome by transcription factors distinct from those active in the pituitary.

of cyclin E, low expression of the cyclin-dependent inhibitor, p27, and a high Ki-67 expression, all indicative of a relatively high proliferative activity *(16)*. The excess number of reproductive-aged women with Cushing's disease, and the fact that there is a male preponderance in prepubertal cases *(20)* suggest a potential etiological role for estrogens.

The Ectopic ACTH Syndrome

Ectopic ACTH secretion causing Cushing's syndrome has been reported across a wide age range, including the elderly and very young, and from a wide range of tumors from different organs (Table 2) *(21–23)*. Tumors may be only a few millimeters in diameter, and the ectopic ACTH syndrome can be broadly classified into "overt," where the source of ACTH is clear on initial diagnostic workup (for example, small cell lung cancer), "covert," where the source is not apparent initially but following repeated investigation is finally disclosed, and "occult," where the source of ACTH is not apparent. Neuroendocrine tumors (carcinoid) causing the ectopic ACTH syndrome, most frequently bronchial, show a molecular phenotype close to that of pituitary corticotrope tumors, and may mimic Cushing's disease in clinical and biochemical features. In contrast, data in small cell lung cancer cells has shown that *POMC* is activated by transcription factors distinct from those in the pituitary, including E2F factors *(24)*, that are able to bind the promoter when it is in an unmethylated state *(25)*, suggesting a different pathogenesis. Moreover in ectopic ACTH syndrome, POMC also appears to be activated from a region in the promoter further 5′ to the transcription start site to produce a transcript of 1,350 nt, although the translated peptide product is the same.

Table 2
Etiology of Ectopic ACTH Secretion

	NIH (21)	*Barts (22)*	*Sao Paulo (23)*
Bronchial carcinoid tumor	35	12	10
Small cell lung carcinoma	3	7	
Pulmonary tumorlets	1		
Thymic carcinoid tumor	5	2	4
Medullary thyroid carcinoma	2	3	
Pancreatic carcinoid tumor	1	3	3
Gastrinoma	6	3	
Appendix	1		
Other GI neuroendocrine tumors (NET)	13		
Mesothelioma			1
Colonic carcinoma		2	
Phaeochromocytoma	5	1	5
Olfactory ethesioneuroblastoma	1		
Disseminated carcinoid tumor		2	
Lymph node NET		2	
Glomus tumor			1
Unknown	17	2	2
Overt	46	26	20
Covert	23	9	3
Occult	17	5	2
Total	90	40	25

Data derived from three major series *(21–23)*

ACTH-Independent Cushing's Syndrome

Adrenal adenomas account for the majority of ACTH-independent causes of clinically apparent Cushing's syndrome, but are by far the largest causes of low-grade autonomous hypercortisolemia (see below "Epidemiology"). Once Cushing's syndrome is confirmed, and plasma ACTH shown to be suppressed, adrenal imaging easily identifies an adrenal adenoma as a small, well-circumscribed lesion, with low Hounsfield units on CT. Any adrenal mass greater than 4 cm in diameter should be considered as potentially malignant, with the likelihood of this increasing with size or any evidence of vascular invasion. The prognosis of adrenocortical carcinoma is frequently very poor, especially if disease is not localized at diagnosis. Any evidence of co-secretion of other steroid hormones increases the likelihood of malignancy.

In ACTH-independent macronodular hyperplasia (AIMAH), excess cortisol secretion may be associated with either ectopically expressed receptors or increased eutopic receptor expression *(26)*, and activation by ligands not usually associated with adrenal steroidogenesis: gastric inhibitory peptide (food-dependent Cushing's), vasopressin, interleukin-1, lutenizing hormone, and serotonin. Activation of receptors increasing intracellular cAMP is thought to cause hyperplasia over many years, and hence Cushing's syndrome. The severity of clinical phenotype may, therefore vary, and can be mild.

Primary pigmented nodular adrenal disease (PPNAD) causes small cortisol-secreting nodules on the adrenal, often not visualized on imaging. PPNAD can be sporadic or part of the Carney complex and most cases occur in late childhood or in young adults, often with a mild or cyclical presentation *(27, 28)*. Germ line mutations of the regulatory subunit R1A of PKA (*PRKAR1A*) are present in approximately 45% of patients with Carney complex *(29, 30)* and as well as in sporadic PPNAD. Interestingly, these patients may show a paradoxical increase in cortisol secretion in response to dexamethasone. In ACTH-independent Cushing's if the adrenal CT scan is within normal limits the most likely explanation is PPNAD, or covert use of hydrocortisone or cortisone acetate, or another synthetic glucocorticoid cross reacting with the cortisol assay.

McCune–Albright syndrome is due to a postzygotic activating mutation in the *GNAS1* gene. The resulting tissue mosaicism results in a varied phenotype and the disease may present in the first few weeks of life. These mutations lead to constitutive steroidogenesis in the affected adrenal nodules *(31)*. Mutations of *GNAS1* have also been found in AIMAH.

EPIDEMIOLOGY

The true prevalence of Cushing's syndrome is difficult to quantify. Earlier data suggest an incidence from 0.7 to 2.4/million population per year *(32)* depending on the population studied *(1)*.

Cortisol excess in the general population is, however, now recognized as being common, and is found frequently in patients with adrenal masses incidentally disclosed on CT scans, so-called adrenal incidentalomas *(33)*. Compared to age, sex, and BMI-matched controls, patients with these cortisol-secreting adrenal adenoma are at significantly increased cardiovascular risk with increases in hypertension, impaired glucose tolerance and diabetes, hyperlipoproteinemia, and increased carotid intima-media thickness *(34–37)*. Although the biochemical cortisol excess is sufficient to causes these changes, it is insufficient to cause the clinical features typically associated with Cushing's syndrome *(1, 2)*. It is for these reasons that the term "Subclinical Cushing's syndrome" (SCS) is often applied to this condition.

Postmortem studies show a prevalence of adrenal adenomas of approximately 10% *(38)*. Approximately 5% of all abdominal CT scans disclose an adrenal incidentaloma *(33, 39)*. The prevalence increases in an age-related fashion and they are found in 0.2% of abdominal CT scans in patients 20–29 years of age, this rising to approximately 10% in those over 70 years of age *(38, 39)*. Between 5 and 20% of these adrenal masses are associated with SCS *(40)*. Thus, SCS is common in the general population (~1% or more of those > 70 years in hospitalized or health-screened populations), and contributes to overall cardiovascular morbidity and mortality. An ever expanding number of patients with adrenal masses are being found due to the increasing use of CT in all areas of medicine: in the past decade, the number of CT scans performed in the United Kingdom has doubled from 1.2 to 2.4 million per year. This huge increase means that the number of patients identified with low-grade cortisol excess is set to rise still further.

The major problem is that management of these patients is *not* established. Approximately, 90% of these patients have hypertension, over 60% have impaired glucose tolerance or diabetes mellitus, and many have osteoporosis *(34, 35, 37, 41–45)*. There is the potential to permanently reduce these risks, and to improve bone health, by adrenalectomy. In terms of the potential benefit from treating these risk factors, meta-analysis of several large prospective studies has shown that a 5–6 mmHg decrease in diastolic blood pressure is associated with a 38% reduction in risk for stroke and a 16% reduction in coronary heart disease events *(46)*, whilst a 10 mmHg reduction in systolic blood pressure is associated with a 31% reduction in risk of stroke *(47)*. Moreover, impaired glucose tolerance is associated with a two-fold risk of cardiovascular death *(48)*. Only a very limited number of individuals with SCS have been subjected to adrenalectomy, with the few reported forming parts of studies investigating the biochemical, cardiovascular, and bone abnormalities of patients with adrenal incidentaloma. In those that have undergone this procedure, improvements have been found in blood pressure (~10 mmHg drop in systolic BP), lipid profiles, fibrinogen levels, and glycemic control *(35–37, 49, 50)*. However, the difficulty facing the clinician is in deciding whether adrenal surgery will be of benefit for a given patient with SCS, and the basis for selection for such permanent and invasive intervention is not established. On follow-up, the majority of incidentalomas remain unchanged in size and malignant transformation is rare *(51)*. In contrast to SCS, the management of other causes in adrenal incidentaloma is not controversial, and the 4.2% that are phaechromocytomas and the 1.6% that are aldosteronomas *(52)* are usually considered for surgical excision. Surgery is also indicated if there is a significant increase in size demonstrated on CT scans repeated at intervals.

A further problem is whether widespread screening for Cushing's in obese and diabetic populations is a cost-effective approach. Large-scale nontargeted screening shows that diagnostic tests used to establish biochemical hypercortisolemia have poor specificity for Cushing's syndrome *(53)*, and this is a major reason why widespread screening in these populations is not recommended *(3)*. For those with vertebral fracture and osteoporosis the pickup rate appears to be higher *(54)*, but as yet there are no formal randomized intervention studies seeking to address whether identification and treatment of clinically nonapparent Cushing's syndrome is of benefit.

APPROACH TO MANAGEMENT

In most circumstances, the mainstay of therapy remains surgery to either an ACTH-secreting tumor or directly to the adrenal glands, but additional treatment with cortisol-lowering drugs and tumor-directed therapy is often needed.

To deliver high-quality treatment to patients with Cushing's syndrome requires a team that includes specialized surgeons and physicians, radiologists, cytologists, histopathologists, and radiotherapists. The sustained hypercortisolemia of Cushing's syndrome, of any etiology, suppresses ACTH secretion from healthy corticotropes and hence hypoadrenalism will be the consequence of complete excision of any tumor causing Cushing's syndrome, be it adrenal, pituitary, or an ectopic source of ACTH secretion, and this may be prolonged.

Most patients initially suspected of possibly having Cushing's syndrome will not have this condition. The complete assessment of a patient known to have some form of Cushing's syndrome is complex, expensive, and often stressful for the patient, who is usually already significantly ill emotionally, psychologically, and physically. Thus, efficient screening procedures are needed to identify the minority who will need intensive and expensive investigation leading to an accurate and precise differential diagnosis *(1, 55)*.

REFERENCES

1. Newell-Price J, Bertagna X, Grossman AB, Nieman LK. Cushing's syndrome. Lancet 2006;367(9522):1605–1617.
2. Newell-Price J, Trainer P, Besser M, Grossman A. The diagnosis and differential diagnosis of Cushing's syndrome and pseudo-Cushing's states. Endocr Rev 1998;19(5):647–672.
3. Nieman LK, Biller BM, Findling JW, et al. The diagnosis of Cushing's syndrome: an Endocrine Society Clinical Practice Guideline. J Clin Endocrinol Metab 2008;93(5):1526–1540.
4. Schteingart DE, Lloyd RV, Akil H, et al. Cushing's syndrome secondary to ectopic corticotropin-releasing hormone-adrenocorticotropin secretion. J Clin Endocrinol Metab 1986;63(3):770–775.
5. Muller OA, von Werder K. Ectopic production of ACTH and corticotropin-releasing hormone (CRH). J Steroid Biochem Mol Biol 1992;43(5):403–408.

6. Bayraktar F, Kebapcilar L, Kocdor MA, et al. Cushing's syndrome due to ectopic CRH secretion by adrenal pheochromocytoma accompanied by renal infarction. Exp Clin Endocrinol Diabetes 2006;114(8):444–447.
7. Rod A, Voicu M, Chiche L, et al. Cushing's syndrome associated with a nested stromal epithelial tumor of the liver: hormonal, immunohistochemical, and molecular studies. Eur J Endocrinol 2009;161(5):805–810.
8. Woo YS, Isidori AM, Wat WZ, et al. Clinical and biochemical characteristics of adrenocorticotropin-secreting macroadenomas. J Clin Endocrinol Metab 2005;90(8):4963–4969.
9. Newell-Price J, Morris DG, Drake WM, et al. Optimal response criteria for the human CRH test in the differential diagnosis of ACTH-dependent Cushing's syndrome. J Clin Endocrinol Metab 2002;87(4):1640–1645.
10. Nieman LK, Oldfield EH, Wesley R, Chrousos GP, Loriaux DL, Cutler GB, Jr. A simplified morning ovine corticotropin-releasing hormone stimulation test for the differential diagnosis of adrenocorticotropin-dependent Cushing's syndrome. J Clin Endocrinol Metab 1993;77(5):1308–1312.
11. de Keyzer Y, Auzan C, Lenne F, et al. Cloning and characterization of the human V3 pituitary vasopressin receptor. FEBS Lett 1994;356(2–3):215–220.
12. Dahia PL, Ahmed-Shuaib A, Jacobs RA, et al. Vasopressin receptor expression and mutation analysis in corticotropin-secreting tumors. J Clin Endocrinol Metab 1996;81(5):1768–1771.
13. de Keyzer Y, Lenne F, Auzan C, et al. The pituitary V3 vasopressin receptor and the corticotroph phenotype in ectopic ACTH syndrome. J Clin Invest 1996;97(5):1311–1318.
14. de Keyzer Y, Rene P, Lenne F, Auzan C, Clauser E, Bertagna X. V3 vasopressin receptor and corticotropic phenotype in pituitary and nonpituitary tumors. Horm Res 1997;47(4–6):259–262.
15. Newell-Price J, Perry L, Medbak S, et al. A combined test using desmopressin and corticotropin-releasing hormone in the differential diagnosis of Cushing's syndrome. J Clin Endocrinol Metab 1997;82(1):176–181.
16. Dahia PL, Grossman AB. The molecular pathogenesis of corticotroph tumors. Endocr Rev 1999;20(2):136–155.
17. Drouin J, Trifiro MA, Plante RK, Nemer M, Eriksson P, Wrange O. Glucocorticoid receptor binding to a specific DNA sequence is required for hormone-dependent repression of pro-opiomelanocortin gene transcription. Mol Cell Biol 1989;9(12):5305–5314.
18. Philips A, Maira M, Mullick A, et al. Antagonism between Nur77 and glucocorticoid receptor for control of transcription. Mol Cell Biol 1997;17(10):5952–5959.
19. Bilodeau S, Vallette-Kasic S, Gauthier Y, et al. Role of Brg1 and HDAC2 in GR trans-repression of the pituitary POMC gene and misexpression in Cushing disease. Genes Dev 2006;20(20):2871–2886.
20. Storr HL, Isidori AM, Monson JP, Besser GM, Grossman AB, Savage MO. Prepubertal Cushing's disease is more common in males, but there is no increase in severity at diagnosis. J Clin Endocrinol Metab 2004;89(8):3818–3820.
21. Ilias I, Torpy DJ, Pacak K, Mullen N, Wesley RA, Nieman LK. Cushing's syndrome due to ectopic corticotropin secretion: twenty years' experience at the National Institutes of Health. J Clin Endocrinol Metab 2005;90(8):4955–4962.
22. Isidori AM, Kaltsas GA, Pozza C, et al. The ectopic adrenocorticotropin syndrome: clinical features, diagnosis, management, and long-term follow-up. J Clin Endocrinol Metab 2006;91(2):371–377.
23. Salgado LR, Fragoso MC, Knoepfelmacher M, et al. Ectopic ACTH syndrome: our experience with 25 cases. Eur J Endocrinol 2006;155(5):725–733.
24. Picon A, Bertagna X, de Keyzer Y. Analysis of the human proopiomelanocortin gene promoter in a small cell lung carcinoma cell line reveals an unusual role for E2F transcription factors. Oncogene 1999;18(16):2627–2633.
25. Newell-Price J, King P, Clark AJ. The CpG island promoter of the human proopiomelanocortin gene is methylated in nonexpressing normal tissue and tumors and represses expression. Mol Endocrinol 2001;15(2):338–348.
26. Lacroix A, Ndiaye N, Tremblay J, Hamet P. Ectopic and abnormal hormone receptors in adrenal Cushing's syndrome. Endocr Rev 2001;22(1):75–110.
27. Storr HL, Mitchell H, Swords FM, et al. Clinical features, diagnosis, treatment and molecular studies in paediatric Cushing's syndrome due to primary nodular adrenocortical hyperplasia. Clin Endocrinol (Oxf) 2004;61(5):553–559.
28. Stratakis CA, Kirschner LS, Carney JA. Clinical and molecular features of the Carney complex: diagnostic criteria and recommendations for patient evaluation. J Clin Endocrinol Metab 2001;86(9):4041–4046.
29 Kirschner LS, Carney JA, Pack SD, et al. Mutations of the gene encoding the protein kinase A type I-alpha regulatory subunit in patients with the Carney complex. Nat Genet 2000;26(1):89–92.
30. Casey M, Vaughan CJ, He J, et al. Mutations in the protein kinase A R1alpha regulatory subunit cause familial cardiac myxomas and Carney complex. J Clin Invest 2000;106(5):R31–38.
31. Weinstein LS, Shenker A, Gejman PV, Merino MJ, Friedman E, Spiegel AM. Activating mutations of the stimulatory G protein in the McCune–Albright syndrome. N Engl J Med 1991;325(24):1688–1695.
32. Etxabe J, Vazquez JA. Morbidity and mortality in Cushing's disease: an epidemiological approach. Clin Endocrinol (Oxf) 1994;40(4):479–484.

33. Young WF, Jr. Clinical practice. The incidentally discovered adrenal mass. N Engl J Med 2007;356(6):601–610.
34. Garrapa GG, Pantanetti P, Arnaldi G, Mantero F, Faloia E. Body composition and metabolic features in women with adrenal incidentaloma or Cushing's syndrome. J Clin Endocrinol Metab 2001;86(11):5301–5306.
35. Rossi R, Tauchmanova L, Luciano A, et al. Subclinical Cushing's syndrome in patients with adrenal incidentaloma: clinical and biochemical features. J Clin Endocrinol Metab 2000;85(4):1440–1448.
36. Tauchmanova L, Rossi R, Biondi B, et al. Patients with subclinical Cushing's syndrome due to adrenal adenoma have increased cardiovascular risk. J Clin Endocrinol Metab 2002;87(11):4872–4878.
37. Terzolo M, Pia A, Ali A, et al. Adrenal incidentaloma: a new cause of the metabolic syndrome? J Clin Endocrinol Metab 2002;87(3):998–1003.
38. Kloos RT, Gross MD, Francis IR, Korobkin M, Shapiro B. Incidentally discovered adrenal masses. Endocr Rev 1995; 16(4):460–484.
39. Mansmann G, Lau J, Balk E, Rothberg M, Miyachi Y, Bornstein SR. The clinically inapparent adrenal mass: update in diagnosis and management. Endocr Rev 2004;25(2):309–340.
40. Terzolo M, Reimondo G, Bovio S, Angeli A. Subclinical Cushing's syndrome. Pituitary 2004;7(4):217–223.
41. Tauchmanova L, Pivonello R, Di Somma C, et al. Bone demineralization and vertebral fractures in endogenous cortisol excess: role of disease etiology and gonadal status. J Clin Endocrinol Metab 2006;91(5):1779–1784.
42. Francucci CM, Pantanetti P, Garrapa GG, Massi F, Arnaldi G, Mantero F. Bone metabolism and mass in women with Cushing's syndrome and adrenal incidentaloma. Clin Endocrinol (Oxf) 2002;57(5):587–593.
43. Chiodini I, Tauchmanova L, Torlontano M, et al. Bone involvement in eugonadal male patients with adrenal incidentaloma and subclinical hypercortisolism. J Clin Endocrinol Metab 2002;87(12):5491–5494.
44. Osella G, Terzolo M, Borretta G, et al. Endocrine evaluation of incidentally discovered adrenal masses (incidentalomas). J Clin Endocrinol Metab 1994;79(6):1532–1539.
45. Terzolo M, Osella G, Ali A, et al. Subclinical Cushing's syndrome in adrenal incidentaloma. Clin Endocrinol (Oxf) 1998;48(1):89–97.
46. Hebert PR, Moser M, Mayer J, Glynn RJ, Hennekens CH. Recent evidence on drug therapy of mild to moderate hypertension and decreased risk of coronary heart disease. Arch Intern Med 1993;153(5):578–581.
47. Lawes CM, Bennett DA, Feigin VL, Rodgers A. Blood pressure and stroke: an overview of published reviews. Stroke 2004;35(4):1024.
48. Glucose tolerance and mortality: comparison of WHO and American Diabetes Association diagnostic criteria. The DECODE study group. European Diabetes Epidemiology Group. Diabetes Epidemiology: Collaborative analysis of diagnostic criteria in Europe. Lancet 1999;354(9179):617–621.
49. Midorikawa S, Sanada H, Hashimoto S, Suzuki T, Watanabe T. The improvement of insulin resistance in patients with adrenal incidentaloma by surgical resection. Clin Endocrinol (Oxf) 2001;54(6):797–804.
50. Terzolo M, Bovio S, Pia A, et al. Midnight serum cortisol as a marker of increased cardiovascular risk in patients with a clinically inapparent adrenal adenoma. Eur J Endocrinol 2005;153(2):307–315.
51. Barzon L, Scaroni C, Sonino N, Fallo F, Paoletta A, Boscaro M. Risk factors and long-term follow-up of adrenal incidentalomas. J Clin Endocrinol Metab 1999;84(2):520–526.
52. Mantero F, Terzolo M, Arnaldi G, et al. A survey on adrenal incidentaloma in Italy. Study Group on Adrenal Tumors of the Italian Society of Endocrinology. J Clin Endocrinol Metab 2000;85(2):637–644.
53. Pecori Giraldi F, Ambrogio AG, De Martin M, Fatti LM, Scacchi M, Cavagnini F. Specificity of first-line tests for the diagnosis of Cushing's syndrome: assessment in a large series. J Clin Endocrinol Metab 2007;92(11):4123–4129.
54. Chiodini I, Mascia ML, Muscarella S, et al. Subclinical hypercortisolism among outpatients referred for osteoporosis. Ann Intern Med 2007;147(8):541–548.
55. Arnaldi G, Angeli A, Atkinson AB, et al. Diagnosis and complications of Cushing's syndrome: a consensus statement. J Clin Endocrinol Metab 2003;88(12):5593–5602.

3 Pathogenesis of Corticotropic Tumors

Anat Ben-Shlomo, Ning-Ai Liu, and Shlomo Melmed

Contents

Summary

Subcellular molecular mechanisms underlying ACTH-secreting pituitary adenomas remain elusive. Genetic and acquired animal and cell models have provided insights into corticotroph cell tumorigenesis, including cell cycle abnormalities and aberrant glucocorticoid feedback mechanisms. Novel peptide therapies targeting somatostatin and/or dopamine (D_2) receptors and emerging microRNA studies may shed light on additional cellular pathways that regulate tumoral corticotroph cell function. Studying human pituitary corticotroph tumor biology is challenging. The rarity of the disease, as well as the small tumor size and commonly encountered specimen contamination with adjacent "normal" pituitary tissue, all represent obstacles to studying disease mechanisms. Moreover, the lack of normal/ non-autopsy derived human pituitary tissue and the inability to separate pure populations of viable corticotroph cells in primary non-human pituitary cultures does not enable easy comparison between normal and abnormal corticotroph cells. Therefore, despite technological and biological advances improving our knowledge of Cushing's disease, the pathophysiology of pituitary corticotroph adenomas remains unclear. This chapter focuses on accumulating knowledge, emphasizing recent progress in identifying molecular and genetic mechanisms contributing to the pathogenesis of Cushing's disease.

Key Words: Corticotroph adenoma, ACTH, Pituitary tumor, POMC gene, T-Pit

Almost 80 years have passed since the American neurosurgeon Harvey Cushing described Cushing's disease, and yet the etiology and pathogenesis of corticotroph cell adenomas remains enigmatic. Corticotroph cell lesions are rare. According to the German Registry of Pituitary Tumors, 405 of 3489

From: *Contemporary Endocrinology: Cushing's Syndrome: Pathophysiology, Diagnosis and Treatment*
Edited by: M.D. Bronstein (ed.), DOI 10.1007/978-1-60327-449-4_3,

Table 1
Corticotroph Cell Tumors

Clinically active	Densely granulated
	Sparsely granulated
	Nelson's tumor
	Extrapituitary parasellar
	Crooke cell
	Carcinoma
Clinically silent	Densely granulated (subtype 1)
	Sparsely granulated (subtype 2)

(11.6%) of pituitary adenomas were clinically active pituitary corticotroph adenomas while 111 (3.2%) were silent *(1)*. As pituitary tumor prevalence is ~200 per million with an annual incidence of ~2 per 100,000, the prevalence of corticotroph tumors is ~10–15% of all pituitary adenomas. Clinicopathological subtypes of corticotroph cell tumors are presented in Table 1.

ANIMAL MODELS OF CUSHING'S DISEASE

Spontaneous disorders mimicking human Cushing's disease (CD) have been described in animal species including dogs, horses, and less commonly cats *(2–5)*. Equine CD usually results from tumors of the intermediate lobe, and rarely from those of the anterior lobe *(2, 3)*. Canine CD is one of the most common endocrine disorders, with an estimated incidence of 1 to 2 cases/1,000 dogs/year *(4 5)*. Approximately 30% of canine CD exhibit tumors of the PI. In addition to typical melanotrophs, the canine PI contains a substantial percentage of a second cell type that stains intensely for ACTH but not for MSH *(6)*. Although the molecular, cellular and genetic make-up of canine corticotroph adenoma remains unclear, the high natural incidence and many clinical similarities to human CD make canine CD a potential spontaneous animal model for both in vitro and in vivo studies to understand CD pathogenesis, as well as to develop and test new therapeutic strategies.

Genetically manipulated mammalian models, such as the mouse, are the most widely used in modeling CD, primarily because of the striking homology between mammalian genomes and the similarities from anatomy to cell biology and physiology. Sophisticated transgenic approaches have allowed the creation of mouse models with overexpression of dominantly acting disease-causing transgenes to recapitulate CD pathology. Furthermore, generation of specific allelic modification through gene targeting by homologous recombination has allowed ablation of single endogenous genes, which have further expanded our knowledge on CD development. Murine models of pituitary POMC-secreting adenomas have been developed using oncogenic viruses, including hormone-promoter targeting of the simian virus (SV)40 T antigen *(7–9)*. These models represent artificial phenomena that offer limited insight into pituitary tumorigenesis. Others were developed by transgenic overexpression of hypothalamic stimulatory hormones or growth factors *(10, 11)*. Furthermore, studies of targeted gene knockout models have implicated cell cycle regulators in CD pathogenesis *(12–14)*.

Transgenic Oncogene Overexpression in CD Models

The first murine CD model induced by genetic manipulation was described in transgenic mice bearing a hybrid gene consisting of the viral polyoma early region promoter linked to the polyoma large T antigen cDNA *(8)*. Transgenic mice developed pituitary microadenomas at 9 months of age, and large adenomas at 13–16 months of age, accompanied by features of Cushing's syndrome that progressed to wasting. Effects of glucocorticoid excess were more pronounced in immunocompetent mice carrying transplants of transgenic pituitary tumors than in the transgenic mice themselves. Mouse is the natural host of polyoma virus, and infection is usually asymptomatic. Inoculation of newborn mice with high titers of virus, however, results in tumor formation in a broad range of tissues, with tumors of the parotid and other salivary glands being the most prevalent *(7)*. One of the two PyLT transgenic lines developed pituitary tumors with 100% penetrance, suggesting that some viral oncogenes exhibit cell specificity in the murine pituitary gland. The latency of tumor formation in PyLT transgenic mice also supports the requirement for additional genetic or epigenetic alterations in corticotroph tumorigenesis *(7, 8)*.

Targeted tumorigenesis utilizing a proopiomelanocortin (POMC) gene promoter (nucleotides –706 to +64) ligated to the simian virus (SV) 40 early gene encoding large T antigen induced large POMC-expressing pituitary tumors arising from the intermediate lobe *(9)*. The tumor contained nuclear SV40 T antigen and POMC peptides, but did not express other pituitary hormones. POMC processing in the pituitary tumors was indistinguishable from normal mouse intermediate lobe melanotrophs and was characterized by high proportions of acetylated and carboxyl-terminal shortened β-endorphins, and amino-terminal acetylated α-melanocyte-stimulating hormone, but virtually no ACTH(1–39), β-lipotropin or POMC. The tumors contained abundant levels of mRNA for the prohormone convertase PC2 and undetectable levels of PC1, similar to wild-type mouse neurointermediate lobe but distinct from the relative abundance of anterior lobe PC1.

Transgenic Alterations of Hormonal and Growth Factor Signals in CD Models

Pituitary tumor growth seems to be promoted by hormones that modulate normal pituitary hormonal activity, and by growth factors implicated in normal fetal pituitary development *(15)*. Several mouse models have validated the roles of these alterations. Transgenic mouse with metallothionine (mMT)-promoter driven overexpression of CRH developed endocrine abnormalities involving the hypothalamic–pituitary–adrenal axis, such as elevated plasma levels of ACTH and glucocorticoids. In addition, transgenic mice display physical changes similar to those of patients with Cushing's syndrome, such as excess fat accumulation, muscle atrophy, thin skin, and alopecia. Although there is no evidence of increased ACTH-expressing cells in the pituitary of mMt-CRH transgenic mice, hypercortisolemia induced by CRH stimulation of ACTH levels may result in inhibitory feedback on pituitary corticotrophs *(10)*.

Arginine-vasopressin is a potent ACTH-releasing hormone which acts synergistically with CRH. Transgenic mice expressing human V3 receptor under the control of rat POMC promoter sequences showed increased basal concentrations of corticosterone, however no corticotroph tumor development *(16)*.

Leukemia inhibitory factor (LIF) is a pleiotropic cytokine that regulates the mature hypothalamic–pituitary–adrenal axis, determines corticotroph cell proliferation, and potently synergizes with CRH to enhance POMC transcription and ACTH secretion *(17)*. Transgenic mice expressing LIF driven by the pituitary glycoprotein hormone α-subunit (aGSU) promoter exhibit corticotroph hyperplasia, thin skin, truncal obesity, and hypercortisolism, consistent with CD. These mice also exhibited central hypogonadism, dwarfism, and mild hypothyroidism, with gonadotroph, somatotroph, lactotroph, and thyrotroph hypoplasia. In the mouse, the initial hormonal evidence of pituitary organ commitment commences with expression of aGSU *(11)*. In the LIF transgenic pituitary, the LIF product diverts progenitor cells to differentiate from Lhx3-dependent cell lineages (gonadotroph, thyrotroph, somatotroph, and lactotroph) to a Lhx3-independent cell lineage, i.e. the corticotroph. Recent studies show that LIF signaling is further potentiated by glucocorticoids *(18)*. These findings imply that neuro-immune-endocrine interfacing molecules act as important players in pituitary corticotroph homeostasis.

GENETIC KNOCKOUT OF CELL CYCLE REGULATORS IN PITUITARY POMC CELL TUMORS

Multiple knockout models of cell cycle regulators exhibit high incidence of pituitary intermediate lobe POMC cell tumors, an otherwise rare tumor type in wild-type mice. Tumor incidence and phenotype are highly dependent on the mouse strain suggesting additional genetic factors involved in tumorigenesis *(19)*. A classical example of the link between cell cycle regulators and pituitary tumorigenesis are manifest in the heterozygous Rb mice *(12–14)*. Rb is a tumor suppressor gene and controls the G1/S checkpoint. Cyclin-dependent kinases (Cdk) phosphorylate Rb to release E2F, enabling S phase progression. Cdk actions are suppressed by Ink4-type inhibitors (p16, p15, p18, p19) and Cip/Kip-type (p21, p27, p57) inhibitors. Sequential activation and inactivation of protein kinase complexes regulate cell-cycle progression including the G1/S phase transition *(20)*. $Rb^{+/-}$ mice develop pituitary intermediate lobe POMC cell tumors at 12 months with 100% penetrance. p27 (Kip1) deletion, like deletion of the Rb gene, caused neoplastic growth of the pituitary pars intermedia. However, p27 deletion leads to intermediate lobe adenomas that is less severe than the intermediate lobe adenocarcinomas arising in $Rb^{+/-}$ animals *(21–23)*. Loss of p27 or p21 enhances intermediate lobe tumorigenesis and shortens the lifespan of $Rb^{+/-}$ animals *(24, 25)*. Additionally, loss of p18 leads to intermediate lobe hyperplasia, which is further enhanced by loss of p27 or p21 *(26, 27)*.

Tumor incidence provoked by the partial deletion of Rb is partially reverted by mutations in Rb effectors such as E2f1 or E2f4 (28, 29), as well as pituitary tumor transforming gene (PTTG) *(30)*. PTTG is a securin that binds separase in the APC complex to regulate sister-chromatid separation, and also plays multiple roles in cell cycle regulation at different stages *(31)*. PTTG deletion decreased pituitary tumor incidence in $Rb^{+/-}$ mice, probably by triggering p53/p21-dependent senescence *(32, 33)*. Therefore, multiple cell cycle pathways are involved in pituitary corticotroph tumorigenesis.

In summary, limited by the low disease incidence and small tumor size in humans, research advancement on studying CD pathogenesis is heavily dependent on studies of animal models. Despite discrepancies in tumor phenotype, genetic and species variations, genetically manipulated mouse models provide important tools for molecular and cellular studies to understand CD pathogenesis. Additionally, animal models with high incidence of spontaneous CD possess potential for in vitro and in vivo studies. Further studies are required to develop model organisms that compliment other animal models to improve the understanding of CD pathogenesis and ultimately lead to new and effective therapies.

PATHOLOGY OF HUMAN PITUITARY CORTICOTROPH ADENOMAS

While 85% of active corticotroph adenomas are microadenomas (up to 10 mm in diameter), most silent corticotroph adenomas and Nelson's tumors are macroadenomas *(1, 34)*.

Active corticotroph adenomas, the hallmark of CD, are slowly growing tumors, mostly in women, located in the center of the gland where the normal corticotroph cells cluster, e.g. central mucoid wedge of the anterior lobe *(35)*. These are the most common pituitary adenomas in the first decade of life *(36)*. Some adenomas are too small to be recognized in the pituitary specimen resected during surgery and only normal pituitary cells and Crooke cells may be detected. These adenomas do not have a capsule and sometimes are intimately associated with non-tumorous cells, yet are distinct from surrounding pituitary tissue *(34)*. These tumors are densely or sparsely granulated ACTH cell adenomas (6.4% and 5.2% of all pituitary adenomas, respectively) or Crooke cell adenomas (0.03%) *(1)*.

Densely granulated ACTH adenoma cells are monomorphic, basophilic, containing PAS-positive granulation and strong ACTH and Tpit immunostaining *(37)*. Immunoreactive α-subunit, FSH/LH, galanin and keratins may also be present *(1, 34, 37)*. Electron microscopy demonstrates monomorphic spherical or ovoid nuclei with nucleoli, moderately developed rough endoplasmic reticulum, medium-sized Golgi and numerous 200–450 nm diameter secretory granules. Cytokeratin filaments and perinuclear bundles are seen in CD but not in Nelson's tumors. *Sparsely granulated ACTH cell adenomas* are weakly basophilic and PAS-positive with somewhat weaker ACTH immunostaining. Cell pleomorphism is more prominent than in densely granulated cells. Electron microscopy demonstrates fewer and smaller secretory granules.

Pituitary Nelson's tumors arise in patients with CD who have undergone bilateral adrenalectomy. Although mostly slowly growing, some tumors can grow rapidly to a large size *(35)*. Crooke hyalinization is usually absent in non-tumorous corticotroph cells derived from pituitary glands harboring Nelson's tumor.

Crooke cell adenomas are extremely rare corticotroph tumors with a typical Crooke cell structure. Expression of cytokeratin microfilaments is variable and 65% are accompanied by hypercortisolism *(1)*. Seventy-two percent of these tumors are invasive *(38)*.

Extrapituitary parasellar corticotroph adenomas are rare and develop in ectopic pituitary tissue. These tumors can be found in the sphenoid sinus, interpeduncular cistern, suprasellar space, and inside the cavernous sinus *(39)*. In some cases, these tumors cannot be localized and bilateral adrenalectomy may reveal subsequent tumor localization as Nelson's tumor developments *(39)*.

Peritumoral non-adenomatous corticotroph cells have characteristic changes termed Crooke hyalinization that occur in most active corticotroph adenoma cases *(1)*. These cells are larger than normal corticotroph cells and exhibit intracytoplasmic hyaline rings composed of keratin intermediate filaments, paranuclear large lysosomes that take up the secretory granules. These changes are attributed to high cortisol levels and appear in other hypercortisolemic states like exogenous high-dose glucocorticoid and extrapituitary tumors secreting ACTH or cortisol. In most Cushing's adenoma patients there is no hyperplasia of non-tumorous corticotroph cells, however, some cases with corticotroph hyperplasia has been reported *(40)*.

There are two major types of clinically *silent ACTH cell adenoma*, densely granulated (subtype 1) and sparsely granulated (subtype 2) *(41)*. These tumors are mostly macroadenomas with more aggressive and invasive characteristics. Subtype 1 comprised 0.06% of 3489 pituitary tumors in the German Pituitary Tumor Registry and subtype 2, 2.6%. Subtype 1 showed higher incidence of hemorrhagic necrosis than in active densely granulated ACTH cell adenomas, and subtype 2 is more common in men. Other than their size and absence of Crooke hyaline changes, these tumors are histologically indistinguishable from densely and sparsely active adenomas *(1)*.

PATHOPHYSIOLOGY

It remains unresolved whether corticotroph tumors arise from a primary defect in the hypothalamus or the pituitary *(42)*. However, currently, most researchers support the primary pituitary origin. Hypothalamic dysfunction was supported by the fact that many CD-associated endocrinopathies suggest hypothalamic dysregulation including inhibition of growth, hypogonadotropic hypogonadism, and hypothyroidism. Moreover, in many cases the pituitary adenoma is not identified on surgery and these tumors often recur after apparently complete resection, and some pituitary glands harboring corticotroph adenomas exhibit corticotroph hyperplasia *(43, 44)*. However, hyperplasia is difficult to detect as differences from normal corticotroph cells are subtle *(40)*. The evidence for a primary pituitary origin is more substantial. High cure rates with reversal of major abnormalities are associated with CD after complete tumor resection and cortisol level normalization. Pituitary hyper-responsiveness to CRH before corticotroph adenoma removal reverses to hypo-responsiveness 1 week after resection *(45)*. Most corticotroph adenomas do not exhibit surrounding hyperplastic corticotrophs *(40)*. Moreover, pituitary tumors were proven to be monoclonal in origin *(46, 47)*.

Corticotroph tumors likely develop from a cell exhibiting a set-point defect rendering it partially resistant to the physiological suppressive effect of glucocorticoids *(48)* hence secreting inappropriately high ACTH levels. When peri-tumoral, presumably normal, and tumoral corticotroph cells were evaluated for dexamethasone responsiveness, dexamethasone reduced both ACTH release and POMC mRNA from peri-tumoral corticotroph cells more effectively than in tumoral corticotroph cells *(49)*. However, as glucocorticoids can still partially suppress ACTH secretion from pituitary corticotroph adenoma cells, these tumors are not completely autonomous *(49–54)*. POMC processing and POMC-derived peptides are similar in normal and tumoral corticotroph cells *(55, 56)* and pituitary glands harboring corticotroph adenomas exhibit increased sensitivity to stimulatory effects of CRH and AVP *(57)*, however, the role of CRH and AVP in pituitary adenoma growth is undetermined. Long-term administration of CRH led to increased corticotroph cell size and number *(58–60)*; however, high CRH cannot explain pituitary corticotroph cell growth in CD as CRH levels are suppressed.

Importantly, human corticotroph tumor studies are difficult to undertake as these are so rare. Moreover, these tumors are small and in many cases the tumor specimen is accompanied by surrounding normal pituitary tissue. In addition, direct comparison of timorous to normal corticotroph cell function is challenging in most of the cases, as normal pituitary tissue from the same patient is usually unavailable, and even if available, the degree of "normalcy" is questionable.

Nelson's tumor was recently demonstrated not to appear de novo but rather to grow from a persistent pituitary corticotroph adenoma *(61)* and therefore exhibits its molecular features. The cause for growth of Nelson's tumor is yet unknown, and causes may include restored tone of CRH and AVP, elimination of the suppressive growth effect of endogenous cortisol and insufficient levels of exogenous cortisone *(62)*.

MOLECULAR PATHOGENESIS ASSOCIATED WITH HUMAN CUSHING'S DISEASE

As comprehensively reviewed, no clear evidence exists regarding consistent corticotroph cell adenoma mutations *(63–65)*. Many protooncogenes were studied as a potential cause for corticotroph adenoma, all showing negative results. These include RAS, c-ERB2/neu, c-MYC, PKC, RET, c-MYB, c-FOS, Gα subunit of the G-protein, p53, Rb1, p16, p18 and p27 *(63)*.

Regulatory receptor genes have also been studied in pituitary corticotroph adenomas. Vesopressin type 3 receptor (V_3R) stimulation enhances ACTH secretion and its mRNA expression is increased in these tumors as a consequence of chronic glucocorticoid exposure, however, no mutation in V_3R was found in 12 corticotroph adenomas *(66)*. No mutations were found in the DNA-binding domain and splice junction region of the glucocorticoid receptor in 17 corticotroph adenomas and 2 Nelson's tumors *(67)*. However, 6 of 22 tumors showed loss of heterozygosity in five known polymorphisms with monoallelic deletion of the GR gene *(68, 69)*. Even though CRH receptor type 1 mRNA is increased in corticotroph adenoma cells, mutations of the coding sequence have not been found in pituitary corticotroph adenomas *(70)*.

ACTH receptor mRNA and melanocortin 2 receptor (MC2) were undetectable in 16 of 22 pituitary corticotroph adenomas. Plasma ACTH levels were significantly higher in tumors that did not express the receptor compared to those that did *(71)*. A mutation in the DAX1 gene that controls HPA axis development was found in a 33-year-old patient with X-linked adrenal hypoplasia congenita and pituitary corticotroph adenoma *(72)*. According to the France-Belgium MEN1 multicenter study, 6 of 136 cases of MEN1 with pituitary adenomas were ACTH-secreting corticotroph adenomas *(73)*. However, expression of MEN1 mRNA is normal in sporadic pituitary corticotroph adenomas *(74, 75)*. Recently pituitary corticotroph microadenomas were reported in two patients with tuberous sclerosis complex, an autosomal dominant neurocutaneous disorder characterized by benign tumors (hamartomas), epilepsy and mental retardation. This complex is a result of mutation in the *TSC1* and *TSC2* genes that encode the proteins hamartin and tuberin, respectively. Mechanisms promoting corticotroph adenoma growth in this disorder are unknown *(76)*.

The most appealing evidence is the discovery that the ATPase subunit of the chromatin remodeling Swi/Snif complex Brg1 and the histone deacetylase HDAC2 may contribute to partial glucocorticoid resistance *(77)*, which is believed to be a central mechanism in the development of pituitary corticotroph adenoma. Brg1 and HDAC2 are nuclear factors responsible for stabilization of the glucocorticoid receptor and eventually repression of *POMC* transcription initiation. Importantly, 50% of pituitary corticotroph adenomas were deficient in nuclear Brg1 or HDAC2. In a subset of these tumors Brg1 was delocalized to the cytoplasm in adenoma cells, while was detected in nuclei of surrounding peri-tumoral corticotroph cells. This observation was apparent in both human and canine pituitary corticotroph adenoma cells *(65, 77)*.

CONCLUSIONS

This chapter highlights current knowledge of tumoral corticotroph cell function, especially in animal models. Unfortunately, a pharmacological cure for this highly morbid and potentially lethal disease remains elusive. New technologies to access these specialized cells will be required to enable understanding of specific molecular alterations in human Cushing's disease.

REFERENCES

1. Saeger W, Ludecke DK, Buchfelder M, Fahlbusch R, Quabbe HJ, Petersenn S. Pathohistological classification of pituitary tumors: 10 years of experience with the German Pituitary Tumor Registry. Eur J Endocrinol 2007;156(2):203–216.
2. Orth DN, Holscher MA, Wilson MG, Nicholson WE, Plue RE, Mount CD. Equine Cushing's disease: plasma immunoreactive proopiolipomelanocortin peptide and cortisol levels basally and in response to diagnostic tests. Endocrinology 1982;110(4):1430–1441.
3. Wilson MG, Nicholson WE, Holscher MA, Sherrell BJ, Mount CD, Orth DN. Proopiolipomelanocortin peptides in normal pituitary, pituitary tumor, and plasma of normal and Cushing's horses. Endocrinology 1982;110(3):941–954.
4. de Bruin C, Meij BP, Kooistra HS, Hanson JM, Lamberts SW, Hofland LJ. Cushing's disease in dogs and humans. Horm Res 2009;71(Suppl 1):140–143.
5. Willeberg PPW. Epidemiological aspects of clinical hyperadrenocorticism in dogs (canine Cushing's syndrome). J Am Anim Hosp Assoc 1982(18):717–724.
6. Halmi NS, Peterson ME, Colurso GJ, Liotta AS, Krieger DT. Pituitary intermediate lobe in dog: two cell types and high bioactive adrenocorticotropin content. Science 1981;211(4477):72–74.
7. Bautch VL, Toda S, Hassell JA, Hanahan D. Endothelial cell tumors develop in transgenic mice carrying polyoma virus middle T oncogene. Cell 1987;51(4):529–537.
8. Helseth A, Siegal GP, Haug E, Bautch VL. Transgenic mice that develop pituitary tumors. A model for Cushing's disease. Am J Pathol 1992;140(5):1071–1080.

9. Low MJ, Liu B, Hammer GD, Rubinstein M, Allen RG. Post-translational processing of proopiomelanocortin (POMC) in mouse pituitary melanotroph tumors induced by a POMC-simian virus 40 large T antigen transgene. J Biol Chem 1993;268(33):24967–24975.
10. Stenzel-Poore MP, Cameron VA, Vaughan J, Sawchenko PE, Vale W. Development of Cushing's syndrome in corticotropin-releasing factor transgenic mice. Endocrinology 1992;130(6):3378–3386.
11. Yano H, Readhead C, Nakashima M, Ren SG, Melmed S. Pituitary-directed leukemia inhibitory factor transgene causes Cushing's syndrome: neuro-immune-endocrine modulation of pituitary development. Mol Endocrinol 1998;12(11): 1708–1720.
12. Lee EY, Chang CY, Hu N, Wang YC, Lai CC, Herrup K, et al. Mice deficient for Rb are nonviable and show defects in neurogenesis and haematopoiesis. Nature 1992;359(6393):288–294.
13. Clarke AR, Maandag ER, van Roon M, van der Lugt NM, van der Valk M, Hooper ML, et al. Requirement for a functional Rb-1 gene in murine development. Nature 1992;359(6393):328–330.
14. Jacks T, Fazeli A, Schmitt EM, Bronson RT, Goodell MA, Weinberg RA. Effects of an Rb mutation in the mouse. Nature 1992;359(6393):295–300.
15. Melmed S. Mechanisms for pituitary tumorigenesis: the plastic pituitary. J Clin Invest 2003;112(11):1603–1618.
16. Rene P, Grino M, Viollet C, Videau C, Jullian E, Bucchini D, et al. Overexpression of the V3 vasopressin receptor in transgenic mice corticotropes leads to increased basal corticosterone. J Neuroendocrinol 2002;14(9):737–744.
17. Auernhammer CJ, Melmed S. Leukemia-inhibitory factor-neuroimmune modulator of endocrine function. Endocr Rev 2000;21(3):313–345.
18. Langlais D, Couture C, Balsalobre A, Drouin J. Regulatory network analyses reveal genome-wide potentiation of LIF signaling by glucocorticoids and define an innate cell defense response. PLoS Genet 2008;4(10):e1000224.
19. Leung SW, Wloga EH, Castro AF, Nguyen T, Bronson RT, Yamasaki L. A dynamic switch in Rb+/- mediated neuroendocrine tumorigenesis. Oncogene 2004;23(19):3296–3307.
20. Quereda V, Malumbres M. Cell cycle control of pituitary development and disease. J Mol Endocrinol 2009; 42(2):75–86.
21. Nakayama K, Ishida N, Shirane M, Inomata A, Inoue T, Shishido N, et al. Mice lacking p27(Kip1) display increased body size, multiple organ hyperplasia, retinal dysplasia, and pituitary tumors. Cell 1996;85(5):707–720.
22. Fero ML, Rivkin M, Tasch M, Porter P, Carow CE, Firpo E, et al. A syndrome of multiorgan hyperplasia with features of gigantism, tumorigenesis, and female sterility in p27(Kip1)-deficient mice. Cell 1996;85(5):733–744.
23. Kiyokawa H, Kineman RD, Manova-Todorova KO, Soares VC, Hoffman ES, Ono M, et al. Enhanced growth of mice lacking the cyclin-dependent kinase inhibitor function of p27(Kip1). Cell 1996;85(5):721–732.
24. Brugarolas J, Bronson RT, Jacks T. p21 is a critical CDK2 regulator essential for proliferation control in Rb-deficient cells. J Cell Biol 1998;141(2):503–514.
25. Park MS, Rosai J, Nguyen HT, Capodieci P, Cordon-Cardo C, Koff A. p27 and Rb are on overlapping pathways suppressing tumorigenesis in mice. Proc Natl Acad Sci U S A 1999;96(11):6382–6387.
26. Franklin DS, Godfrey VL, Lee H, Kovalev GI, Schoonhoven R, Chen-Kiang S, et al. CDK inhibitors p18(INK4c) and p27(Kip1) mediate two separate pathways to collaboratively suppress pituitary tumorigenesis. Genes Dev 1998;12(18): 2899–2911.
27. Franklin DS, Godfrey VL, O'Brien DA, Deng C, Xiong Y. Functional collaboration between different cyclin-dependent kinase inhibitors suppresses tumor growth with distinct tissue specificity. Mol Cell Biol 2000;20(16):6147–6158.
28. Yamasaki L, Bronson R, Williams BO, Dyson NJ, Harlow E, Jacks T. Loss of E2F-1 reduces tumorigenesis and extends the lifespan of Rb1(+/-)mice. Nat Genet 1998;18(4):360–364.
29. Lee EY, Cam H, Ziebold U, Rayman JB, Lees JA, Dynlacht BD. E2F4 loss suppresses tumorigenesis in Rb mutant mice. Cancer Cell 2002;2(6):463–472.
30. Chesnokova V, Kovacs K, Castro AV, Zonis S, Melmed S. Pituitary hypoplasia in Pttg-/- mice is protective for Rb+/- pituitary tumorigenesis. Mol Endocrinol 2005;19(9):2371–2379.
31. Vlotides G, Eigler T, Melmed S. Pituitary tumor-transforming gene: physiology and implications for tumorigenesis. Endocr Rev 2007;28(2):165–186.
32. Chesnokova V, Zonis S, Kovacs K, Ben-Shlomo A, Wawrowsky K, Bannykh S, et al. p21(Cip1) restrains pituitary tumor growth. Proc Natl Acad Sci U S A 2008;105(45):17498–17503.
33. Chesnokova V, Zonis S, Rubinek T, Yu R, Ben-Shlomo A, Kovacs K, et al. Senescence mediates pituitary hypoplasia and restrains pituitary tumor growth. Cancer Res 2007;67(21):10564–10572.
34. Lloyd R, Kovacs K, Young WF Jr., Farrel WE, Asa SL, Trouillas J, Kontogeorgos G, Sano T, Scheithauer BW, Horvath E. World Health Organization classification of tumours: pathology and genetics of tumours of endocrine organs. In: DeLellis R, Lloyd RV, Heitz PU, Eng C, eds. Lyon, France: International Agency for Research on Cancer (IRAC); 2004.

35. Challa VR, Marshall RB, Hopkins MB 3rd, Kelly DL, Jr., Civantos F. Pathobiologic study of pituitary tumors: report of 62 cases with a review of the recent literature. Hum Pathol 1985;16(9):873–884.
36. Mindermann T, Wilson CB. Age-related and gender-related occurrence of pituitary adenomas. Clin Endocrinol (Oxf) 1994;41(3):359–364.
37. Al-Shraim M, Asa SL. The 2004 World Health Organization classification of pituitary tumors: what is new? Acta Neuropathol 2006;111(1):1–7.
38. George DH, Scheithauer BW, Kovacs K, Horvath E, Young WF, Jr., Lloyd RV, et al. Crooke's cell adenoma of the pituitary: an aggressive variant of corticotroph adenoma. Am J Surg Pathol 2003;27(10):1330–1336.
39. Pluta RM, Nieman L, Doppman JL, Watson JC, Tresser N, Katz DA, et al. Extrapituitary parasellar microadenoma in Cushing's disease. J Clin Endocrinol Metab 1999;84(8):2912–2923.
40. Kovacs K. The pathology of Cushing's disease. J Steroid Biochem Mol Biol 1993;45(1–3):179–182.
41. Kovacs KH, E. Tumors of the Pituitary Gland. Washington DC: Armed Forces Institute of Pathology; 1986.
42. Burch WM. Cushing's disease. A review. Arch Intern Med 1985;145(6):1106–1111.
43. Lamberts SW, Klijn JG, de Quijada M, Timmermans HA, Uitterlinden P, de Jong FH, et al. The mechanism of the suppressive action of bromocriptine on adrenocorticotropin secretion in patients with Cushing's disease and Nelson's syndrome. J Clin Endocrinol Metab 1980;51(2):307–311.
44. Lamberts SW, Stefanko SZ, de Lange SA, Fermin H, van der Vijver JC, Weber RF, et al. Failure of clinical remission after transsphenoidal removal of a microadenoma in a patient with Cushing's disease: multiple hyperplastic and adenomatous cell nets in surrounding pituitary tissue. J Clin Endocrinol Metab 1980;50(4):793–795.
45. Orth DN, DeBold CR, DeCherney GS, Jackson RV, Alexander AN, Rivier J, et al. Pituitary microadenomas causing Cushing's disease respond to corticotropin-releasing factor. J Clin Endocrinol Metab 1982;55(5):1017–1019.
46. Alexander JM, Biller BM, Bikkal H, Zervas NT, Arnold A, Klibanski A. Clinically nonfunctioning pituitary tumors are monoclonal in origin. J Clin Invest 1990;86(1):336–340.
47. Herman V, Fagin J, Gonsky R, Kovacs K, Melmed S. Clonal origin of pituitary adenomas. J Clin Endocrinol Metab 1990;71(6):1427–1433.
48. Wolfsen AR, Odell WD. The dose–response relationship of ACTH and cortisol in Cushing's disease. Clin Endocrinol (Oxf) 1980;12(6):557–568.
49. Suda T, Tozawa F, Yamada M, Ushiyama T, Tomori N, Sumitomo T, et al. Effects of corticotropin-releasing hormone and dexamethasone on proopiomelanocortin messenger RNA level in human corticotroph adenoma cells in vitro. J Clin Invest 1988;82(1):110–114.
50. Oosterom R, Verleun T, Uitterlinden P, Hackeng WH, Burbach JP, Wiegant VM, et al. ACTH and beta-endorphin secretion by three corticotrophic adenomas in culture. Effects of culture time, dexamethasone, vasopressin and synthetic corticotrophin releasing factor. Acta Endocrinol (Copenh) 1984;106(1):21–29.
51. White MC, Adams EF, Loizou M, Mashiter K, Fahlbusch R. Ovine corticotrophin releasing factor stimulates ACTH release from human corticotrophinoma cells in culture; interaction with hydrocortisone and arginine vasopressin. Clin Endocrinol (Oxf) 1985;23(3):295–302.
52. Mashiter K, Adams EF, Gillies G, Van Noorden S, Ratter S. Adrenocorticotropin and lipotropin secretion by dispersed cell cultures of a human corticotropic adenoma: effect of hypothalamic extract, arginine vasopressin, hydrocortisone, and serotonin. J Clin Endocrinol Metab 1980;51(3):566–572.
53. Gillies G, Ratter S, Grossman A, Gaillard R, Lowry PJ, Besser GM, et al. Secretion of ACTH, LPH and beta-endophin from human pituitary tumours in vitro. Clin Endocrinol (Oxf) 1980;13(2):197–205.
54. Lamberts SW, Bons EG, Uitterlinden P. Studies on the glucocorticoid-receptor blocking action of RU 38486 in cultured ACTH-secreting human pituitary tumour cells and normal rat pituitary cells. Acta Endocrinol (Copenh) 1985;109(1): 64–69.
55. de Keyzer Y, Bertagna X, Lenne F, Girard F, Luton JP, Kahn A. Altered proopiomelanocortin gene expression in adrenocorticotropin-producing nonpituitary tumors. Comparative studies with corticotropic adenomas and normal pituitaries. J Clin Invest 1985;76(5):1892–1898.
56. Raffin-Sanson ML, de Keyzer Y, Bertagna X. Proopiomelanocortin, a polypeptide precursor with multiple functions: from physiology to pathological conditions. Eur J Endocrinol 2003;149(2):79–90.
57. Bertagna X. Unrestrained production of proopiomelanocortin (POMC) and its peptide fragments by pituitary corticotroph adenomas in Cushing's disease. J Steroid Biochem Mol Biol 1992;43(5):379–384.
58. Westlund KN, Aguilera G, Childs GV. Quantification of morphological changes in pituitary corticotropes produced by in vivo corticotropin-releasing factor stimulation and adrenalectomy. Endocrinology 1985;116(1):439–445.
59. Gertz BJ, Contreras LN, McComb DJ, Kovacs K, Tyrrell JB, Dallman MF. Chronic administration of corticotropin-releasing factor increases pituitary corticotroph number. Endocrinology 1987;120(1):381–388.

60. Horacek MJ, Campbell GT, Blake CA. Effects of corticotrophin-releasing hormone on corticotrophs in anterior pituitary gland allografts in hypophysectomized, orchidectomized hamsters. Cell Tissue Res 1989;258(1):65–68.
61. Assie G, Bahurel H, Coste J, Silvera S, Kujas M, Dugue MA, et al. Corticotroph tumor progression after adrenalectomy in Cushing's Disease: a reappraisal of Nelson's Syndrome. J Clin Endocrinol Metab 2007;92(1):172–179.
62. Assie G, Bahurel H, Bertherat J, Kujas M, Legmann P, Bertagna X. The Nelson's syndrome… revisited. Pituitary 2004;7(4):209–215.
63. Dahia PL, Grossman AB. The molecular pathogenesis of corticotroph tumors. Endocr Rev 1999;20(2):136–155.
64. Suhardja AS, Kovacs KT, Rutka JT. Molecular pathogenesis of pituitary adenomas: a review. Acta Neurochir (Wien) 1999;141(7):729–736.
65. Drouin J, Bilodeau S, Vallette S. Of old and new diseases: genetics of pituitary ACTH excess (Cushing) and deficiency. Clin Genet 2007;72(3):175–182.
66. Dahia PL, Ahmed-Shuaib A, Jacobs RA, Chew SL, Honegger J, Fahlbusch R, et al. Vasopressin receptor expression and mutation analysis in corticotropin-secreting tumors. J Clin Endocrinol Metab 1996;81(5):1768–1771.
67. Dahia PL, Honegger J, Reincke M, Jacobs RA, Mirtella A, Fahlbusch R, et al. Expression of glucocorticoid receptor gene isoforms in corticotropin-secreting tumors. J Clin Endocrinol Metab 1997;82(4):1088–1093.
68. Huizenga NA, de Lange P, Koper JW, Clayton RN, Farrell WE, van der Lely AJ, et al. Human adrenocorticotropin-secreting pituitary adenomas show frequent loss of heterozygosity at the glucocorticoid receptor gene locus. J Clin Endocrinol Metab 1998;83(3):917–921.
69. Huizenga NA, Koper JW, De Lange P, Pols HA, Stolk RP, Burger H, et al. A polymorphism in the glucocorticoid receptor gene may be associated with and increased sensitivity to glucocorticoids in vivo. J Clin Endocrinol Metab 1998;83(1):144–151.
70. Dieterich KD, Gundelfinger ED, Ludecke DK, Lehnert H. Mutation and expression analysis of corticotropin-releasing factor 1 receptor in adrenocorticotropin-secreting pituitary adenomas. J Clin Endocrinol Metab 1998;83(9):3327–3331.
71. Morris DG, Kola B, Borboli N, Kaltsas GA, Gueorguiev M, McNicol AM, et al. Identification of adrenocorticotropin receptor messenger ribonucleic acid in the human pituitary and its loss of expression in pituitary adenomas. J Clin Endocrinol Metab 2003;88(12):6080–6087.
72. De Menis E, Roncaroli F, Calvari V, Chiarini V, Pauletto P, Camerino G, et al. Corticotroph adenoma of the pituitary in a patient with X-linked adrenal hypoplasia congenita due to a novel mutation of the DAX-1 gene. Eur J Endocrinol 2005;153(2):211–215.
73. Verges B, Boureille F, Goudet P, Murat A, Beckers A, Sassolas G, et al. Pituitary disease in MEN type 1 (MEN1): data from the France-Belgium MEN1 multicenter study. J Clin Endocrinol Metab 2002;87(2):457–465.
74. Asa SL, Somers K, Ezzat S. The MEN-1 gene is rarely down-regulated in pituitary adenomas. J Clin Endocrinol Metab 1998;83(9):3210–3212.
75. Satta MA, Korbonits M, Jacobs RA, Bolden-Dwinfour DA, Kaltsas GA, Vangeli V, et al. Expression of menin gene mRNA in pituitary tumours. Eur J Endocrinol 1999;140(4):358–361.
76. Dworakowska D, Grossman AB. Are neuroendocrine tumours a feature of tuberous sclerosis? A systematic review. Endocr Relat Cancer 2009;16(1):45–58.
77. Bilodeau S, Vallette-Kasic S, Gauthier Y, Figarella-Branger D, Brue T, Berthelet F, et al. Role of Brg1 and HDAC2 in GR trans-repression of the pituitary POMC gene and misexpression in Cushing disease. Genes Dev 2006;20(20):2871–2886.

4 Pathogenesis of Adrenocortical Tumors

Madson Q. Almeida, Emilia M. Pinto, and Ana Claudia Latronico

CONTENTS

SUMMARY

Adrenocortical carcinomas are rare malignant tumors. However, the high incidence of the adrenocortical tumors in pediatric and adult patients from the Southern region of Brazil is particularly remarkable, since it has been estimated to be approximately ten times greater than the worldwide incidence. Adrenocortical tumors occur as a component of several hereditary tumor syndromes, which include the Li–Fraumeni syndrome, Beckwith–Wiedemann syndrome, multiple endocrine neoplasia 1, Carney complex, and congenital adrenal hyperplasia. The study of these rare genetic syndromes has greatly contributed to the elucidation of sporadic adrenocortical tumorigenesis. This chapter summarizes the molecular alterations likely involved in the multistage tumorigenesis of familial or sporadic adrenocortical adenomas and carcinomas.

Key Words: Adrenal, tumors, pathogenesis, tumorigenesis

From: *Contemporary Endocrinology: Cushing's Syndrome: Pathophysiology, Diagnosis and Treatment*
Edited by: M.D. Bronstein (ed.), DOI 10.1007/978-1-60327-449-4_4,

INTRODUCTION

Adrenocortical carcinomas account for only 0.05–0.2% of all cancers, with an estimated incidence of 0.5–2 per million per year in adults *(1)*. In the USA, only about 25 new cases of adrenocortical carcinoma occur each year and constitute about 0.2% of all pediatric malignancies *(2)*. However, the incidence of adrenocortical tumors is remarkably high in Southern Brazil, where it is estimated to be 10–15 times greater than the worldwide incidence *(1, 3)*. A bimodal age distribution has been reported, with the first peak occurring before the age of five years, and the second between the fourth and fifth decade *(1)*. At presentation, virilization is the most common syndrome in children with adrenocortical tumors. Isolated signs of Cushing syndrome are infrequent, occurring most often in combination with signs of increased androgen secretion *(3)*. In adults, adrenocortical tumors are classically discovered under two circumstances: firstly, in symptomatic patients with steroid excess (Cushing syndrome, Conn syndrome, or hyperandrogenism in women) or with symptoms related to the tumor mass; secondly, and more frequently, they are discovered as incidentalomas *(1)*.

Adrenocortical tumors in children appear to behave differently than histologically similar tumors in adult individuals. Pathological criteria for malignancy in the adult population are well established in the literature *(4)*. Otherwise, childhood adrenocortical neoplasms with apparently poor prognosis based on histopathological features have often a good clinical outcome *(5, 6)*.

Adrenocortical carcinoma remains a disease of poor prognosis, with little expectation of long-term survival if complete surgical removal is not achieved *(7)*. In the last decade, considerable advances toward understanding the molecular mechanisms of adrenocortical tumorigenesis have mainly been made in adrenocortical tumors of patients from distinct ethnicities *(3)*. The study of rare genetic syndromes associated with adrenocortical tumors has greatly contributed to the elucidation of sporadic adrenocortical tumorigenesis (Table 1). Here, we reviewed some of the molecular aspects of sporadic adrenocortical tumors arising in children and adults.

Table 1
Hereditary Syndromes Associated with Adrenocortical Tumors and Somatic Genetic Defects in Sporadic Adrenocortical Tumors Diagnosed in Adult Patients

Hereditary syndrome	*Gene, chromosomal locus*	*Prevalence of adrenocortical tumors*	*Somatic defects in sporadic adrenocortical tumors*
Li–Fraumeni syndrome	*P53* (17p13)	Adrenocortical carcinoma (3%)	*p53* mutations (30%) and 17p13 LOH (> 80%) in adrenocortical carcinomas
Multiple endocrine neoplasia type 1 (MEN1)	*MEN1* (11q13)	Hyperplasia, adrenocortical adenoma (25–40%) and, rarely, carcinoma (< 1%)	Rare somatic *MEN1* mutations; 11q13 LOH in sporadic adrenocortical carcinomas (> 80%)
Beckwith–Wiedemann syndrome	11p15 locus	Adrenocortical carcinoma (3%)	11p15 LOH and/or *IGF-II* overexpression in sporadic adrenocortical carcinomas (93%)
Familial adenomatous polyposis coli	*APC* (5q12–22)	Rare cases of adrenocortical adenomas and carcinomas (< 1%)	β-catenin somatic mutations in sporadic adrenocortical adenomas (27%) and carcinomas (31%)

LOH loss of heterozygosity, *APC* adenomatous polyposis coli

p53 TUMOR SUPPRESSOR GENE AND LOCUS 17p13

The P53 tumor suppressor is a phosphoprotein that acts as a transcription factor in the cell cycle regulation, inducing cell cycle arrest or cell death in response to DNA-damaging agents, such as virus, radiation, and chemotherapeutics *(8–11)*. Inactivation of p53 by mutations is a key molecular event that can be detected in more than half of all human cancers. The *p53* gene is located on the short arm of human chromosome 17. Loss of heterozygosity (LOH) at chromosomal *locus* 17p has been consistently observed in adrenocortical carcinomas *(12)*.

Reincke et al. *(13)* investigated *p53* mutations in exons 5–8, a highly conserved region, in 16 human adrenocortical tumors (five adenomas and 11 carcinomas) from adult European patients and two adrenocortical tumor cell lines. Single point mutations were detected in three adrenocortical carcinomas and in both cell lines *(13)*. Interestingly, Lin et al. *(14)* reported a new mutational hot spot within exon 4 in benign adrenal tumors (60% of adrenocortical adenomas and 50% of pheochromocytomas) from adult Taiwanese patients. However, these findings were not confirmed in a larger series of Caucasians from the USA and Europe, suggesting that ethnic and environmental factors may be responsible for p53 mutational spectrum *(15)*.

More recently, a high incidence of a *p53* germline mutation was demonstrated in 35 of 36 children with adrenocortical tumors originated from Southern Brazil *(16)*. This mutation was located outside the highly conserved DNA binding domain, resulting in the substitution of arginine for histidine at position 337 of the tetramerization domain of p53 protein (Fig. 1). This missense mutation was also present in 76% of children with benign and malignant sporadic adrenocortical tumors in another Brazilian series, confirming the high incidence of the Arg337His mutation in Brazilian children with adrenocortical tumors (Table 2) *(17)*. Furthermore, the Arg337His mutation was not restricted to the pediatric group, as it was also found in 14% of adult patients with adrenocortical tumors *(17)*.

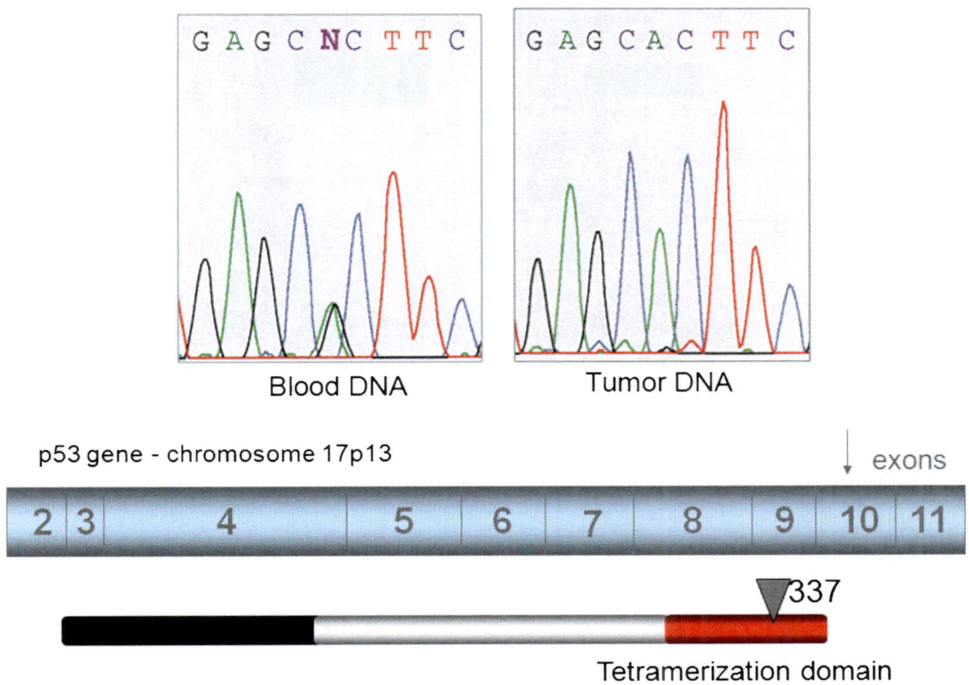

Fig. 1. The automatic sequencing of the exon 10 of *p53* gene (genomic DNA extracted from blood and tumor tissue). The nucleotide change (G>A) results in the germinative Arg337His mutation in one Brazilian children with adrenocortical adenoma. This missense mutation is located within the tetramerization domain of the P53.

Table 2
Frequent Genetic Alterations of Sporadic Adrenocortical Tumors in Children

Gene	*Locus*	*Genetic alterations*	*No. of children studied*	*References*
p53	17q13	Germline Arg337His mutation	35/36 (97%)	Ribeiro et al. (2001) *(16)*
			14/18 (78%)	Latronico et al. (2001) *(17)*
		Somatic Arg337His mutation	1/14 (7%)	Varley et al. (1999) *(76)*
		Germline Pro152Leu mutation	6/14 (43%)	
		Germline Arg158His mutation	3/14 (21%)	
		Chromosome 17 deletion	13 (3 ad., 10 ca.)/15 (87%)	Pinto et al. (2005) *(25)*
ACTH-R	18p11.2	Somatic mutation	0/2	Latronico et al. (1995) *(31)*
		Deletion	0/1	Reincke et al. (1997) *(33)*
PKC	17q22/13p21	Normal activity	0/4	Latronico et al. (1994) *(37)*
IGF-II	11q15	LOH	4/4 (100%)	Wilkin et al. (2000) *(55)*
		Overexpression	3 (2 ad., 1 ca.)/4 (75%)	
		Overexpression	20 (15 ad., 5 ca.)/22 (91%)	Almeida et al. (2008) *(56)*
		Overexpression	22 (5 ad., 17 ca.)/23 (96%)	West et al. (2007) *(65)*
IGF-IR	15q25	Overexpression	2/17 adenomas (12%)	Almeida et al. (2008) *(56)*
			6/6 carcinomas (100%)	
	9q34	Gain	8/9 (89%)	Figueiredo et al. (1999) *(59)*
			13/20 (65%)	James et al. (1999) *(60)*
		Chromosome 9 deletion	3 (2 ad., 1 ca.)/13 (23%)	Pinto et al. (2005) *(25)*
HSD3B2	1p13.1	Low expression	15 (5 ad., 10 ca.)/23 (65%)	West et al. (2007) *(65)*
SF-1	9q33	Amplification	8/9 (89%)	Figueiredo et al. (2005) *(70)*
		Overexpression	8/10 (80%)	Pianovski et al. (2006) *(71)*

LOH loss of heterozygosity, *ad* adenoma, *ca* carcinoma

The germline Arg337His mutation of *p53* was inherited in the vast majority of cases, indicating that this mutation apparently increases predisposition to childhood adrenocortical tumors *(17)*. The inherited forms of p53 mutations are commonly described in Li–Fraumeni syndrome (Table 1) *(18–20)*. This rare familial cancer syndrome is characterized by a high incidence of sarcoma diagnosed early in life and at least two first-degree relatives with cancer occurring before the age of 45 years.

such as breast cancer and other diverse neoplasms, particularly brain tumors, leukemia, and adrenocortical carcinomas *(18)*. In contrast with these features, the germline Arg337His mutation was found in patients with sporadic adrenocortical tumors and in their first-degree relatives with no evidence of bearing a tumor *(15, 16)*. Therefore, it is important to stress that the inherited p53 mutation is not a sure predictor of the occurrence of adrenocortical tumors. Indeed, the estimated penetrance of adrenocortical tumors associated with the Arg337His mutation was 10% in a large cohort of individuals from Southern Brazil *(21)*.

Given the high frequency of the inherited Arg337His mutation in Brazilian children with adrenocortical tumors, it is most likely that this p53 mutation has originated from a single founder. In according with this hypothesis, a strong evidence of co-segregation between two distinct polymorphic alleles within the *p53* gene and the Arg337His mutation was demonstrated in this population *(22)*. In addition, the allelic frequencies were significantly different between patients harboring the Arg337His mutation and normal individuals, suggesting that this p53 mutation originated from a common ancestral *(22)*.

p53 mutations are rarely observed in benign tumors and are generally associated with poor prognosis in several types of cancer *(23, 24)*. However, only one of 13 Brazilian children with adrenocortical tumors harboring the Arg337His mutation developed metastasis, suggesting that this mutation was not related to an unfavorable prognosis in most children with adrenocortical tumors *(17)*. A high frequency (79%) of loss of the entire chromosome 17 was also evidenced in patients with benign or malignant adrenocortical tumors associated with the Arg337His mutation *(25)*.

Gicquel et al. *(26)*, in search of a reliable molecular marker for malignancy, assessed three markers, including 17p13 LOH, in a large series of adult patients with sporadic adrenocortical tumors. It was demonstrated that 17p13 LOH was a strong predictor of shorter disease-free survival and had independent prognostic significance *(26)*. Nevertheless, these findings were not confirmed in childhood adrenocortical tumors associated with Arg337His mutation. Loss of the entire chromosome 17 was observed in both benign and malignant tumors, being even more prevalent in adenomas, showing a lack of correlation between chromosome 17 loss and tumor aggressiveness in Brazilian children and adolescents *(25)*. In addition, losses of chromosomes 2 and 11 were seen in both benign and malignant lesions. In contrast, the concomitant loss of chromosomes 2, 9, 11, and 17 was exclusively found in adrenocortical carcinomas, demonstrating that chromosome instability involving three or more chromosomes may contribute to define malignancy in the pediatric group *(25)*.

The loss of chromosome 17 harboring the normal *p53* allele in most of affected patients with the Arg337His mutation is crucial for adrenocortical tumor development *(25)*. However, the etiologic factor for the occurrence of this second event in childhood remains unknown. Interestingly, the peak age of occurrence of adrenocortical tumors in Brazilian children is under four years of age, suggesting that this second event occurs very early in life or even during fetal life. In addition, the stability of the p53 tetramerization domain containing the Arg337His mutation is highly sensitive to pH in the physiological range, suggesting that the contribution of this mutation in a tissue-specific manner to adrenocortical tumors may be associated with an elevated pH within fetal adrenal cells *(27)*.

More recently, p53 mutations were also screened in 45 Brazilian unrelated individuals with family histories fulfilling the clinical definitions of Li–Fraumeni-like syndrome *(28)*. The germline Arg337His mutation was identified in 46% of the patients harboring p53 mutations. Families with the Arg337His mutation presented a wide spectrum of tumors, including breast cancers (30%), brain cancers (11%), soft tissue sarcomas (10.7%), and adrenocortical tumors (8.9%) *(28)*. Overall, these observations suggest that the Arg337His mutation may confer a higher susceptibility to adrenocortical tumors, but does not in an exclusive form, as previously reported *(16)*.

ACTH RECEPTOR, GSα GENES, AND PKC ACTIVITY

That hyperstimulation of the adrenals by ACTH could result in adrenocortical tumors was suggested by isolated case reports of carcinomas arising after the diagnosis of classic congenital adrenal hyperplasia *(29, 30)*. However, the direct sequencing of ACTH receptor gene did not reveal constitutively activating mutations in two series of sporadic adrenocortical tumors. Both studies incorporated adults and children with adrenocortical tumors, but with a small proportion of the later group. These findings indicated that ACTH receptor activation is not a frequent mechanism in human adrenocortical tumorigenesis (Table 2) *(31–33)*.

Activating mutations of the Gsα gene were described in affected tissues from patients with the McCune–Albright syndrome, and these included hyperfunctioning adrenocortical adenomas *(34)*. These findings raised the hypothesis that overactivity of the G protein signaling pathway might occasionally lead to the development of adrenocortical tumors. Nevertheless, defects in the Gsα and Giα_2 were not found in large series of adults with sporadic benign or malignant adrenocortical tumors *(35, 36)*.

Protein kinase C activity, a potential marker for human malignant diseases, was described as not increased in Brazilian patients (14 adults and four children) with benign or malignant adrenocortical tumors, as well as in diffuse and macronodular adrenal hyperplasia when compared to levels in normal adrenal tissue, suggesting that this molecular mechanism is not related to adrenocortical tumorigenesis (Table 2) *(37)*.

A N-*ras* activating mutation, resulting in a substitution of glutamine by arginine at codon 61, was described in seven of 56 adults with adrenocortical tumors with equal prevalence in benign and malignant tumors *(38)*. However, Moul et al. *(39)* failed to find any *ras* mutations in 11 adrenocortical tumors. Combined, these findings suggest that activating *ras* mutations are rare events in adults with adrenocortical tumors.

MULTIPLE ENDOCRINE NEOPLASIA TYPE I, *MEN1* GENE, AND LOCUS 11q13

Adrenocortical tumors are present in 25–40% of the patients with multiple endocrine neoplasia type I (MEN1), a dominantly inherited syndrome characterized by parathyroid (95%), endocrine pancreas (45%), and pituitary (45%) tumors. A heterozygous germline mutation of *MEN1* occurs in about 90% of families with MEN1 *(40)*. Somatic mutation of the *MEN1* gene is extremely rare in adult sporadic adrenocortical tumors (Tabel 4.1). By contrast, LOH at 11q13 is present in 10–14% of adrenocortical adenomas and almost always found in sporadic adrenocortical carcinomas *(41)*. This discrepancy suggests that another tumor suppressor gene, at the same locus, could be involved in sporadic adrenocortical tumors.

IGF SYSTEM AND LOCUS 11p15

The IGF signaling pathway has many important roles in normal cell growth and development. All of the components of the IGF system (IGFs, receptors, and binding proteins) are expressed by human fetal adrenals *(42)*. IGF-II is thought to be involved in the regulation of fetal development because its circulating and tissue levels are highest during fetal life and decrease postnatally *(43)*. Weber et al. *(44)* demonstrated that postnatal overexpression of IGF-II in the adrenal gland of adult transgenic mice was associated with adrenocortical hyperplasia.

The *IGF-II* gene maps to the *locus* 11p15, which is organized in two different clusters: a telomeric domain, including the *IGF-II (45)* and *H19 (46)* genes, and a centromeric domain, including *p57kip2*, a cyclin-dependent kinase inhibitor involved in the cell cycle arrest *(47)*. The *IGF-II* gene is maternally imprinted and is, therefore, expressed only from the paternal allele *(45)*. The *H19* is a microRNA gene and modulate *IGF-II* overexpression *(48)*. The *H19* and *p57kip2* genes are also controlled by functional imprinting, but unlike *IGF-II* these genes are expressed from the maternal allele *(49, 50)*. Uniparental paternal isodisomy at the *locus* 11p15 was associated with the Beckwith–Wiedmann syndrome *(51)* (Table 1). This structural abnormality is characterized by loss of maternal allele with duplication of the paternal allele, leading to biallelic expression of *IGF-II* gene and decrease in the *H19* and *p57kip2* expression *(52)*. The Beckwith–Wiedmann syndrome is an overgrowth disorder characterized by macroglossia, abdominal well defects, gigantism, and an increase risk of developing Wilms' tumor, hepatoblastoma, rhabdomyosarcoma, and adrenocortical carcinoma *(51)*.

Structural abnormalities at the 11p15 *locus*, particularly uniparental paternal isodisomy, were initially described in 37% of adults with sporadic adrenocortical tumors *(53)*. Gicquel et al. *(53)* also detected very high *IGF-II* mRNA contents in five of six (83%) adrenocortical carcinomas. Four of these carcinomas showed abnormalities at the *locus* 11p15.5, suggesting that there is a strong relation between *IGF-II* overexpression and rearrangements at the 11p15 *locus* in adrenocortical carcinomas of adult patients. In a large adult series of 82 adrenocortical tumors, abnormalities of the 11p15 region and/or *IGF-II* gene overexpression were confirmed as frequent features of the malignant state, being found in 27 of 29 (93.1%) malignant tumors and in only three of 35 (8.6%) benign tumors *(54)*.

Molecular events leading to *IGF-II* overexpression were studied in only four pediatric adrenocortical tumors (three adenomas and one carcinoma) *(55)*. Structural abnormalities at the *locus* 11p15 were detected in all cases, and elevated *IGF-II* mRNA contents were detected in 75% of the adrenocortical tumors (two adenomas and one carcinoma). Although these genetic alterations seem to correlate with poor outcome in adults, conclusions concerning prognosis in children could not be stated because of the small number of patients included in this study *(55)*. Recently, we studied the *IGF-II* expression in a larger cohort of 23 Brazilian children with adrenocortical tumors (17 adenomas and six carcinomas) *(56)*. In contrast with adult adrenocortical tumors, IGF-II transcripts were overexpressed in both adrenocortical adenomas and carcinomas, demonstrating that a high *IGF-II* expression was not associated with a poor clinical outcome in children with adrenocortical tumors (Table 2) *(56)*.

The mitogenic effects of IGF-II are mediated on the IGF receptor type 1 (IGF-IR) *(57)*. Interaction of IGF-II with IGF-IR plays a pivotal role in tumorigenesis, proliferation, and spread of many cancers *(58)*. Recently, a strong increase in *IGF-IR* expression was identified only in pediatric adrenocortical carcinomas (Table 2). Additionally, a selective IGF-IR kinase inhibitor had antitumor effects in adult and pediatric adrenocortical tumor cell lines, suggesting that IGF-IR inhibitors represent a promising therapy for human adrenocortical carcinoma *(56)*.

COMPARATIVE GENOMIC HYBRIDIZATION ANALYSIS

Figueiredo et al. *(59)* reported gain of 9q34 in eight of nine sporadic adrenocortical tumors (six carcinomas and three adenomas) of Brazilian children, in addition to gains at many other chromosomes as well as losses at 2q, 3, 4, 9p, 11, 13q, 18, 20p, and Xq. Limitations of this study concern the small number of patients and the unclear malignancy classification, which was not based on the presence of metastasis, but on histopathological criteria. A high level amplification of chromosome 9q34 was also demonstrated in 13 of 20 adrenocortical tumors in an England series *(60)*. These findings of numerous gains and losses in benign and malignant childhood adrenocortical tumors stand in contrast to adrenocortical tumors in adults, in which chromosomal gain and losses occur mainly in carcinomas *(61, 62)*.

MICROARRAY ANALYSIS

Two microarray studies identified that upregulation of *IGF-II* expression was the dominant change in malignant adrenocortical tumors *(63, 64)*. In addition, the study of Giordano et al. *(77)* reported upregulation of proliferation-related genes such as TOP2A (topoisomerase) and Ki-67. No other growth factor receptors were increased, with the exception of the fibroblast growth factor receptor type 1 (FGFR1). They also suggested enhanced Wnt signaling, as evidenced by increased transcription of some of the downstream targets of this pathway *(63)*.

More recently, West et al. *(65)* performed the first microarray analysis of childhood adrenocortical tumors. *FGFR4* and *IGF-II* genes were found to be upregulated, but their expression levels were not useful to predict malignant potential in children with adrenocortical tumors. In addition, *HSD3B2* gene was significantly underexpressed in childhood adrenocortical tumors when compared to normal controls. Concerning the differences between pediatric adrenocortical carcinomas and adenomas, a marked decrease in the expression of major histocompatibility class II (HLA class II) genes was evidenced in carcinomas *(65)*.

STEROIDOGENIC FACTOR 1

Several molecules are important for the specific development of the adrenogonadal primordium. In particular, two transcription factors, steroidogenic factor 1 (SF-1) and dosage-sensitive sex reversal, adrenal hypoplasia congenital X-linked (DAX-1), are essential for the development and differentiation of the adrenal cortex and gonads *(66)*.

SF-1 is an orphan member of the nuclear receptor family of transcription factors and plays an important role in endocrine function, including the regulation of steroid hydroxylases, male sexual differentiation, and the development and function of the adrenal cortex *(67, 68)*. *SF-1* maps to 9q33.3, a chromosomal region associated with amplification in childhood adrenocortical tumors *(59, 60)*. SF-1 was shown to be essential for compensatory adrenal growth following unilateral adrenalectomy in adult *SF-1*$^{+/-}$ mice *(69)*. Using fluorescence in situ hybridization, Figueiredo et al. *(70)* detected an amplification of the *SF-1* gene in eight of nine childhood adrenocortical tumors with 9q gain, suggesting an association between the *SF-1* increased copy numbers and adrenocortical tumorigenesis. Furthermore, SF-1 protein was found to be overexpressed in these cases (Table 2) *(71)*.

WNT-β-CATENIN PATHWAY

Genetic alterations in the Wnt signaling pathway were initially identified in familial adenomatous polyposis coli. Notably, patients with this condition due to inactivating mutations of the adenomatous polyposis coli gene (*APC*), which lead to activation of the Wnt signaling pathway, may develop adrenocortical tumors (Table 1) *(72)*. Wnt binds to its receptor complex, which is composed of members of the frizzled family and low-density lipoprotein receptor related proteins. The Wnt activation results in the inhibition of the axin–adenomatous polyposis coli–glycogen synthase kinase 3β (GSK-3) complex, leading to a block in β-catenin phosphorylation by GSK-3 and accumulation of β-catenin in the cytoplasm. β-catenin. The accumulated β-catenin translocates into the nucleus where it interacts with the T cell-specific transcription factor/lymphoid enhancer-binding factor 1 family of transcription factors to regulate transcription of Wnt target genes. In the absence of Wnt signaling activation, GSK-3 phosphorylates β-catenin, resulting in its ubiquitination and degradation by proteosomes *(73)*.

The Wnt pathway was analyzed in 26 adrenocortical adenomas and 13 carcinomas from adult patients. Abnormal cytoplasmic and/or nuclear accumulation of β-catenin was detected in 10 of 26 (38%) adenomas and 11 of 13 (77%) carcinomas, with a focal pattern in adrenocortical adenomas and a diffuse pattern in carcinomas. The β-catenin gene was screened for mutations, with similar frequencies of mutations found in both adrenocortical adenomas (27%) and carcinomas (31%) *(74)*. The frequency of β-catenin mutations in adrenocortical tumors from children and adolescents was not yet determined.

CONCLUSIONS AND PERSPECTIVES

Several acquired capabilities of malignant cells can be recognized in the adrenocortical carcinomas (Fig. 2). They represent essential alterations in cell physiology that collectively dictate malignant growth *(75)*. Elucidation of the molecular etiology of rare genetic syndromes associated with adrenocortical tumors has greatly increased our understanding of sporadic adrenocortical tumors. Studies targeting cellular oncogenes and tumor suppressor genes, as well as genes involved in normal senescence, apoptosis, and differentiation might provide not only knowledge of the mechanisms of adrenocortical tumorigenesis, but also may help to find reliable molecular diagnostic and prognostic markers. Finally, advances toward the molecular pathogenesis of adrenocortical tumors may contribute to the development of new treatment strategies that can effectively target the molecular abnormalities driving this cancer.

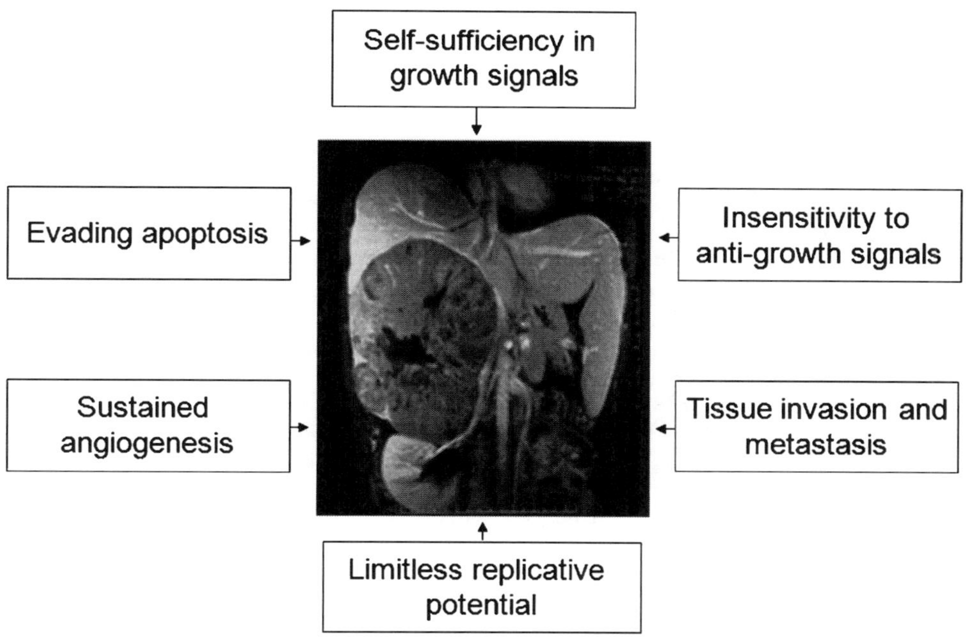

Fig. 2. Acquired capabilities observed in cancer cells. Several alterations in cell physiology that collectively dictate malignant growth in a large unilateral adrenocortical carcinoma with multiple necrosis areas detected by magnetic resonance (*sagittal view*) *(75)*.

REFERENCES

1. Latronico AC, Chrousos GP. Extensive personal experience: adrenocortical tumors. J Clin Endocrinol Metab 1997;82(5):1317–1324.
2. Young JL, Jr., Miller RW. Incidence of malignant tumors in U.S. children. J Pediatr 1975;86(2):254–258.
3. Sandrini R, Ribeiro RC, DeLacerda L. Childhood adrenocortical tumors. J Clin Endocrinol Metab 1997;82(7):2027–2031.
4. Weiss LM. Comparative histologic study of 43 metastasizing and nonmetastasizing adrenocortical tumors. Am J Surg Pathol 1984;8(3):163–169.
5. Mendonca BB, Lucon AM, Menezes CA, et al. Clinical, hormonal and pathological findings in a comparative study of adrenocortical neoplasms in childhood and adulthood. J Urol 1995;154(6):2004–2009.
6. Wieneke JA, Thompson LD, Heffess CS. Adrenal cortical neoplasms in the pediatric population: a clinicopathologic and immunophenotypic analysis of 83 patients. Am J Surg Pathol 2003;27(7):867–881.
7. Allolio B, Fassnacht M. Clinical review: adrenocortical carcinoma: clinical update. J Clin Endocrinol Metab 2006;91(6):2027–2037.
8. Levine AJ. The p53 tumor-suppressor gene. N Engl J Med 1992;326(20):1350–1352.
9. Hollstein M, Sidransky D, Vogelstein B, Harriss CC. p53 mutations in human cancers. Science 1991;253(5015):49–53.
10. Harris CC, Hollstein M. Clinical implications of the p53 tumor-suppressor gene. N Engl J Med 1993;329(18):1318–1327.
11. Kern SE, Kinzler KW, Bruskin A, et al. Identification of p53 as a sequence-specific DNA-binding protein. Science 1991;252(5013):1708–1711.
12. Yano T, Linehan M, Anglard P, et al. Genetic changes in human adrenocortical carcinomas. J Natl Cancer Inst 1989;81(7):518–523.
13. Reincke M, Karl M, Travis WH, et al. p53 mutations in human adrenocortical neoplasms: immunohistochemical and molecular studies. J Clin Endocrinol Metab 1994;78(3):790–794.
14. Lin SR, Lee YJ, Tsai JH. Mutations of the p53 gene in human functional adrenal neoplasms. J Clin Endocrinol Metab 1994;78(2):483–491.
15. Reincke M, Wachenfeld C, Mora P, et al. p53 mutations in adrenal tumors: Caucasian patients do not show the exon 4 "hot spot" found in Taiwan. J Clin Endocrinol Metab 1996;81(10):3636–3638.
16. Ribeiro RC, Sandrini F, Figueiredo B, et al. An inherited p53 mutation that contributes in a tissue-specific manner to pediatric adrenal cortical carcinoma. Proc Natl Acad Sci USA 2001;98(16):9330–9335.
17. Latronico AC, Pinto EM, Domenice S, et al. An inherited mutation outside the highly conserved DNA-binding domain of the p53 tumor suppressor protein in children and adults with sporadic adrenocortical tumors. J Clin Endocrinol Metab 2001;86(10):4970–4973.
18. Malkin D, Li FP, Strong LC, et al. Germ line p53 mutations in a familial syndrome of breast cancer, sarcomas, and other neoplasms. Science 1990;250(4985):1233–1238.
19. Srivastava S, Zou ZQ, Pirollo K, Blattner W, Chang EH. Germ-line transmission of a mutated p53 gene in a cancer-prone family with Li–Fraumeni syndrome. Nature 1990;348(6303):747–749.
20. Malkin D, Jolly KW, Barbier N, et al. Germline mutations of the p53 tumor-suppressor gene in children and young adults with second malignant neoplasms. N Engl J Med 1992;326(20):1309–1315.
21. Figueiredo BC, Sandrini R, Zambetti GP, et al. Penetrance of adrenocortical tumours associated with the germline TP53 R337H mutation. J Med Genet 2006;43(1):91–96.
22. Pinto EM, Billerbeck AE, Villares MC, Domenice S, Mendonca BB, Latronico AC. Founder effect for the highly prevalent R337H mutation of tumor suppressor p53 in Brazilian patients with adrenocortical tumors. Arq Bras Endocrinol Metabol 2004;48(5):647–650.
23. Esrig D, Elmajian D, Groshen S, et al. Accumulation of nuclear p53 and tumor progression in bladder cancer. N Engl J Med 1994;331(19):1259–1264.
24. Ichikawa A, Kinoshita T, Watanabe T, et al. Mutations of the p53 gene as a prognostic factor in aggressive B-cell lymphoma. N Engl J Med 1997;337(8):529–534
25. Pinto EM, Billerbeck AE, Fragoso MC, Mendonca BB, Latronico AC. Deletion mapping of chromosome 17 in benign and malignant adrenocortical tumors associated with the Arg337His mutation of the p53 tumor suppressor protein. J Clin Endocrinol Metab 2005;90(5):2976–2981.
26. Gicquel C, Bertagna X, Gaston V, et al. Molecular markers and long-term recurrences in a large cohort of patients with sporadic adrenocortical tumors. Cancer Res 2001;61(18):6762–6767.
27. DiGiammarino EL, Lee AS, Cadwell C, et al. A novel mechanism of tumorigenesis involving pH-dependent destabilization of a mutant p53 tetramer. Nat Struct Biol 2002;9(1):12–16.
28. Achatz MI, Olivier M, Calvez FL, et al. The TP53 mutation, R337H, is associated with Li–Fraumeni and Li–Fraumeni-like syndromes in Brazilian families. Cancer Lett 2007;245(1):96–102.

29. Barzilay JI, Pazianos AG. Adrenocortical carcinoma. Urol Clin North Am 1989;16(3):457–468.
30. Gicquel C, Bertagna X, Le Bouc Y. Recent advances in the pathogenesis of adrenocortical tumours. Eur J Endocrinol 1995;133(2):133–144.
31. Latronico AC, Reincke M, Mendonca BB, et al. No evidence for oncogenic mutations in the adrenocorticotropin receptor gene in human adrenocortical neoplasms. J Clin Endocrinol Metab 1995;80(3):875–877.
32. Light K, Jenkins PJ, Weber A, et al. Are activating mutations of the adrenocorticotropin receptor involved in adrenal cortical neoplasia? Life Sci 1995;56(18):1523–1527.
33. Reincke M, Mora P, Beuschlein F, Arlt W, Chrousos GP, Allolio B. Deletion of the adrenocorticotropin receptor gene in human adrenocortical tumors: implications for tumorigenesis. J Clin Endocrinol Metab 1997;82(9):3054–3058.
34. Weinstein LS, Shenker A, Gejman PV, Merino MJ, Friedman E, Spiegel AM. Activating mutations of the stimulatory G protein in the McCune–Albright syndrome. N Engl J Med 1991;325(24):1688–1695.
35. Reincke M, Karl M, Travis W, Chrousos GP. No evidence for oncogenic mutations in guanine nucleotide-binding proteins of human adrenocortical neoplasms. J Clin Endocrinol Metab 1993;77(5):1419–1422.
36. Gicquel C, Dib A, Bertagna X, Amselem S, Le Bouc Y. Oncogenic mutations of alpha-Gi2 protein are not determinant for human adrenocortical tumourigenesis. Eur J Endocrinol 1995;133(2):166–172.
37. Latronico AC, Mendonca BB, Bianco AC, et al. Calcium-dependent protein kinase-C activity in human adrenocortical neoplasms, hyperplastic adrenals, and normal adrenocortical tissue. J Clin Endocrinol Metab 1994;79(3):736–739.
38. Yashiro T, Hara H, Fulton NC, Obara T, Kaplan EL. Point mutations of ras genes in human adrenal cortical tumors: absence in adrenocortical hyperplasia. World J Surg 1994;18(4):455–460; discussion 60–61.
39. Moul JW, Bishoff JT, Theune SM, Chang EH. Absent ras gene mutations in human adrenal cortical neoplasms and pheochromocytomas. J Urol 1993;149(6):1389–1394.
40. Brandi ML, Gagel RF, Angeli A, et al. Guidelines for diagnosis and therapy of MEN type 1 and type 2. J Clin Endocrinol Metab 2001;86(12):5658–5671.
41. Schulte KM, Mengel M, Heinze M, et al. Complete sequencing and messenger ribonucleic acid expression analysis of the MEN I gene in adrenal cancer. J Clin Endocrinol Metab 2000;85(1):441–448.
42. Ilvesmaki V, Blum WF, Voutilainen R. Insulin-like growth factor binding proteins in the human adrenal gland. Mol Cell Endocrinol 1993;97(1–2):71–79.
43. Mesiano S, Jaffe RB. Developmental and functional biology of the primate fetal adrenal cortex. Endocr Rev 1997;18(3):378–403.
44. Weber MM, Fottner C, Schmidt P, et al. Postnatal overexpression of insulin-like growth factor II in transgenic mice is associated with adrenocortical hyperplasia and enhanced steroidogenesis. Endocrinology 1999;140(4):1537–1543.
45. DeChiara TM, Robertson EJ, Efstratiadis A. Parental imprinting of the mouse insulin-like growth factor II gene. Cell 1991;64(4):849–859.
46. Hao Y, Crenshaw T, Moulton T, Newcomb E, Tycko B. Tumour-suppressor activity of H19 RNA. Nature 1993;365(6448):764–767.
47. Matsuoka S, Edwards MC, Bai C, et al. p57KIP2, a structurally distinct member of the p21CIP1 Cdk inhibitor family, is a candidate tumor suppressor gene. Genes Dev 1995;9(6):650–662.
48. Brannan CI, Dees EC, Ingram RS, Tilghman SM. The product of the H19 gene may function as an RNA. Mol Cell Biol 1990;10(1):28–36.
49. Ferguson-Smith AC, Sasaki H, Cattanach BM, Surani MA. Parental-origin-specific epigenetic modification of the mouse H19 gene. Nature 1993;362(6422):751–755.
50. Hatada I, Mukai T. Genomic imprinting of p57KIP2, a cyclin-dependent kinase inhibitor, in mouse. Nat Genet 1995;11(2):204–206.
51. Ping AJ, Reeve AE, Law DJ, Young MR, Boehnke M, Feinberg AP. Genetic linkage of Beckwith–Wiedemann syndrome to 11p15. Am J Hum Genet 1989;44(5):720–723.
52. Henry I, Jeanpierre M, Couillin P, et al. Molecular definition of the 11p15.5 region involved in Beckwith–Wiedemann syndrome and probably in predisposition to adrenocortical carcinoma. Hum Genet 1989;81(3):273–277.
53. Gicquel C, Bertagna X, Schneid H, et al. Rearrangements at the 11p15 locus and overexpression of insulin-like growth factor-II gene in sporadic adrenocortical tumors. J Clin Endocrinol Metab 1994;78(6):1444–1453.
54. Gicquel C, Raffin-Sanson ML, Gaston V, et al. Structural and functional abnormalities at 11p15 are associated with the malignant phenotype in sporadic adrenocortical tumors: study on a series of 82 tumors. J Clin Endocrinol Metab 1997;82(8):2559–2565.
55. Wilkin F, Gagne N, Paquette J, Oligny LL, Deal C. Pediatric adrenocortical tumors: molecular events leading to insulin-like growth factor II gene overexpression. J Clin Endocrinol Metab 2000;85(5):2048–2056.
56. Almeida MQ, Fragoso MC, Lotfi CF, et al. Expression of insulin-like growth factor-II and its receptor in pediatric and adult adrenocortical tumors. J Clin Endocrinol Metab 2008;93(9):3524–3531.

57. Logie A, Boulle N, Gaston V, et al. Autocrine role of IGF-II in proliferation of human adrenocortical carcinoma NCI H295R cell line. J Mol Endocrinol 1999;23(1):23–32.
58. Wang Y, Sun Y. Insulin-like growth factor receptor-1 as an anti-cancer target: blocking transformation and inducing apoptosis. Curr Cancer Drug Targets 2002;2(3):191–207.
59. Figueiredo BC, Stratakis CA, Sandrini R, et al. Comparative genomic hybridization analysis of adrenocortical tumors of childhood. J Clin Endocrinol Metab 1999;84(3):1116–1121.
60. James LA, Kelsey AM, Birch JM, Varley JM. Highly consistent genetic alterations in childhood adrenocortical tumours detected by comparative genomic hybridization. Br J Cancer 1999;81(2):300–304.
61. Kjellman M, Kallioniemi OP, Karhu R, et al. Genetic aberrations in adrenocortical tumors detected using comparative genomic hybridization correlate with tumor size and malignancy. Cancer Res 1996;56(18):4219–4223.
62. Dohna M, Reincke M, Mincheva A, Allolio B, Solinas-Toldo S, Lichter P. Adrenocortical carcinoma is characterized by a high frequency of chromosomal gains and high-level amplifications. Genes Chromosomes Cancer 2000;28(2):145–153.
64. de Fraipont F, El Atifi M, Cherradi N, et al. Gene expression profiling of human adrenocortical tumors using complementary deoxyribonucleic acid microarrays identifies several candidate genes as markers of malignancy. J Clin Endocrinol Metab 2005;90(3):1819–1829.
65. West AN, Neale GA, Pounds S, et al. Gene expression profiling of childhood adrenocortical tumors. Cancer Res 2007;67(2):600–608.
66. Keegan CE, Hammer GD. Recent insights into organogenesis of the adrenal cortex. Trends Endocrinol Metab 2002;13(5):200–208.
67. Ikeda Y, Lala DS, Luo X, Kim E, Moisan MP, Parker KL. Characterization of the mouse FTZ-F1 gene, which encodes a key regulator of steroid hydroxylase gene expression. Mol Endocrinol 1993;7(7):852–860.
68. Parker KL, Schimmer BP. Steroidogenic factor 1: a key determinant of endocrine development and function. Endocr Rev 1997;18(3):361–377.
69. Beuschlein F, Mutch C, Bavers DL, et al. Steroidogenic factor-1 is essential for compensatory adrenal growth following unilateral adrenalectomy. Endocrinology 2002;143(8):3122–3135.
70. Figueiredo BC, Cavalli LR, Pianovski MA, et al. Amplification of the steroidogenic factor 1 gene in childhood adrenocortical tumors. J Clin Endocrinol Metab 2005;90(2):615–619.
71. Pianovski MA, Cavalli LR, Figueiredo BC, et al. SF-1 overexpression in childhood adrenocortical tumours. Eur J Cancer 2006;42(8):1040–1043.
72. Kikuchi A. Tumor formation by genetic mutations in the components of the Wnt signaling pathway. Cancer Sci 2003;94(3):225–229.
73. Gordon MD, Nusse R. Wnt signaling: multiple pathways, multiple receptors, and multiple transcription factors. J Biol Chem 2006;281(32):22429–22433.
74. Tissier F, Cavard C, Groussin L, et al. Mutations of beta-catenin in adrenocortical tumors: activation of the Wnt signaling pathway is a frequent event in both benign and malignant adrenocortical tumors. Cancer Res 2005;65(17):7622–7627.
75. Hanahan D, Weinberg RA. The hallmarks of cancer. Cell 2000;100(1):57–70.
76. Varley JM, McGown G, Thorncroft M, et al. Are there low-penetrance TP53 Alleles? Evidence from childhood adrenocortical tumors. Am J Hum Genet 1999;65(4):995–1006.
77. Giordano TJ, Thomas DG, Kuick R, et al. Distinct transcriptional profiles of adrenocortical tumors uncovered by DNA microarray analysis. Am J Pathol 2003;162(2):521–531.

5 Clinical Features of Cushing's Syndrome

Oscar D. Bruno

Contents

INTRODUCTION

In spite of its low frequency, endogenous Cushing's syndrome (CS) is not an exceptional clinical entity. A growing number of cases are currently derived to specialized centers suggesting an increasing knowledge of the clinical features of hypercortisolism from the part of general practitioners, internists, cardiologists, gynecologists, dermatologists, and specialists of other branches of clinical medicine. Since the first description of this syndrome by Harvey Cushing in 1912, we have learnt to recognize the many faces through which it can manifest itself. Disturbed cortisol hypersecretion leads to an exaggeration of the well-known physiological actions of this hormone inducing protein breakdown, hyperglycemia, fat mobilization, dyslipidemia, hydrosaline retention, immunosuppression, and increased susceptibility to infection. Despite its low specificity for being highly prevalent in the general population, cardinal symptoms such as recent and/or unexplained development of central obesity, mood changes, fatigue, weakness, myopathy, easy bruisability, skin atrophy and red striae, arterial hypertension, diabetes, and hyperlipidemia, generally combined in different ways are suggestive of the diagnosis. From a clinical epidemiological point of view, the possibility of existence of CS is to be suspected and

From: *Contemporary Endocrinology: Cushing's Syndrome: Pathophysiology, Diagnosis and Treatment*
Edited by: M.D. Bronstein (ed.), DOI 10.1007/978-1-60327-449-4_5,

consequently searched for among patients with uncontrolled high blood pressure (HBP) or diabetes mellitus despite treatment, metabolic syndrome, polycystic ovarian syndrome, osteoporosis, depression, or adrenal incidentaloma. True CS has to be differentiated from pseudo syndromes mimicking it. Most sensitive physical signs for discriminating CS from pseudo-Cushing states are the presence of supraclavicular fat pads, myopathy, thin skin, and easy bruising.

The recognition of the clinical manifestations of CS and of the subpopulations at risk of contracting the disease should be improved through medical education at the medical school and at postgraduate levels. Clinical detection of CS must be performed mainly by nonendocrinologists, yet its etiological diagnosis and therapeutic management is to be carried out in highly experienced and specialized centers, to ensure the best results in the treatment of this really challenging endocrine disturbance.

From a semiological point of view, CS is one of the most expressive disorders in clinical endocrinology. Since the original report of the syndrome by Harvey Cushing in 1912 *(1)* followed by a more comprehensive description in 1932 *(2)*, the knowledge about its typical features and different modes of presentation has been progressively enriched so the many faces with which this interesting and challenging syndrome can manifest itself are much better known nowadays. Briefly, CS can be ACTH-dependent in about 80–85% of the cases, usually caused by a pituitary adenoma and much less frequently by an ACTH or CRH secreting extra-pituitary tumor- or ACTH-independent mainly due to an adrenal tumor; these and other infrequent etiologies are thoroughly analyzed in other chapters of this book. Regardless of its origin, the clinical signs of CS are usually quite similar. The impressive development of biochemical and imaging technologies that we have witnessed in the last 40 years has also contributed to a better understanding of the varied traits that the syndrome can bear, allowing demonstrating its existence in different clinical settings.

The manifestations of CS are induced by the chronic exposure of tissues to excessive cortisol blood concentrations derived from an increased cortisol production rate *(3)* followed by an enhancement of the biological actions of glucocorticoids (GC) (Table 1) *(4)*. Among these, the impact on protein and glucose metabolism is crucial. The clinical signs of CS are variable and differ widely depending on several factors such as age, duration of the disease, and severity of hypercortisolism. It is usually reported by patients and their relatives that significant "unexplained" physical and psychological changes occurred over a relatively short period of time (months or few years) and comparing pictures of the patient taken at different moments over the last years can help to testify the syndrome development. The relative frequency of the cardinal signs of CS reported in the literature is somewhat variable depending on the observer. Table 2 represents the main manifestations of the disorder in a group of

Table 1
Main Biological Actions of Cortisol

Increase	*Decrease*
Protein/collagen breakdown	LH and FSH secretion
Gluconeogenesis	TSH release
Liver glycogen deposition	GH secretion
Insulin resistance	Vitamin D and calcium intestinal absorption
Free fatty acid production	Osteocalcin formation
Sodium and water retention	Inflammatory response
PTH secretion	Immune system activity
Osteoclast activity	

Table 2
Frequency of Initial Signs Leading to Consultation in 156 Patients with CS

Clinical Sign	%
Obesity/overweight	46.2
Hypertension/edema	30.8
Hyperandrogenic signs	23.7
Psychological changes	22.0
Menstrual disturbance	17.9
Skin signs	16.6
Facial changes	15.4
Muscular signs	8.3
Neurologic disorders	6.4
Diabetes	5.8
Other/miscellaneous	5.8

patients studied in our hospital. In the following paragraphs, we will describe the main signs and symptoms of CS as well as its pathogenetic mechanisms.

Key Words: Hypercortisolism clinical signs, Cushing's syndrome features, Cushing's syndrome diagnosis

OBESITY AND LIPID METABOLISM

Obesity or overweight is one of the most frequent complaints of patients affected by CS. The degree of fat accumulation is variable and depends – among others factors – on (a) the duration of the diseased condition, (b) individual characteristics probably related to variation in affinity of GC for its receptor *(5)*, and (c) premorbid conditions (e.g., some patients may have already been obese or overweight when CS development started). Weight increase develops over a relatively short period of time without any apparent change in diet and physical activity. Grade III obesity is attained only exceptionally (Fig. 1); however, in some cases only fat distribution occurs, with no significant increase or even an initial decrease in weight redundant. The distribution of fat is quite typical with particular predilection for trunk and abdomen. Fat pads develop in the supraclavicular area with disappearance of normal fossae, and fat deposition at the level of the spinal apophysis of the first dorsal vertebra gives the typical "buffalo hump" appearance (Fig. 2). At the same time, the reduction of limbs fat stores, gives, along with the accompanying muscle atrophy, a particular physical appearance (Fig. 3).

Body fat accrual and change in its distribution are mainly due to increased cortisol-induced central (trunk-abdominal) depots along with augmented lipolysis in peripheral fat depots (limbs), which can be explained by greater sensitivity to GC than to insulin in the latter, as opposed to the reverse effect in the former. Increase in the Bichat's protuberance (buccal fat pad) contributes to rounding of the face which, together with its red appearance and conjunctiva injection, makes up the characteristic cushingoid plethoric facies. A moderate exophthalmus may also be seen in patients with CS.

Mobilization of lipids gives origin to disturbed serum lipid concentrations, with higher levels of triglycerides, total and LDL cholesterol and lower levels of HDL cholesterol.

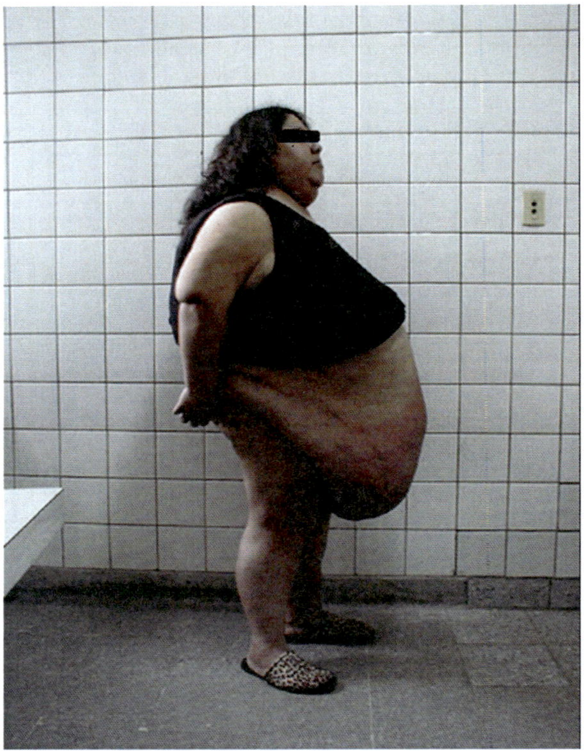

Fig. 1. Morbid obesity in CS: a 23-year-old woman who complained about an abrupt change in weight from 80 to 170 kg for a height of 154 cm (BMI from 31.7 to 71.7) in one year. She was successfully operated on of a corticotrophic adenoma.

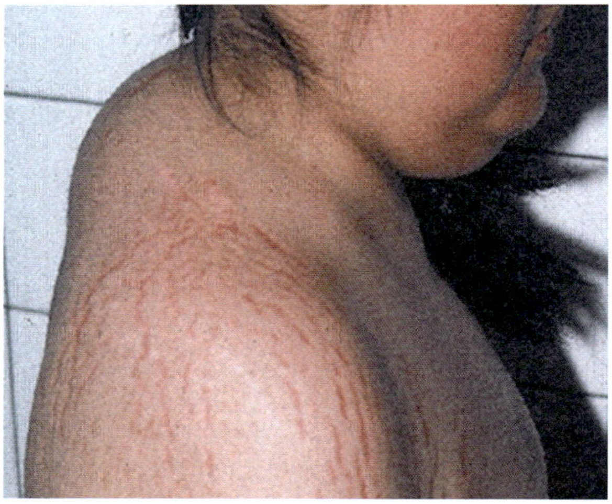

Fig. 2. Classic aspect of Cushing's syndrome (CS). Note the plethoric facies, supraclavicular fat pads, "buffalo" hump, and red striae in a 16-year-old girl.

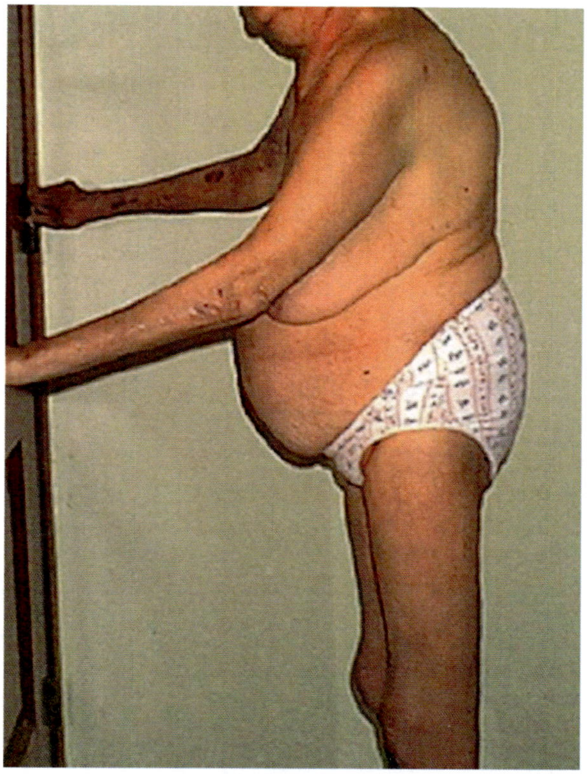

Fig. 3. A 64-year-old woman with typical traits of CS. Observe the prominent abdomen and the clear atrophy of thigh (quadricipital) muscles.

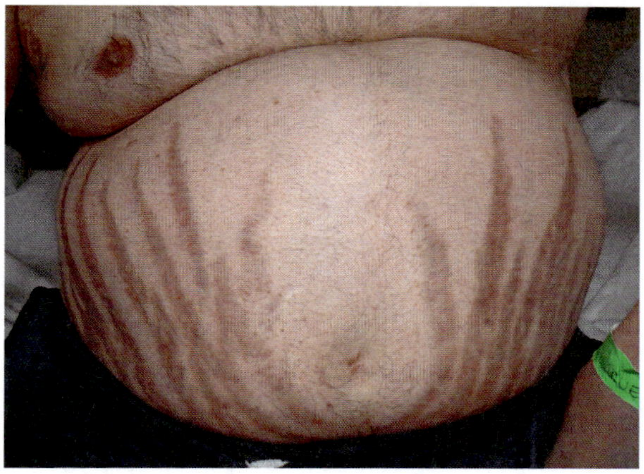

Fig. 4. Abdominal red striae in a young woman affected by CS.

SKIN CHANGES

The deleterious hypercatabolic effects of hypercortisolism are notorious on the skin surface. Atrophy of the skin is easily noticed – especially in younger patients – by slightly pinching a skin folder on the patient's forearm and comparing it with that of the observer (old age may mislead conditions). Thinner, and therefore transparent skin, allows seeing the subcutaneous blood vessels giving a characteristic reddish-purple aspect. Atrophy and disruption of collagenous subcutaneous fibers lead to the development of red striae, typically – yet not always – wider than 1 cm, mainly on the abdomen and flanks (Fig. 4); striae can also develop in other sites such as in lower and upper limbs and shoulders (Fig. 2); they are more frequently seen and particularly marked in young patients with CS. Attention must be paid to differentiate this kind of striae in CS, from those seen in young girls at the time of the pubertal spurt *(6)* (Fig. 5). Easy bruising is another frequent sign. This is mainly evident on the extension surface of arms and legs where ecchymosis and hematomas develop following minimal blows or after blood sampling. Stumbling and hitting a piece of furniture can injure and cause wounds in the anterior tibial face with torpid evolution and delayed cicatrization; some of these patients consult dermatologists for chronic ulceration of the legs in the absence of disturbed arterial or venous circulation. Pityriasis versicolor and other dermatomycosis can be found in patients with CS. As a consequence of concomitant androgen hypersecretion in ACTH-dependent forms or in adrenocortical cancer causing CS, hirsutism with frontal balding and acne can also occur and in some cases, constitute the first and main sign of abnormality in female patients. Acanthosis nigricans with acrochordons (skin tags) in correlation with severe insulin resistance can be found mainly in the region of the neck (Fig. 6). Finally, although it has

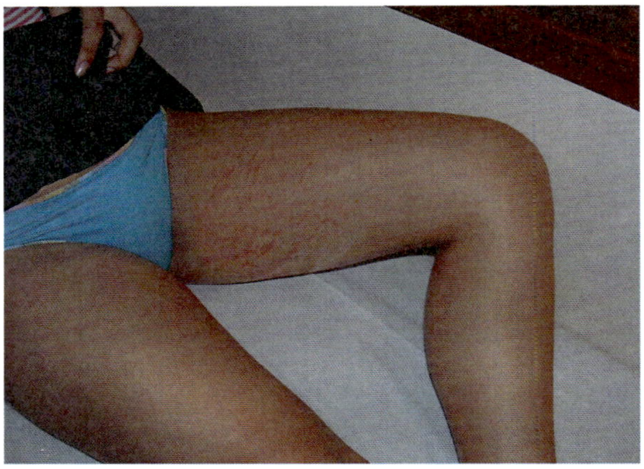

Fig. 5. Cushing's-like reddish striae on the inner surface of thighs in a 14-year-old girl; biochemical tests were negative for hypercortisolism.

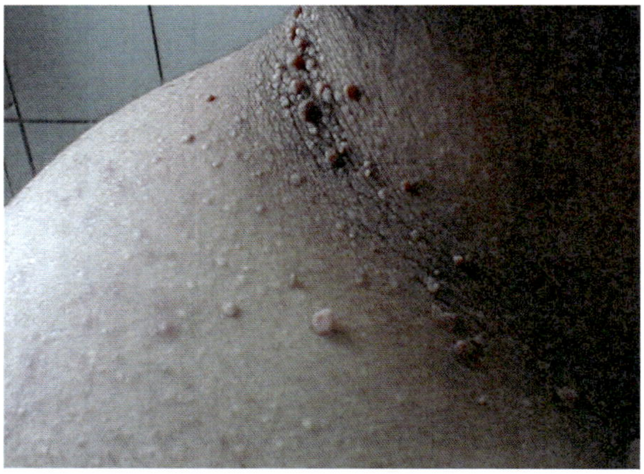

Fig. 6. Acrochordons in a 26-year-old male patient with CS and severe insulin resistance.

been more frequently ascribed to the ectopic variants, hyperpigmentation can also be found in cases of pituitary CS (Cushing's disease).

MUSCLE CHANGES

Fatigue is a common complaint in Cushing's patients. In well-developed CS, muscle atrophy is evident especially in the lower limbs. Loss of strength affects mainly muscles of the pelvic girdle. Patients complain of not being able to climb a ladder or even to take a short walk; physical examination shows that they are not capable of rising from the recumbent (Plummer's maneuver) or from the squatting position without helping themselves with their hands. The existence of hypokalemia can certainly aggravate the muscular feebleness. Weakness may also involve respiratory muscles, being one of the many factors involved in the surgical risk of CS patients.

CARDIOVASCULAR SYSTEM

Cardiovascular disease, in particular hypertension, is a major factor of morbidity and mortality in patients with CS, more than 70% of whom having HBP at diagnosis *(7)*. Arterial hypertension involves both systolic and diastolic measurements and can lead to cerebrovascular or cardiovascular complications. The pathogenetic mechanism of hypertension is related to several factors. A very relevant one is the mineralocorticoid effect of excess cortisol at kidney level (see below) which leads to sodium retention and expansion of the extracellullar space. Edema of ankles and legs is frequently found and can be attributed to the positive sodium and water balance. Vasodilatation inhibitory activity, enhanced cardiovascular response to vasoactive substances, and a direct effect of ACTH on vascular tone are also involved in the pathogenesis of HBP *(8–10)*. In addition, GC excess can accelerate the development of atherosclerosis by promoting direct endothelial cell injury and by inducing hyperlipidemia and glucose intolerance, both factors contributing to blood vessels damage *(11–13)*. Dilated cardiomyopathy, cardiac failure, or brain stroke may result from persistent hypercortisolism.

NERVOUS SYSTEM, NEUROPSYCHOLOGICAL AND PSYCHIATRIC CHANGES

Patients affected with CS usually complain of easy fatigability, irritability, anxiety, insomnia, memory disorders, lack of concentration, appetite change, lack of sexual desire, and hallucinations; in some cases, mental changes are so severe that psychotic crises and suicidal tendencies can develop requiring urgent hospitalization and specialized management. The relative frequency of all these manifestations is variably reported in the literature depending on the interest of different observers to record it systematically but can amount to 66.7% of the patients, with a predominance of atypical depressive disorder in 51.5% and/or major affective disorders in 12% *(14)*.

ELECTROLYTE AND WATER BALANCE

Cortisol has affinity for mineralocorticoid receptors in the kidney but, in healthy people, normal amounts of this hormone are inactivated to cortisone by the enzyme 11β-hydroxysteroid dehydrogenase type 2. Hypercortisolism of CS overcomes the enzyme capacity and binds to the receptor so inducing an increased expoliation of potassium and retention of sodium at the tubular level which leads to the already mentioned expansion of the extracellular compartment. Therefore, hypercortisolism can be accompanied by hypokalemia in all forms of CS, but specially in the ectopic ACTH-dependent form, in which low potassium levels have been described in up to 57% of patients *(15, 16)*.

GLUCOSE METABOLISM

Cortisol increases synthesis of hepatic glycogen by augmentation of the breakdown of proteins. So, hepatic output of glucose is increased and hyperglycemia ensues with a concomitant stimulation of insulin secretion and development of a state of insulin resistance, since cortisol inhibits the entry of glucose into the cells. About 80–90% of patients with CS have undue levels of plasma glucose when explored by a glucose tolerance test and some 20% develop overt type 2 diabetes or, less frequently, insulin-dependent diabetes *(17)*.

BONE METABOLISM: OSTEOPOROSIS

The osseous tissue is severely affected by the chronic exposure to unduly high amounts of GC which usually lead to different degrees of osteoporosis *(18)*. The pathophysiological mechanisms of damage are multiple and influence almost all the factors that normally intervene in the regulation of bone metabolism. Excess cortisol decreases the formation of the osseous matrix through diminished synthesis and increased breakdown of proteins. Osteoblastic function is significantly inhibited by GC as indicated by great decreases in serum osteocalcin concentrations. Conversely, osteoclastic function and bone resorption are enhanced while in addition, increased PTH secretion can been found in chronic hypercortisolism *(19)*. Mobilization of calcium from bone to the extracellular space is not sufficient to induce hypercalcemia, but hypercalciuria is a frequent finding; nephrolithiasis can be found in as much as 50% of patients with CS although there is no clear explanation for that *(20)*. In parallel with these direct actions on bone, other indirect alterations induced by cortisol contribute to the development of osteoporosis. At the intestinal level, both calcium and vitamin D2 absorption is decreased by GC, the conversion of 25-OH-cholecalciferol to 1,25-OH-cholecalciferol is diminished due to inhibition of the renal 1-hydroxylase and, in both sexes, a decrease in gonadal steroids (see below) additionally aggravates bone loss. Osteoporosis especially affects cancellous bone. Densitometric values are frequently decreased to less than 2.5 standard deviations and rib and vertebral fractures can ensue with significant reduction in stature in some cases. The typical finding in sagittal imaging thoracic views is that of the so-called fish-mouth vertebrae produced by the crushing of the frontal vertebral bodies mainly at the level of the last dorsal and first lumbar vertebrae (Fig. 7). Although less frequent than in the iatrogenic variant, aseptic necrosis of the femoral head has also been reported in endogenous CS *(21)*.

GONADAL CHANGES

Loss of libido in both sexes, menstrual irregularity with oligomenorrhea or amenorrhea in women and sexual dysfunction in men are very frequent manifestations of gonadal dysfunction in CS *(22, 23)*. GC in excess are not only inhibitory of hypothalamic GnRH and pituitary gonadotrophic cell secretion, but also affect steroid synthesis at the gonads and their peripheral action at target cells level. Impaired estradiol or testosterone synthesis highly contributes to osteoporosis development. Due to this steroid-induced hypogonadotropic hypogonadism, followed by amenorrhea in up to 70–80% of patients, pregnancy is a rare event in women with CS occurring in those who keep ovulatory cycles in spite of hypercortisolism *(24)* (see Chap. 21).

GROWTH RETARDATION

Chronic hypercortisolism inhibits GHRH synthesis at hypothalamic level and GH formation at pituitary level. Growth hormone induced IGF-1 synthesis is also decreased with the resulting lack of stimulation of the cartilage plate leading to growth arrest *(25)*. In children, weight gain associated

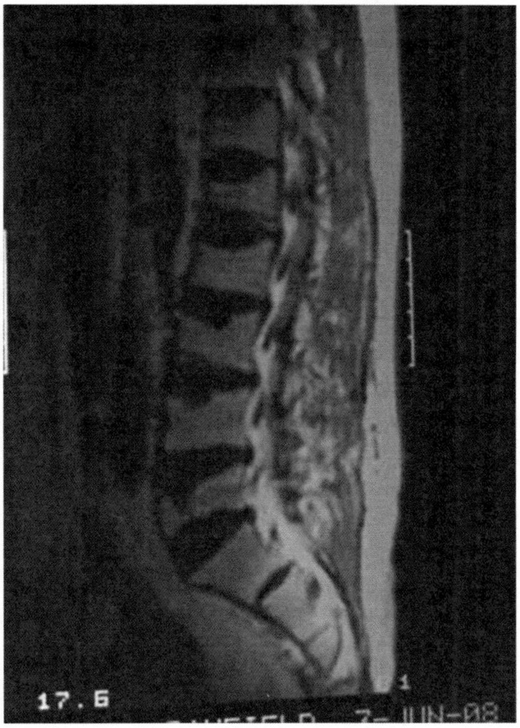

Fig. 7. Lateral MRI view of the dorsolumbar spine showing vertebral crushing in a 28-year-old man with Cushing's disease.

with growth retardation should include CS in the differential diagnosis. However, this clinical picture is interpreted erroneously as hypothyroidism in many cases. The CS in children is thoroughly discussed in Chap. 22 of this book.

THYROID GLAND

Classically, thyroid dysfunction in CS has been attributed to a state of steroid-induced central hypothyroidism with inhibition of TRH, TSH, and T4 to T3 peripheral conversion. However, an increased frequency of primary thyroid abnormalities (up to 30%) has been found in patients with CS as compared with the general population *(26, 27)*. Autoimmune thyroid disease frequency further increases after resolution of hypercortisolism *(26, 27)*.

IMMUNE SYSTEM

Physiologically, there exists an interaction between the hypothalamic pituitary adrenal axis and the immune system. Immune molecules such as cytokines are stimulatory of the activation of the hypothalamic-pituitary structures resulting in secretion of ACTH. Alternatively, cortisol modulates cytokine production *(28)*. The GC in excess are strong inhibitors of the immune and inflammatory responses to diverse noxae. Patients with CS are severely immunocompromised and at high risk of acquiring infections caused by usual and unusual germs. Opportunistic infections in endogenous CS are associated with severe cortisol excess and carry a high mortality. They are most prevalent in the ectopic

ACTH syndrome explained by the very high plasma cortisol concentrations in this condition in which infections with *Cryptococcus neoformans*, *Aspergillus fumigatus*, *Herpes simplex*, *Pneumocystis carinii*, and *Nocardia asteroides* predominate *(29)*.

IN WHAT CLINICAL SETTINGS SHOULD CUSHING'S SYNDROME BE SUSPECTED?

The different signs through which CS is manifested as well as its pathogenesis have been described in the preceding paragraphs. However, they do not usually present themselves all together but regrouped in different ways according to the relative predominance of one or the other and depending on diverse factors such as age, sex, previous disease, and genetic background (Table 3). In the experience of the author, the signs that are most sensitive in discriminating CS from pseudo-Cushing states are the presence of supraclavicular fat pads, myopathy, thin skin, and easy bruising. Frequently, these manifestations are not initially well interpreted, and therefore diagnosis is delayed sometimes for many months or years. This is probably due to the fact that many of the main signs of CS leading to

Table 3
Clinical Settings in Which CS Should Be Suspected

Recently developed truncal obesity with plethora
Recently discovered arterial hypertension
Recent neuropsychiatric changes (depression, anxiety, insomnia)
Polycystic ovarian syndrome
Metabolic syndrome
Type 2 diabetes
Osteoporosis
Adrenal incidentaloma

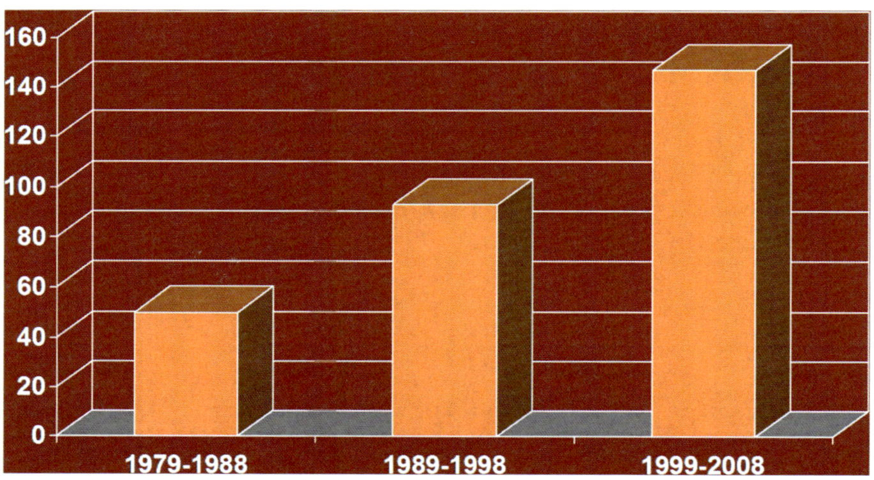

Fig. 8. Increasing number of new cases of CS derived over a 30-year span to the Division of Endocrinology, Hospital de Clínicas, University of Buenos Aires.

consultation are of high prevalence in the general population: overweight or obesity, arterial hypertension, menstrual cycle disturbances, diabetes, dyslipidemia, osteoporosis, or depression; therefore, the probability that two or more of those signs present themselves in a combined manner is also very high. A growing number of cases are presently derived to specialized centers (Fig. 8) suggesting an increase in the knowledge of the clinical features of hypercortisolism by general practitioners, internists, cardiologists, gynecologists, dermatologists, and specialists of other branches of clinical medicine who, after evoking the possibility of hypercortisolism, indicate the initial studies aiming to confirm or reject the diagnosis. Afterwards, etiologic diagnosis and therapeutic management must be conducted by experienced endocrinologists in a multidisciplinary team.

REFERENCES

1. Cushing H. The pituitary body and its disorders: clinical states produced by disorders of the hypophysis cerebri. Philadelphia: J.B. Lipincott 1912.
2. Cushing H. The basophil adenomas of the pituitary body and their clinical manifestations (pituitary basophilism). Bull John Hopkins Hosp 1932; 50:137–195.
3. Esteban NV, Loughlin T, Yergey AL, et al. Daily cortisol production rate in man determined by stable isotope dilution/ mass spectrometry. J Clin Endocrinol Metab 1991; 72:39–45.
4. Stewart PM. The adrenal cortex; corticosteroid hormone action. In: Kronenberg HM, Melmed S, Polonsky KS, Reed Larsen P, eds. Williams Textbook of Endocrinology. 11th ed. Philadelphia, PA: Saunders Elsevier, 2008:453–458.
5. Ruscscher H, Smit P, van den Akker EL, et al. Two polymorphisms of the glucocorticoid receptor gene directly affect glucocorticoid-regulated gene expression. J Clin Endocrinol Metab 2005;90:5804–5810.
6. Cohen HA, Matalon A, Mezger A, et al. Striae in adolescents mistaken for physical abuse. J Fam Pract 1997;45:84–85.
7. Magiakou MA, Smyrnaki P, Chrousos GP. Hypertension in Cushing's syndrome. Best Pract Res Clin Endocrinol Metab 2006;20:467–482.
8. Saruta T, Suzuki H, Handa M, et al. Multiple factors contribute to the pathogenesis of hypertension in Cushing's syndrome. J Clin Endocrinol Metab 1986;62:275–279.
9. Hatakeyama H, Inaba S. Miyamori I. 11 ß Hydroxysteroid dehydrogenase in cultured human vascular cells: possible role in the development of hypertension. Hypertension 1999;33:1179–1184.
10. Hatakeyama H, Inaba S, Taniguch N, et al. Functional adrenocorticotropic hormone receptor in cultured human vascular endothelial cells. Hypertension 2000;36:862–865.
11. Nashel DJ. Is atherosclerosis a complication of long-term corticosteroid treatment? Am J Med 1986;80:925–929.
12. Colao A, Pivonello R, Spiezia S, et al. Persistence of increased cardiovascular risk in patients with Cushing's disease after five years of successful cure. J Clin Endocrinol Metab 1999;84:2664–2672.
13. Faggiano A, Pivonello R, Spiezia S, et al. Cardiovascular risk factors and common carotid artery caliber and stiffness in patients with Cushing's disease and 1 year after disease remission. J Clin Endocrinol Metab 2003;88:2527–2533.
14. Dorn LD, Burgess ES, Friedman TC, et al. The longitudinal course of psychopathology in Cushing's syndrome after correction of hypercortisolism. J Clin Endocrinol Metab 1997;82:912–919.
15. Howlett TA, Drury PL, Perry L, et al. Diagnosis and management of ACTH-dependent Cushing's syndrome: comparison of the features in ectopic and pituitary ACTH production. Clin Endocrinol (Oxf) 1986;24:699–713.
16. Torpy DJ, Mullen N, Ilias I, et al. Association of hypertension and hypokalemia with Cushing's syndrome caused by ectopic ACTH secretion: a series of 58 cases. Ann NY Acad Sci 2002;970:134–144.
17. Nestler JE, McClanahan MA. Diabetes and adrenal disease. Baillieres Clin Endocrinol Metab 1992;6:829–847.
18. Magiakou MA, Mastorakos G, Webster E, et al. The hypothalamic-pituitary-adrenal axis and the female reproductive system. Ann NY Acad Sci 1997;816:42–56.
19. Lanna CM, Paula FJ, Montenegro RM Jr, et al. Parathyroid hormone secretion in chronic human endogenous hypercortisolism. Braz J Med Biol Res 2002;35:229–236.
20. Faggiano A, Pivonello R, Melis D, et al. Nephrolithiasis in Cushing's disease: prevalence, etiopathogenesis, and modification after disease cure. J Clin Endocrinol Metab 2003;88:2076–2080.
21. Koch CA., Tsigos C, Patronas NJ, et al. Cushing's disease presenting with avascular necrosis of the hip: an orthopedic emergency. J Clin Endocrinol Metab 1999;84:3010–3012.
22. Mazziotti G, Giustina A, Canalis E, et al. Glucocorticoid-induced osteoporosis: clinical and therapeutic aspects. Arq Bras Endocrinol Metab 2007;51:1404–1412.

23. Luton JP, Thieblot P, Valcke JC, et al. Reversible gonadotropin deficiency in male Cushing's disease. J Clin Endocrinol Metab 1977;45:488–495.
24. Lindsay JR, Jonklaas J, Oldfield EH, et al. Cushing's syndrome during pregnancy: personal experience and review of the literature. J Clin Endocrinol Metab 2005;90:3077–3083.
25. Magiakou MA, Mastorakos G, Gomez MT, et al. Suppressed spontaneous and stimulated growth hormone secretion in patients with Cushing's disease before and after surgical cure. J Clin Endocrinol Metab 1994;78:131–137.
26. Colao A, Pivonello R, Faggiano A, et al. Increased prevalence of thyroid autoimmunity in patients successfully treated for Cushing's disease. Clin Endocrinol 2000;53:13–19.
27. Niepomniczcze H, Pitoia F, Katz S, et al. Primary thyroid disorders in endogenous Cushing's syndrome. Eur J Endocrinol 2002;147:305–311.
28. Elenkov IJ. Neurohormonal-cytokine interactions: implications for inflammation, common human diseases and well-being. Neurochem Int 2008;52:40–51.
29. Graham BS, Tucker WS Jr. Opportunistic infections in endogenous Cushing's syndrome. Ann Intern Med 1984;101:334–338.

6 Laboratorial Diagnosis of Cushing's Syndrome: Differential Diagnosis with Pseudo Cushing's Conditions as Obesity, Alcoholism and Depression

Martina De Martin, Francesca Pecori Giraldi, and Francesco Cavagnini

CONTENTS

SUMMARY

The diagnosis of Cushing's syndrome requires a high degree of suspicion and this may lead to testing of patients with some, but not all, features of hypercortisolism due to causes other than adrenal/pituitary dysfunction. Indeed, conditions such as depression, alcoholism, obesity and polycystic ovary syndrome may be accompanied by Cushing's-like physical and biochemical changes and are therefore grouped under the heading of "pseudoCushing".

This review will summarize clinical and biochemical findings in pseudoCushing's states and describe the differential diagnosis with Cushing's syndrome.

Key Words: Cushing's syndrome, pseudoCushing, alcoholism, obesity, depression, polycystic ovary syndrome, diagnosis, urinary free cortisol, dexamethasone suppression test, cortisol circadian rhythm

The diagnosis of Cushing's syndrome may not be obvious. Indeed, one of the major difficulties in the diagnostic work-up of these patients lies in the distinction between Cushing's syndrome and pseudoCushing's states. PseudoCushing is a condition due to causes other than those responsible for

From: *Contemporary Endocrinology: Cushing's Syndrome: Pathophysiology, Diagnosis and Treatment*
Edited by: M.D. Bronstein (ed.), DOI 10.1007/978-1-60327-449-4_6,

TESTS for the DIAGNOSIS of CUSHING'S SYNDROME

First tier tests for Cushing's syndrome	Criteria for Cushing's syndrome*
Urinary free cortisol: 2-3 collections	above normal range; >250 μg/24h (*1*)
Midnight cortisol: - salivary	assay dependent
- serum	>1.8 μg/dl (*9*); >5 μg/dl (*146*); >7.5 μg/dl (*10*)
Low dose dexamethasone suppression tests:	
- 1 mg dexamethasone at 11 PM, measure cortisol at 8 AM	>1.8 μg/dl (*17*); >5 μg/dl (*110*)
- 0.5 mg dexamethasone every 6 h for 2 days, measure UFC on 2nd day or cortisol at 8 AM on 3rd day	>20 μg/24h (*146*) >1.4 μg/dl (*26*); >1.8 μg/dl (*9*)

Tests for distinction between PseudoCushing and Cushing's syndrome

Currently used	
Dexamethasone-suppressed CRH test: 0.5 mg dexamethasone every 6 h for 2 days followed by CRH testing on 3rd day (2h after last dexamethasone tablet): measure cortisol 15 minutes after CRH injection	>1.4 μg/dl (26); >3.98 μg/dl (*30*)
Desmopressin test: 10 μg i.v.; measure ACTH for 2 hours	increase by at least 27 pg/ml (*32*)
Rarely used	
Insulin-induced hypoglycemia: 0.15-0.3 UI/kg body weight i.v.; measure cortisol and glycemia for 2 hours (blood glucose must fall below 46 mg/dl)	impaired increase (< 20 μg/dl) (*84*)
Hexarelin: 2 μg/kg body weight i.v., measure ACTH and cortisol for 90 minutes	marked ACTH/cortisol increase (*49*)
Naloxone: 125 μg/kg body weight i.v., measure cortisol for 2 hours	diminshed ACTH/cortisol increase (*51*)
Loperamide: 16 mg p.o.; measure cortisol after 3.5 hours	absent ACTH/cortisol suppression (*52*)

Fig. 1. Tests for the diagnosis of Cushing's syndrome. * Different cut-off values yield different diagnostic accuracy.

Cushing's syndrome, characterized by milder clinical features and laboratory alterations reminiscent of Cushing's syndrome, all of which resolve after cure of the underlying disease *(1)*. The most frequent causes of pseudoCushing are depression, alcoholism, obesity and polycystic ovary syndrome, which may occur in the same patient. The differential diagnosis between mild Cushing's syndrome and pseudoCushing may be difficult, time-consuming and requires multiple tests and extended follow-up. This review will summarize clinical findings and canvass diagnostic procedures used to distinguish between the two conditions (Fig. 1), and then discuss individual causes of pseudoCushing.

CLINICAL ASSESSMENT

Both Cushing's syndrome and pseudoCushing commonly feature truncal obesity, hypertension, impaired glucose tolerance or frank diabetes, psychiatric disturbances and dyslipidemia, whereas other features are more distinctive between the two states. In particular, thinning of the skin, proximal myopathy, easy bruising and early onset osteoporosis characterize true Cushing's syndrome but are less common in pseudoCushing. Irregular menses or amenorrhea may accompany polycystic ovary syndrome or simple obesity or be secondary to true endogenous hypercortisolism, thus do not differentiate between the two states. In children, simple obesity is commonly associated with normal or even above normal growth, whereas children with Cushing's syndrome are obese but growth stunted. Lumbar *striae rubrae* are not uncommon in children with rapid weight gain and, thus, do not help in the distinction. Rapidly progressing features are usually indicative of Cushing's syndrome, whereas pseudoCushing usually does not worsen over time; indeed, prolonged follow-up and symptomatic treatment may prove a reliable means to distinguish between Cushing's syndrome and pseudoCushing in difficult cases.

LABORATORIAL DIAGNOSIS OF CUSHING'S SYNDROME

Urinary Free Cortisol

As a rule, urinary free cortisol (UFC) levels above 250 µg/24 h (690 nmol/24 h) are clearly indicative of Cushing's syndrome but mildly elevated or even occasionally normal UFC levels may occasionally be registered among patients who subsequently prove themselves to be true Cushing's syndrome *(2)*. On the other hand, falsely elevated UFC values are registered in only 9% of Cushing's syndrome suspects, i.e., patients with features suggestive of hypercortisolism who proved not to be affected by Cushing's syndrome *(3)*, thus this procedure is sufficiently accurate (Fig. 2). Impaired kidney function (i.e., creatinine clearance <20 ml/min) may lead to spuriously low UFC measurements and other diagnostic procedures should be performed in patients with high serum creatinine or reduced creatinine clearance *(4)*. Physiological urine volumes (500—2500 ml/24 h) are unrelated to UFC levels *(5)*; UFC appears correlated to urine volume only during water loading as the attendant increase in water diuresis allows more free cortisol to escape proximal tubule reabsorption *(6)*.

Methodology of UFC assay should also be taken into account as some laboratories measure unextracted UFC, some use radioimmunoassays or simple ELISA and others use HPLC or tandem mass spectrometry. The latter, though vulnerable to interference by some agents, e.g., fenofibrate and carbamazepine *(7, 8)*, offers the greatest specificity but is currently costly and not feasible in everyday clinical setting; for the field endocrinologist, reliability of the UFC assay is a prerequisite to accurate diagnosis.

Midnight Cortisol

Measurement of midnight serum/salivary cortisol has proven a sensitive means to identify patients with Cushing's syndrome, although the highest sensitivity is associated with a considerable proportion of false positives. Indeed, a recent study showed that over 80% of Cushing's syndrome suspects present midnight serum cortisol greater than 1.8 µg/dl (50 nmol/l) *(3)*, the threshold which assures 100% sensitivity for Cushing's syndrome *(9)*. Adopting a higher cut-off (7.5 µg/dl, 207 nmol/l) raised specificity to 87% at a small expense of sensitivity, i.e., 90–96% *(2, 10)* (Fig. 2). Patients with pseudoCushing often fall within the gray area between these two cut-offs and will require further testing. Of note, midnight cortisol increases with age *(3, 11)*and this should be taken into account for older patients although age-related normative values are not available.

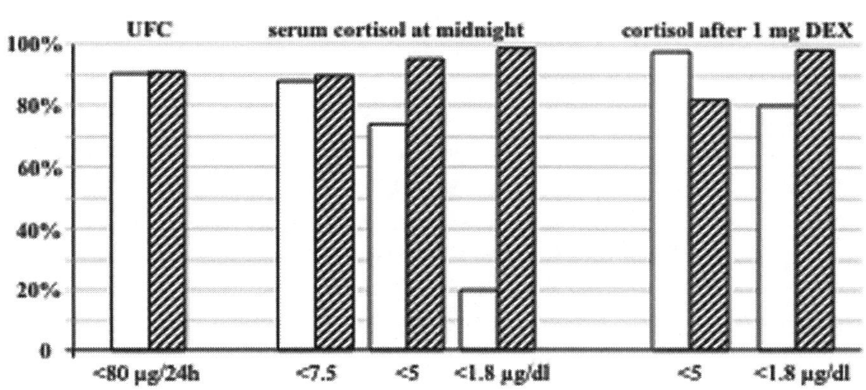

Fig. 2. Mean specificity (white boxes) and sensitivity (dashed boxes) of tests used for the diagnosis of Cushing's syndrome.

Salivary cortisol has gained increasing acceptance as a first-line test for Cushing's syndrome as it combines evaluation of cortisol circadian rhythm with the assessment of biologically active free cortisol. Indeed, salivary cortisol closely reflects blood cortisol levels *(12)* and is unaffected by changes in cortisol-binding globulin *(13)*. Assays for salivary cortisol differ considerably and validation on a large number of normal subjects is required to establish the upper reference range; indeed, these differ considerably among assays, i.e., from 0.13 μg/dl *(14)* to 0.43 μg/dl *(15)* or even 0.55 μg/dl *(16)*. In our experience *(17)*, salivary cortisol levels above 0.35 μg/dl (9.7 nmol/l) offer a good sensitivity (93%), especially for those patients with Cushing's syndrome in whom UFC values overlap with those observed in pseudoCushing. As with serum midnight cortisol, salivary cortisol increases with age *(18)*.

Assessment of midnight cortisol, in serum or saliva, may be the only useful test to exclude Cushing's syndrome in patients on drugs such as anticonvulsants, fenofibrate, rifampicin, licorice and carbenoxolone, which interfere with UFC measurement and/or dexamethasone suppression *(8, 19–21)*.

Low Dose Dexamethasone Suppression Tests

Both 1 mg overnight (Nugent's test) and 48 h 2 mg/day (Liddle's low dose test) dexamethasone suppression tests are among the mainstays of the diagnostic work-up of Cushing's syndrome. Diagnostic criteria achieving maximal sensitivity are obviously somewhat lower than those ensuring greater specificity but, on balance, both 1.8 μg/dl (50 nmol/l) and 5 μg/dl (135 nmol/l) offer good diagnostic accuracy (Fig. 2) *(3, 22, 23)*. In keeping with the age-related increase in serum cortisol, older patients may fail to suppress below 1.8 μg/dl *(3)*. These tests should not be used in patients on drugs which alter hepatic dexamethasone clearance, most notably CYP 3A4 enhancers such as phenobarbital, carbamazepine, phenytoin, rifampicin and pioglitazone, or inhibitors, e.g., itraconazole, fluoxetine, diltiazem, cimetidine *(24)*, and women on contraceptives in whom increased synthesis of cortisol-binding globulin leads to higher serum cortisol concentrations *(25)*. Liver or kidney failure may also alter results of suppression tests and yield false results *(21)*.

SECOND TIER TESTS TO EXCLUDE/CONFIRM CUSHING'S SYNDROME

Additional tests (Fig. 1) are available to help distinguish Cushing's syndrome from pseudoCushing's states although none, not even the dexamethasone-suppressed CRH test *(26)*, achieves absolute diagnostic accuracy. These tests are particularly useful for those patients with persistently discordant findings in whom clinical options, e.g., symptomatic treatment, re-evaluation after follow-up, appear unfeasible.

The *dexamethasone-suppressed CRH test* was first proposed in the 1990s *(26)* and is still recommended *(24)* although several more recent studies have shown that diagnostic accuracy and in particular, specificity is far from absolute *(27–31)*. Rationale for this test is the resistance to glucocorticoid negative feedback in patients harboring an ACTH- or cortisol-secreting tumor, who will therefore be able to mount a cortisol response to CRH (100 μg administered 2 h after the last dexamethasone tablet of the Liddle low dose test). Conversely, if cortisol hypersecretion is due to causes other than endocrine tumors then enhancement of glucocorticoid negative feedback will blunt the cortisol response to CRH. One drawback of this test is that the majority of patients with Cushing's syndrome *(1)* will present serum cortisol levels higher than the recommended cut-off (1.4 μg/dl; 38 nmol/l at 15 min after CRH) prior to CRH injection, thereby rendering the administration of this costly drug quite useless. Further, some 35% of patients with pseudoCushing will exceed the established cut-off yielding false-positive responses *(29, 31)*. Raising the diagnostic threshold to 3.98 μg/dl (110 nmol/l) increased specificity without affecting sensitivity and might prove a better criterion *(30, 31)*.

The *desmopressin test* was developed more recently *(32)* and is based on the observation by Malerbi and colleagues that patients with Cushing's disease display an enhanced response to this long-acting vasopressin agonist *(33)* due to an overexpression of the pituitary AVP receptor, the V3 subtype *(34, 35)*, as well as possible extrapituitary mechanisms *(36)*. The authors initially recommended its use in the differential diagnosis of ACTH-dependent Cushing's syndrome, i.e., between pituitary and ectopic ACTH-secreting tumors, but diagnostic accuracy proved too low in larger series *(37)* given the number of extrapituitary neuroendocrine tumors which exhibited an ACTH response. Conversely, desmopressin may help distinguish pituitary Cushing's syndrome from pseudoCushing as the former but not the latter respond to the AVP analogue. In fact, patients with Cushing's disease exhibit a marked ACTH response after 10 μg desmopressin i.v. bolus, and increases by at least 27 pg/ml (6 pmol/l) are a hallmark of pituitary ACTH-secreting adenomas *(32)*. On the contrary, the ACTH/cortisol increase is negligible in patients with pseudoCushing due to alcoholism, obesity or depression *(32, 38–40)*, as well as in normal subjects *(41, 42)*. As with the standard CRH test, not all patients with Cushing's disease respond *(32, 33, 43, 44)*, but false-positive responses among pseudoCushing patients are rare *(38–40)* and, in our hands, this test offers higher specificity than the dexamethasone-suppressed CRH test *(31)*. Contreras and colleagues proposed, along the same line of the dexamethasone-suppressed CRH test, a dexamethasone-.suppressed lysine-vasopressin test (1 mg dexamethasone at midnight followed by 10 UI LVP the following morning) which reportedly achieved excellent specificity and 89% sensitivity for absolute cortisol values >138 nmol/l (5 μg/dl) and incremental cortisol values >166 nmol/l (5 μg/dl) *(45)*.

Insulin-induced hypoglycemia (ITT) was extensively used in the past to diagnose Cushing's syndrome as the hypoglycemic stress obtained with 0.15–0.2 U/kg body weight regular insulin usually evoked a blunted ACTH and cortisol increase in these patients compared with normal subjects *(46)*, depressed *(47)* and obese patients *(48)*.

Other dynamic tests. Patients with Cushing's syndrome exhibit a marked ACTH release after *hexarelin*, the synthetic GH-releasing peptide, injected at 2 μg/kg body weight, an effect also observed in normal subjects but not in obese *(49)* or alcoholic patients *(39)*. Hexarelin appears to act at suprapituitary level, possibly via CRH or other, as yet unknown, hypothalamic mediators *(50)*. Opiates also modulate the HPA axis at hypothalamic or suprahypothalamic level; indeed, *naloxone*, an opiate antagonist (125 μg/kg body weight infused i.v. over 2 minutes), stimulates ACTH release via activation of CRH neurons *(51)*, whereas the opiate agonist *loperamide* (16 mg p.o.) potentiates tonic opiate inhibiton of CRH secretion causing a decrease in cortisol levels *(52)* in normal and obese subjects but not in patients with Cushing's syndrome. None of these tests is currently used for diagnostic purposes.

DEPRESSION

Hyperactivity of the HPA axis is a typical feature of depression and, indeed, there is a large body of evidence attesting to this alteration in both human and experimental models. Changes in HPA secretion reverse upon resolution of depressive symptoms and the bidirectional link between HPA axis and depression is strengthened by the fact that depression is a common occurrence in Cushing's disease. Along this line, adrenal glands are enlarged in depressive patients *(53)* and their size normalizes after successful treatment *(54)*. In the past, the adrenal gland was believed to be an independent contributor to HPA hyperactivity in depression *(55, 56)*, but this mechanism is currently deemed less relevant.

Most studies on HPA hyperactivity in depression focused on CRH as cerebrospinal fluid (CSF) CRH levels are increased in depressed patients *(57, 58)*. Indeed, pharmacological trials – as yet in initial phases – with CRH receptor antagonists have been shown to ameliorate depressive symptoms *(59)*. CRH hypersecretion in depression is believed to result from an imbalance between the two central cortisol receptors, the hippocampal mineralocorticoid receptor (MR) and the hypothalamic glucocorticoid receptor (GR). The former is mainly involved in regulating the HPA axis at trough cortisol levels, for example, during the night, whereas GR is responsible for negative feedback at high cortisol concentrations, e.g., in the morning or during stress. Increased MR activity *(60)* accompanied by reduced GR number or sensitivity *(61, 62)* would lead to increased nocturnal cortisol levels and impaired sensitivity to glucocorticoid feedback, respectively, two hallmarks of HPA dysregulation in depression. Support for the role of MR/GR imbalance was obtained by studies showing changes in MR and GR expression in rats *(63, 65)* and reduced CRH synthesis and secretion in humans *(63, 66)* following antidepressant treatment. Other factors could contribute to CRH hypersecretion, most notably biogenic amines such as norepinephrine *(66)*, or even leptin, which is increased in depressed patients *(67)*. Another determinant of HPA hyperactivity in depression is vasopressin; indeed, the proportion of paraventricular hypothalamic CRH neurons that co-express vasopressin is increased in depressed patients *(68)*; both CRH and vasopressin would then act on the pituitary to stimulate ACTH secretion. ACTH secretion itself is altered in depressed patients, as the pituitary responds less to CRH *(69)*, and the reduced responsiveness appears linked to reduced dexamethasone suppressiveness *(70)*. Indeed, removal of negative glucocorticoid feedback by pretreatment with metyrapone (2 g p.o.) restores the ACTH response to CRH *(71)* and increases evening ACTH levels *(72)*. The importance of HPA hyperactivity in depression is strengthened by the administration of steroid synthesis inhibitors in addition to traditional antidepressants to patients with drug-refractory depression *(73, 74)*.

Depressed patients present elevated serum and urinary cortisol levels *(75–77)*, altered cortisol daily rhythm, especially in patients with psychotic major depression (PMD) *(78, 79)*, and resistance to glucocorticoid negative feedback *(80)*. This latter alteration is closely associated with disease activity and, indeed, a variant of the dexamethasone-suppressed CRH test, using 1.5 mg dexamethasone administered at 11 PM and CRH injected at 3 PM the day after, is routinely used to predict beneficial effects of antidepressant therapy *(81, 82)* as well as susceptibility to depression in healthy relatives of depressed subjects *(83)*. As mentioned above, the ACTH response to insulin-induced hypoglycemia is preserved in depressed patients *(84)*, whereas opiate agonists or antagonists proved of little diagnostic use in this context *(85)*. On the other hand, several antidepressants, such as reboxetin and serotonin-reuptake inhibitors *(86)*, stimulate ACTH and cortisol secretion in the short term and should therefore be avoided during diagnostic procedures. Remission of depression is accompanied by reversal of HPA axis alterations, both as regards basal hormone levels and responsiveness to DEX-CRH test *(82, 87–89)* and repeat testing can therefore aid to distinguish between primary depression and Cushing's syndrome.

ALCOHOLISM

In ethanol-induced pseudoCushing, clinical features are usually more pronounced than those occurring in depressed patients; indeed, some patients present full blown Cushingoid habitus with truncal obesity, facial plethora and peripheral muscle atrophy *(90, 91)*. Conversely, hormonal alterations are less clear cut and depend on the degree of alcohol intake, the duration of alcoholism and any abstinence. Acute, excessive alcohol intake activates CRH and, possibly, AVP neurons *(92, 93)*, leading to increased ACTH and cortisol secretion *(94–96)*. Increased serum cortisol levels are observed with blood ethanol levels >30 mg/dl in naïve subjects and levels greater than 50—150 mg/dl in chronic alcohol consumers *(97)*. Cortisol elevation with the attendant increased negative feedback upon the hypothalamus is followed by a reversible decrease in hypothalamic CRH *(98)* and down-regulation of pituitary CRH receptors *(99)*, which translates into a blunted ACTH response to CRH *(100)* and a reduced ACTH and 11deoxycortisol increase after metyrapone *(90)*. Concurrently, hepatic cortisol activation is enhanced by the increase in 11ßhydroxysteroid dehydrogenase type 1 (11ßHSD1) synthesis and activity *(101)* and, indeed, the urinary cortisol–cortisone metabolite ratio is elevated in alcoholic disease *(102)*.

Drinkers often temporarily interrupt alcohol consumption and undergo abstinence-related stress, associated with increased ACTH and cortisol levels *(91)*. Indeed, high CSF levels can be detected on the first day of alcohol withdrawal *(103)*. Chronic alcoholism is often characterized by an irregular pattern of alcohol consumption and withdrawal and the attendant activity of the HPA axis is equally irregular. Of note, alcoholics are also frequently depressed and malnourished, two conditions that may directly affect the HPA axis.

Serum cortisol levels in the upper normal range or frankly increased are commonly observed in active drinkers *(104, 105)* and cortisol circadian rhythmicity is set at a higher setpoint *(106–108)*. Urinary free cortisol levels are also increased *(90, 107, 109)* and reflect the abovementioned changes in 11ßHSD1 in addition to increased cortisol secretion. Increased dexamethasone hepatic clearance *(110)* may also contribute to the high percentage of non-suppressors after low-dose dexamethasone, up to 40% of alcoholics in some series *(104, 107, 111, 112)*. Alcoholics commonly do not respond to desmopressin nor hexarelin *(39)*. Several alterations in the HPA axis have been reported in children of alcoholic parents *(113)*, suggesting that some HPA disruptive mechanisms may be an inherited trait *(114, 115)*.

Prolonged abstinence, e.g., 2–4 months, usually leads to amelioration of Cushingoid features and laboratory parameters, although normalization may require longer time. Indeed, altered cortisol circadian rhythm, absent suppression after low-dose dexamethasone and after the short variant of the DEX-CRH test as well as absence of response to insulin-induced hypoglycemia are still commonly encountered during short-term abstinence, i.e., within 2–4 months *(91, 116)*.

OBESITY

Excess body weight is associated with a varied pattern of HPA alterations, mostly depending on adipose tissue distribution. In fact, most changes in HPA hormones occur in patients with truncal obesity rather than generalized or peripheral fat accumulation, and abdominal adipose tissue appears to play a pivotal role. Indeed, in contrast to other causes of pseudoCushing, excess cortisol secretion in obesity seems due, to a large extent, to peripheral causes.

Reports of increased UFC levels in obese patients date back to the 1960s *(117)* and are nowadays believed to be partly due to an increased cortisol clearance via the 5alfa reductase pathway *(118)*. Elevated UFC measurements can be detected in 5% of patients with simple obesity *(119, 120)* and are higher in subjects with central compared to peripheral obesity *(121)*. In obese children, UFC secretion should be corrected for body surface area *(122)* keeping in mind that children with Cushing's syndrome have increased body weight but stunted height velocity, whereas height increases together with body weight in children with simple obesity *(123)*. Cortisol secretion is increased in order to compensate for accelerated cortisol clearance and, indeed, the daily cortisol production rate in obese subjects is 36% higher than in normal weight individuals *(124)*. The increased cortisol metabolic clearance may lead to an overdrive of the hypothalamic-pituitary-axis, as documented by the enhanced ACTH/cortisol response to CRH described by some *(125, 126)* though not all *(127, 128)* investigators, and the increased adrenal responsiveness to exogenous ACTH *(129)*. Of note, responses to CRH were linked to measures of central adiposity *(125, 130)* and BMI *(131)*. In addition to these changes, generation of cortisol from cortisone through 11ßHSD1 in the abdominal adipose tissue is enhanced in obese subjects *(132)*, leading to the concept of "Cushing's disease of the omentum" *(133)*. The role of the adipose tissue enzyme as a determinant of abdominal obesity has been elegantly proven by studies on transgenic and knock-out mice *(134, 135)*. Further, 11ßHSD1 expression in omental adipose tissue is positively correlated with BMI and greater in subjects with simple obesity compared with patients with Cushing's syndrome *(136)*. Obesity is also accompanied by excessive insulin secretion *(137)* and hyperinsulinemia has been shown to activate HPA activity *(138, 139)*. Finally, obese women often present polycystic ovaries and hyperandrogenism may have additional, deleterious effects on cortisol secretion. Indeed, androgens increase 5 alfa reductase activity *(140)* and reduce cortisol binding globulin concentrations *(141)*, leading to an increased and deranged ACTH and cortisol circadian pulsatility *(142)*.

Overall, the cortisol daily circadian pattern is maintained in patients with simple obesity, as shown by measurements of serum and salivary midnight cortisol *(3, 17, 143)* and by the limited overlap in evening UFC between patients with Cushing's syndrome and obese subjects *(144)*. As regards dexamethasone suppression tests, false-positive responses are observed in 2–13% of obese patients *(145–147)*. Non-alcoholic hepatic steatosis *(148)* and abdominal obesity *(149)* appear associated with impaired cortisol suppression after dexamethasone. Conversely, the two-day low-dose dexamethasone suppression test yielded a consistent cortisol suppression in the obese pediatric population *(27)*. Regarding second tier tests, obese subjects respond to insulin-induced hypoglycemia, indeed responses are correlated with body weight *(48)*, and, as expected, fail to respond to desmopressin *(40)* and hexarelin *(49)*, thereby qualifying these tests as good means to exclude Cushing's syndrome in obese patients. Finally, it is worth to recall that occult Cushing's syndrome has been reported in a few obese patients seeking bariatric surgery *(150)* or affected by uncontrolled or even newly diagnosed diabetes *(151–154)*, thus careful case-study evaluation is mandatory even in such a high prevalence disease.

CONCLUSION

Patients with pseudoCushing usually present with mild alterations of one or more laboratory test. These patients require through hormonal evaluation and follow-up before the definite diagnosis, before Cushing's syndrome or any condition associated with pseudoCushing, can be safely established. Additional work-up may comprise repeating tests that yielded abnormal results after symptomatic treatment, e.g., antidepressives, weight loss, or other, second-tier tests. None of these procedures achieves absolute diagnostic accuracy and the definite distinction between Cushing's syndrome and pseudoCushing cannot rely on endocrine tests alone but requires skilful clinical judgement.

REFERENCES

1. Newell-Price J, Trainer PJ, Besser GM, Grossman AB. The diagnosis and differential diagnosis of Cushing's syndrome and Pseudo-Cushing's states. Endocrine Rev. 1998;19:647–672.
2. Invitti C, Pecori Giraldi F, De Martin M, Cavagnini F, and the Study Group of the Italian Society of Endocrinology on the Pathophysiology of the Hypothalamic-Pituitary-Adrenal Axis. Diagnosis and management of Cushing's syndrome: results of an Italian multicentre study. J Clin Endocrinol Metab. 1999;84:440–448.
3. Pecori Giraldi F, Ambrogio AG, De Martin M, Fatti LM, Scacchi M, Cavagnini F. Specificity of first-line tests for the diagnosis of Cushing's syndrome: assessment in a large series. J Clin Endocrinol Metab 2007;92:4123–4129.
4. Chan KCA, Lit LCW, Law ELK, Tai MHL, Yung CU, Chan MHM, et al. Diminished urinary free cortisol excretion in patients with moderate and severe renal impairment. Clin Chem 2004;50:757–759.

5. Putignano P, Dubini A, Cavagnini F. Urinary free cortisol is unrelated to physiological changes in urine volume in healthy women. Clin Chem 2000;46:879.
6. Fenske M. Urinary free cortisol and cortisone excretion in healthy individuals: influence of water loading. Steroids 2006;71:1014–1018.
7. Findling JW, Pinkstaff SM, Shaker JL, Raff H, Nelson JC. Pseudohypercortisoluria: spurious elevation of urinary cortisol due to carbamazepine. Endocrinologist 1998;8:51–54.
8. Meikle AW, Findling J, Kushnir MM, Rockwood AL, Nelson GJ, Terry AH. Pseudo-Cushing syndrome caused by fenofibrate interference with urinary cortisol assayed by high-performance liquid chromatography. J Clin Endocrinol Metab 2003;88:3521–3524.
9. Newell-Price J, Trainer PJ, Perry L, Wass JAH, Grossman AB, Besser GM. A single sleeping midnight cortisol has 100% sensitivity for the diagnosis of Cushing's syndrome. Clin Endocrinol 1995;43:545–550.
10. Papanicolaou DA, Yanovski, JA, Cutler GBJr., Chrousos GP, Nieman LK. A single midnight serum cortisol measurement distinguishes Cushing's syndrome from pseudo-Cushing states. J Clin Endocrinol Metab 1998;83:1163–1167.
11. van Cauter E, Leproult R, Kupfer DJ. Effects of gender and age on the levels and circadian rhythmicity of plasma cortisol. J Clin Endocrinol Metab 1996;81:2468–2473.
12. Viardot A, Huber P, Puder JJ, Zulewski H, Keller U, Müller B. Reproducibility of nighttime salivary cortisol and its use in the diagnosis of hypercortisolism compared with urinary free cortisol and overnight dexamethasone suppression test. J Clin Endocrinol Metab 2005;90:5730–5736.
13. Brien TG. Human corticosteroid binding globulin. Clin Endocrinol 1981;14:193–212.
14. Raff H, Raff JL, Findling JW. Late-night salivary cortisol as a screening test for Cushing's syndrome. J Clin Endocrinol Metab 1998;83:2681–2686.
15. Nunes ML, Vattaut S, Corcuff JB, Rault A, Loiseau H, Gatta B, et al. Late-night salivary cortisol for diagnosis of overt and subclinical Cushing's syndrome in hospitalized and ambulatory patients. J Clin Endocrinol Metab 2009;94:456–462.
16. Papanicolaou DA, Mullen N, Kyrou I, Nieman LK. Nighttime salivary cortisol: a useful test for the diagnosis of Cushing's syndrome. J Clin Endocrinol Metab 2002;87:4515–4521.
17. Putignano P, Toja PM, Dubini A, Pecori Giraldi F, Corsello SM, Cavagnini F. Midnight salivary cortisol versus urinary free and midnight cortisol as screening tests for Cushing's syndrome. J Clin Endocrinol Metab 2003;88:4153–4157.
18. Liu H, Bravata DM, Cabaccan J, Raff H, Ryzen E. Elevated late-night salivary cortisol levels in elderly male type 2 diabetic veterans. Clin Endocrinol 2005;63:642–649.
19. Tiong K, Falhammar H. Carbamazepine and falsely positive screening tests for Cushing's syndrome. N Z Med J 2009;122:100–102.
20. Jubiz W, Meikle AW, Levison RA, Mizutani S, West CD, Tyler FH. Effect of diphenylhydantoin on the metabolism of dexamethasone. N Engl J Med 1970;2:11–14.
21. Reimondo G, Pia A, Bovio S, Allasino B, Daffara F, Paccotti P, et al. Laboratory differentiation of Cushing's syndrome. Clin Chim Acta 2008;388:5–14.
22. Wood PJ, Barth JH, Freedman DB, Perry L, Sheridan B. Evidence of the low dose dexamethasone suppression test to screen for Cushing's syndrome - recommendations for a protocol for biochemistry laboratories. Ann Clin Biochem 1997;34:222–229.
23. Fok ACK, Tan KT, Jacob E, Sum CF. Overnight (1 mg) dexamethasone suppression testing reliably distinguishes non-cushingoid obesity from Cushing's syndrome. Steroids 1991;56:549–561.
24. Nieman LK, Biller BMK, Findling JW, Newell-Price J, Savage MO, Stewart PM, et al. Diagnosis of Cushing's syndrome: an Endocrine Society Clinical Practice Guideline. J Clin Endocrinol Metab 2008;93:1526–1540.
25. Coenen CM, Thomas CM, Borm GF, Hollanders JM, Rolland R. Changes in androgens during treatment with four low-dose contraceptives. Contraception 1996;53:171–176.
26. Yanovski JA, Cutler, GBJr, Chrousos GP, Nieman LK. Corticotropin-releasing hormone stimulation following low-dose dexamethasone administration. JAMA 1993;269: 2232–2238.
27. Batista D, Courkoutsakis NA, Riar J, Keil MF, Stratakis CA. Severe obesity confounds the interpretation of low dose dexamethasone test with the administration of ovine corticotrophin releasing hormone in childhood Cushing syndrome. J Clin Endocrinol Metab 2008;93:4323–4330.
28. Erickson D, Natt N, Nippoldt TB, Young WFJr, Carpenter PC, Petterson T, et al. Dexamethasone-suppressed corticotropin-releasing hormone stimulation test for diagnosis of mild hypercortisolism. J Clin Endocrinol Metab 2007;92:2972–2976.
29. Martin NM, Dhillo WS, Banerjee A, Abdulali A, Jayasena CN, Donaldson M, et al. Comparison of the dexamethasone-suppressed corticotrophin-releasing hormone test and low-dose dexamethasone suppression test in the diagnosis of Cushing's syndrome. J Clin Endocrinol Metab 2006;91:2582–2586.

30. Gatta B, Chabre O, Cortet C, Martinie M, Corcuff JB, Roger P, et al. Reevaluation of the combined dexamethasone suppression-corticotropin-releasing hormone test for differentiation of mild Cushing's disease from pseudo-Cushing's syndrome. J Clin Endocrinol Metab 2007;92:4290–4293.
31. Pecori Giraldi F, Pivonello R, Ambrogio AG, De Martino MC, De Martin M, Scacchi M, et al. The dexamethasone-suppressed corticotropin-releasing hormone stimulation test and the desmopressin test to distinguish Cushing's syndrome from pseudo-Cushing's states. Clin Endocrinol 2006;66:251–257.
32. Moro M, Putignano P, Losa M, Invitti C, Maraschini C, Cavagnini F. The desmopressin test in the differential diagnosis between Cushing's disease and pseudoCushing states. J Clin Endocrinol Metab 2000;85:3569–3574.
33. Malerbi DA, Bilharinho de Mendonça B, Liberman B, Toledo SPA, Corradini MCM, Cunha-Neto MB, et al. The desmopressin stimulation test in the differential diagnosis of Cushing's syndrome. Clin Endocrinol 1993;38: 463–472.
34. Dahia PLM, Ahmed-Shuaib A, Jacobs RA, Chew SL, Honegger J, Fahlbusch R, et al. Vasopressin receptor expression and mutation analysis in corticotropin-secreting tumors. J Clin Endocrinol Metab 1996;81:1768–1771.
35. De Keyzer Y, René P, Beldjord C, Lenne F, Bertagna X. Overexpression of vasopressin (V3) and corticotrophin-releasing hormone receptor genes in corticotroph tumours. Clin Endocrinol 1998;49:475–482.
36. Pecori Giraldi F, Marini E, Torchiana E, Mortini P, Dubini A, Cavagnini F. Corticotrophin-releasing activity of desmopressin in Cushing's disease. Lack of correlation between in vivo and in vitro responsiveness. J Endocrinol 2003;177:373–379.
37. Terzolo M, Reimondo G, Alì A, Borretta G, Cesario F, Pia A, et al. The limited value of the desmopressin test in the diagnostic approach to Cushing's syndrome. Clin Endocrinol 2001;54:609–616.
38. Malerbi DA, Villares Fragoso MCB, Vieira Filho AHG, Brenlha EML, Bilharinho de Mendonça B. Cortisol and adrenocorticotropin response to desmopressin in women with Cushing's disease compared with depressive illness. J Clin Endocrinol Metab 1996;81: 2233–2237.
39. Coiro V, Volpi R, Capretti L, Caffarri G, Chiodera P. Desmopressin and hexarelin tests in alcohol-induced pseudo-Cushing's syndrome. J Intern Med 2000;247:667–673.
40. Tsagarakis S, Vasiliou V, Kokkoris P, Stavropoulos G, Thalassinos N. Assessment of cortisol and ACTH responses to the desmopressin test in patients with Cushing's syndrome and simple obesity. Clin Endocrinol 1999;51:473–477.
41. Andersson KE, Arner B, Hedner P, Mulder JL. Effects of 8-lysine-vasopressin and synthetic analogues on release of ACTH. Acta Endocrinol (Copenh) 1972;69:640–648.
42. Gaillard RC, Riondel AM, Ling N, Muller AF. Corticotropin releasing factor activity of CRF-41 in normal man is potentiated by angiotensin II and vasopressin but not by desmopressin. Life Sci 1988;43:1935–1944.
43. Colombo P, Passini E, Re T, Faglia G, Ambrosi B. Effect of desmopressin on ACTH and cortisol secretion in states of ACTH excess. Clin Endocrinol 1997;46:661–668.
44. Sakai Y, Horiba N, Tozawa F, Sakai K, Kuwayama A, Demura H, et al. Desmopressin stimulation test for diagnosis of ACTH-dependent Cushing's syndrome. Endocr J 1997;44: 687–695.
45. Contreras P, Araya V. Overnight dexamethasone pre-treatment improves the performance of the lysine-vasopressin test in the diagnosis of Cushing's syndrome. Clin Endocrinol 1996;44:703–710.
46. Besser GM, Edwards CRW. Cushing's syndrome. Clin Endocrinol Metab 1972;1:451–490.
47. Lopez JF, Kathol RG, Jaeckle RS, Meiler W. The HPA axis response to insulin hypoglycemia in depression. Biol Psychiatry 1987;22:153–166.
48. Weaver JU, Kopelman PG, McLoughlin L, Forsling ML, Grossman AB. Hyperactivity of the hypothalamo pituitary adrenal axis in obesity - a study of ACTH, AVP, beta-lipotrophin and cortisol responses to insulin-induced hypoglycaemia. Clin Endocrinol 1993;39:345–350.
49. Grottoli S, Arvat E, Gauna C, Maccagno B, Ramunni J, Giordano R, et al. Effects of alprazolam, a benzodiazepine, on the ACTH-, GH- and PRL-releasing activity of hexarelin, a synthetic peptidyl GH secretagogue (GHS), in patients with simple obesity and in patients with Cushing's disease. Pituitary 1999;2:197–204.
50. Hickey GJ, Drisko J, Faidley T, Chang C, Anderson LL, Nicolich S, et al. Mediation by the central nervous system is critical to the in vivo activity of the GH secretagogue L-692,585. J Endocrinol 1996;148:371–380.
51. Jackson RV, Hockings GI, Torpy DJ, Grice JE, Crosbie GV, Walters MM, et al. New diagnostic tests for Cushing's syndrome: uses of naloxone, vasopressin and alprazolam. Clin Exp Pharmacol Physiol 1996;23:579–581.
52. Ambrosi B, Bochicchio D, Ferrario R, Colombo P, Faglia G. Effects of the opiate agonist loperamide on pituitary adrenal function in patients with supected hypercortisolism. J Endocrinol Invest 1989;12:31–35.
53. Nemeroff CB, Krishnan KRR, Reed D, Leder R, Beam C, Dunnick NR. Adrenal gland enlargement in major depression. A computed tomographic study. Arch Gen Psychiatry 1992;49:384–387.
54. Rubin RT, Phillips JJ, Sadow TF, McCracken JT. Adrenal gland volume in major depression. Increase during the depressive episode and decrease with successful treatment. Arch Gen Psychiatry 1995;52:213–218.

55. Jaeckle RS, Kathol RG, Lopez JF, Meller WH, Krummel SJ. Enhanced adrenal sensitivity to exogenous cosyntropin (ACTH alfa 1–24) stimulation in major depression. Relationship to dexamethasone suppression test results. Arch Gen Psychiatry 1987;44:233–240.
56. Ehrhart-Bornstein M, Hinson JP, Bornstein SR, Scherbaum WA, Vinson GP. Intraadrenal interactions in the regulation of adrenocortical steroidogenesis. Endocrine Rev 1998;19:101–143.
57. Kling MA, Roy A, Doran AR, Calabrese JR, Rubinow DR, Whitfield HJ, et al. Cerebrospinal fluid immunoreactive corticotropin-releasing hormone and adrenocorticotropin secretion in Cushing's disease and major depression: potential clinical implications. J Clin Endocrinol Metab 1991;72:260–271.
58. Nemeroff CB, Widerlöv E, Bissette G, Walléus H, Karlsson I, Eklund K, et al. Elevated concentrations of CSF corticotropin-releasing factor-like immunoreactivity in depressed patients. Science 1984;226:1342–1344.
59. Zobel AW, Nickel T, Künzel HE, Ackl N, Sonntag A, Ising M, et al. Effects of the high-affinity corticotropin-releasing hormone receptor 1 antagonist R121919 in major depression: in the first 20 patients treated. J Psychiat Res 2000;34:171–181.
60. Young EA, Lopez JF, Murphy-Weinberg V, Watson SJ, Akil H. Mineralcorticoid receptor function in major depression. Arch Gen Psychiatry 2003;60:24–28.
61. Calfa G, Kademian S, Ceschin D, Vega G, Rabinovich GA, Volosin M. Characterization and functional significance of glucocorticoid receptors in patients with major depression: modulation by antidepressant treatment. Psychoneuroendocrinology 2003;28:687–701.
62. Pariante CM, Miller AH. Glucocorticoid receptors in major depression: relevance to pathophysiology and treatment. Biol Psychiatry 2009;49:391–404.
63. Brady LS, Whitfield HJ, Fox RJ, Gold PW, Herkenham M. Long-term antidepressant administration alters corticotropin-releasing hormone, tyrosine hydroxylase, and mineralcorticoid receptor gene expression in rat brain. J Clin Invest 1991;87:831–837.
64. Seckl JR, Fink G. Antidepressants increase glucocorticoid and mineralcorticoid receptor mRNA expression in rat hippocampus in vivo. Neuroendocrinology 1992;55:621–626.
65. Reul JM, Stec I, Soder M, Holsboer F. Chronic treatment of rats with the antidepressant amitriptyline attenuates the activity of the hypothalamic-pituitary-adrenocortical system. Endocrinology 1993;133:312–320.
66. Schüle C. Neuroendocrinological mechanisms of actions of antidepressant drugs. J Neuroendocrinol 2006;19:213–226.
67. Antonijevic IA, Murck H, Frieboes RM, Horn R, Brabant G, Steiger A. Elevated nocturnal profiles of serum leptin in patients with depression. J Psychiat Res 1998;32:403–410.
68. Raadsheer FC, Hoogendijk WJG, Stam FC, Tilders FJH, Swaab DF. Increased numbers of corticotropin-releasing hormone expressing neurons in the hypothalamic paraventricular nucleus of depressed patients. Neuroendocrinology 1994;60:436–444.
69. Gold PW, Loriaux DL, Roy A, Kling MA, Calabrese JR, Kellner CH, et al. (1986) Responses to corticotropin-releasing hormone in the hypercortisolism of depression and Cushing's disease. Pathophysiologic and diagnostic implications. N Engl J Med 1986;314:1329–1335.
70. Krishnan KR, Rayasam K, Reed DR, Smith M, Chappell P, Saunders WB, et al. The corticotropin-releasing factor stimulation test in patients with major depression: relationship to dexamethasone suppression test results. Depression 1993;1:133–136.
71. von Bardeleben U, Stalla GK, Müller OA, Holsboer F. Blunting of ACTH response to human CRH in depressed patients is avoided by metyrapone pretreatment. Biol Psychiatry 1988;24:782–786.
72. Young EA, Haskett RF, Grunhaus L, Pande A, Weinberg MV, Watson SJ, et al. Increased evening activation of the hypothalamic-pituitary-adrenal axis in depressed patients. Arch Gen Psychiatry 1994;51:701–707.
73. Murphy BEP. Antiglucocorticoid therapies in major depression: a review. Psychoneuroendocrinology 1997;22:S125–S132.
74. Kling MA, Coleman VH, Schulkin J. Glucocorticoid inhibition in the treatment of depression: can we think outside the endocrine hypothalamus? Depress Anxiety 2009;doi, 10.1002/da.20546.
75. Young EA, Carlson NE, Brown MB. Twenty-four-hour ACTH and cortisol pulsatility in depressed women. Neuropsychopharmacology 2001;25:267–276.
76. Carroll BJ, Curtis GC, Davies BM, Mendels J, Sugerman AA. Urinary free cortisol excretion in depression. Psychol Med 1976;6:43–50.
77. Anton RF. Urinary free cortisol in psychotic depression. Biol Psychiatry 1987;22:24–34.
78. Keller J, Flores B, Gomez RG, Sovason HB, Kenna H, Williams GH, et al. Cortisol circadian rhythm alterations in psychotic major depression. Biol Psychiatry 2005;60:275–281.
79. Nelson JC, Davis JM. DST studies in psychotic depression: a meta-analysis. Am J Psychiatry 1997;154:1497–1503.

80. Young EA, Haskett RF, Murphy-Weinberg V, Watson SJ, Akil H. Loss of glucocorticoid fast feedback in depression. Arch Gen Psychiatry 1991;48:693–699.
81. Zobel AW, Nickel T, Sonntag A, Uhr M, Holsboer F, Ising M. Cortisol response in the combined dexamethasone/CRH test as predictor of relapse in patients with remitted depression: a prospective study. J Psychiat Res 2001;35:83–94.
82. Appelhof BC, Huyser J, Verweij M, Brouwer JP, van Dyck R, Fliers E, et al. Glucocorticoids and relapse of major depression. Biol Psychiatry 2006;59:696–701.
83. Holsboer F, Lauer CJ, Schreiber W, Krieg JC. Altered hypothamic-pituitary-adrenocortical regulation in healthy subjects at high familial risk for affective disorders. Neuroendocrinology 1995;62:340–347.
84. Kathol RG, Gehris TL, Carroll BT, Samuelson SD, Pitts AF, Meller WH, et al. Blunted ACTH response to hypoglycemic stress in depressed patients but not in patients with schizophrenia. J Psychiat Res 1992;26:103–116.
85. Bernini GP, Argenio GF, Cerri F, Franchi F. Comparison between the suppressive effects of dexamethasone and loperamide on cortisol and ACTH secretion in some pathological conditions. J Endocrinol Invest 1994;17:799–804.
86. Ambrogio AG, Pecori Giraldi F, Cavagnini F. Drugs and the HPA axis. Pituitary 2008;11:219–229.
87. Gibbons L. Cortisol secretion rate in depressive illness. Arch Gen Psychiatry 1964;10: 572–575.
88. Heuser I, Yassouridis A, Holsboer F. The combined dexamethasone/CRH test: a refined laboratory test for psychiatric disorders. J Psychiat Res 1994;28:341–356.
89. Zobel AW, Yassouridis A, Frieboes RM, Holsboer F. Prediction of medium-term outcome by cortisol response to the combined dexamethasone-CRH test in patients with remitted depression. Am J Psychiatry 1999;156:949–951.
90. Wand GS, Dobs AS. Alterations in the hypothalamic-pituitary-adrenal axis in actively drinking alcoholics. J Clin Endocrinol Metab 1991;72:1290–1295.
91. Groote Veldman R, Meinders AE. On the mechanism of alcohol-induced pseudo-Cushing's syndrome. Endocrine Rev 1996;17:262–268.
92. Rivier C. Alcohol stimulates ACTH secretion in the rat: mechanisms of action and interactions with other stimuli. Alcohol Clin Exp Res 1996;20:240–254.
93. Ogilvie K, Lee S, Weiss B, Rivier C. Mechanisms mediating the influence of alcohol on the hypothalamic-pituitary-adrenal axis responses to immune and nonimmune signals. Alcohol Clin Exp Res 1998;22:243S–247S.
94. Ellis F. Effect of ethanol on plasma corticosterone levels. J Pharmacol Exp Ther 1966;153: 121–128.
95. Rivier C, Bruhn T, Vale W. Effect of ethanol on the hypothalamic-pituitary axis in the rat: role of CRH. J Pharmacol Exp Ther 1984;229:127–131.
96. Wand G, Froehlich J. Alterations in hypothalamo-hypophyseal function by ethanol. In: McCleod, R, Müller, EE, eds. Neuroendocrine perspectives., New York: Spinger Verlag, 1990;45–122.
97. Mendelson JH, Ogata M, Mello NK. Adrenal function and alcoholism. I. Serum cortisol. Psychosom Med 1971;33:145–157.
98. Dave JR, Eiden LE, Karanian JW, Eskay RL. Ethanol exposure decreases pituitary corticotropin-releasing factor binding, adenylate cyclase activity, proopiomelanocortin biosyntesis, and plasma beta-endorphin levels in the rat. Endocrinology 1986;118:280–286.
99. Rivier C, Lee S. Acute alcohol administration stimulates the activity of hypothalamic neurons that express corticotropin-releasing factor and vasopressin. Brain Res 1996;726:1–10.
100. Costa A, Bono G, Martignoni E, Merlo P, Sances G, Nappi G. An assessment of hypothalamo-pituitary-adrenal axis functioning in non-depressed, early abstinent alcoholics. Psychoneuroendocrinology 1996;21:263–275.
101. Ahmed A, Saksena S, Sherlock M, Olliff SP, Elias E, Stewart PM. Induction of hepatic 11 -hydroxysteroid dehydrogenase type 1 in patients with alcoholic liver disease. Clin Endocrinol 2008;68:898–903.
102. Stewart PM, Burra P, Shackleton CHL, Sheppard MC, Elias E. 11 hydroxysteroid dehydrogenase deficiency and glucocorticoid status in patients with alcoholic and non-alcoholic chronic liver disease. J Clin Endocrinol Metab 1993;76:748–751.
103. Adinoff B, Anton R, Linnoila M, Guidotti A, Nemeroff CB, Bissette G. Cerebrospinal fluid concentrations of corticotropin-releasing hormone (CRH) and diazepam-binding inhibitor (DBI) during alcohol withdrawal and abstinence. Neuropsychopharmacology 1996;15:288–295.
104. Wilkins JN, Gorelick DA, Nademanee K, Taylor A, Herzberg DS. Hypothalamic-pituitary function during alcohol exposure and withdrawal and cocaine exposure. Recent Dev Alcohol 1992;10:57–71.
105. Berman JD, Cook DM, Buchman M, Keith LD. Diminished adrenocorticotropin response to insulin-induced hypoglycemia in nondepressed, actively drinking male alcoholics. J Clin Endocrinol Metab 1990;71:712–717.
106. Stokes PE. Adrenocortical activation in alcoholics during chronic drinking. Ann NY Acad Sci 1973;215:77–83.
107. Fonzi S, Murialdo G, Bo P, Filippi U, Costelli P, Parodi C, et al. The neuroendocrine aspects of chronic alcoholism: the effect of alcohol intake and its withdrawal. Ann Ital Med Int 1992;7:87–94.

108. Bertello P, Agrimonti F, Gurioli L, Frairia R, Fornaro D, Angeli A. Circadian patterns of plasma cortisol and testosterone in chronic male alcoholics. Alcohol Clin Exp Res 1982;6:475–481.
109. Hasselbach H, Selmer J, Sestoft L, Kehlet H. Hypothalamic-pituitary-adrenocortical function in chronic alcoholism. Clin Endocrinol 1982;16:73–76.
110. Meikle AW. Dexamethasone suppression tests: usefulness of simultaneous measurement of plasma cortisol and dexamethasone. Clin Endocrinol 1982;16:401–408.
111. Kirkman S, Nelson DH. Alcohol-induced pseudo-Cushing's disease: a study of prevalence with review of the literature. Metabolism 1988;37:390–394.
112. Jeffcoate WJ. Alcohol-induced pseudo-Cushing's syndrome. Lancet 1993;341:676–677.
113. Waltman C, McCaul ME, Wand GS. Adrenocorticotropin responses following administration of ethanol and ovine corticotropin-releasing hormone in the sons of alcoholics and control subjects. Alcohol Clin Exp Res 1994;18:826–830.
114. Sher L, Cooper TB, Mann JJ, Oquendo MA. Modified dexamethasone suppression-corticotropin-releasing hormone stimulation test: a pilot study of young healthy volunteers and implications for alcoholism research in adolescents and young adults. Int J Adolesc Med Health 2006;18:133–137.
115. Dai X, Thavundayil J, Santella S, Gianoulakis C. Response of the HPA-axis to alcohol and stress as a function of alcohol dependence and family history of alcoholism. Psychoneuroendocrinology 2007;32:293–305.
116. Ehrenreich H, Schuck J, Stender N, Pilz J, Gefeller O, Schilling L, et al. Endocrine and hemodynamic effects of stress versus systemic CRF in alcoholics during early and medium term abstinence. Alcohol Clin Exp Res 1997;21:1285–1293.
117. Dunkelman SS, Fairhurst B, Plager J, Waterhouse C. Cortisol metabolism in obesity. J Clin Endocrinol Metab 1964;24:832–841.
118. Andrew R, Phillips DIW, Walker BR. Obesity and gender influence cortisol secretion and metabolism in man. J Clin Endocrinol Metab 1998;83:1806–1809.
119. Copinschi G, Cornil A, Leclercq R, Franckson JR. Cortisol secretion rate and urinary corticoid excretion in normal and obese subjects. Acta Endocrinol 1966;51:186–192.
120. Trainer PJ, Grossman AB. The diagnosis and differential diagnosis of Cushing's syndrome. Clin Endocrinol 1991;34:317–330.
121. Pasquali R, Cantorelli S, Casimirri F, Capelli M, Bortoluzzi L, Flamia R, et al. The hypothalamic-pituitary-adrenal axis in obese women with different patterns of body fat distribution. J Clin Endocrinol Metab 1993;77:341–346.
122. Gomez MT, Malozowski S, Winterer J, Vamvakopoulos NC, Chrousos GP. Urinary free cortisol values in normal children and adolescents. J Pediatr 1991;118:256–258.
123. Jones KL. The Cushing syndrome. Pediatr Clin North Am 1990;37:1313–1329.
124. Migeon CJ, Green OC, Eckert JP. Study of adrenocortical function in obesity. Metabolism 1963;12:718–739.
125. Vicennati V, Pasquali R. Abnormalities of the hypothalamic-pituitary-adrenal axis in nondepressed women with abdominal obesity and relations with insulin resistence: evidence for a central and a peripheral alteration. J Clin Endocrinol Metab 2000;85:4093–4098.
126. Lanzone A, Cucinelli F, Fulghesu AM, Caruso A, Guido M, Mancuso S. Somatostatin treatment reduces the exaggerated response of adrenocorticotropin hormone and cortisol to corticotropin- releasing hormone in polycystic ovary syndrome. Fertil Steril 1997;67:34–39.
127. Ljung T, Holm G, Friberg P, Andersson B, Bengtsson BA, Svensson J, et al. The activity of the hypothalamic-pituitary-adrenal axis and the sympathetic nervous system in relation to waist/hip circumference ratio in men. Obes Res 2000;8:487–495.
128. Kopelman PG, Grossman A, Lavender P, Besser GM, Rees LH, Coy D. The cortisol response to corticotrophin-releasing factor is blunted in obesity. Clin Endocrinol 1988;28: 15–18.
129. Luboshitzky R, Ishai A, Shen-Or Z, Herer P. Evaluation of the pituitary-adrenal axis in hyperandrogenic women with polycystic ovary syndrome. Neuro Endocrinol Lett 2003;24: 249–254.
130. Katz JR, Taylor NF, Goodrick S, Perry L, Yudkin JS, Coppack SW. Central obesity, depression and the hypothalamo-pituitary-adrenal axis in men and postmenopausal women. Int J Obes Relat Metab Disord 2000;24:246–251.
131. Ward AMV, Syddall HE, Wood PJ, Dennison EM, Phillips DIW. Central hypothalamic-pituitary-adrenal activity and the metabolic syndrome: studies using the corticotropin-releasing hormone test. Metab›lism 2004;53:720–726.
132. Putignano P, Pecori Giraldi F, Cavagnini F. Tissue-specific dysregulation of 11 -hydroxysteroid dehydrogenase type 1 and pathogenesis of the metabolic syndrome. J Endocrinol Invest 2004;27:969–974.
133. Bujalska IK, Kumar S, Stewart PM. Does central obesity reflect "Cushing's disease of the omentum"? Lancet 1997;349:1210–1213.

134. Masuzaki H, Paterson J, Shinyama H, Morton NM, Mullins JJ, Seckl JR, et al. A transgenic model of visceral obesity and the metabolic syndrome. Science 2001;294:2166–2170.
135. Morton NM, Paterson JM, Masuzaki H, Holmes MC, Staels B, Fievet C, et al. Novel adipose tissue-mediated resistance to diet-induced visceral obesity in 11 beta-hydroxysteroid dehydrogenase type 1-deficient mice. Diabetes 2004;53:931–938.
136. Mariniello B, Ronconi C, Rilli S, Bernante P, Boscaro M, Mantero F, et al. Adipose tissue 11 -hydroxysteroid dehydrogenase type 1 expression in obesity and Cushing's syndrome. Eur J Endocrinol 2006;155:435–441.
137. Ferrannini E, Natali A, Bell P, Cavallo-Perin P, Lalic N, Mingrone G, et al. Insulin resistance and hypersecretion in obesity. J Clin Invest 1997;100:1166–1173.
138. Fruehwald-Schultes B, Kern W, Born J, Fehm HL, Peters A. Hyperinsulinemia causes activation of the hypothalamus-pituitary-adrenal axis in humans. Int J Obes Relat Metab Disord 2001;25:S38–S40.
139. Chan O, Inouye K, Akirav E, Park E, Riddell MC, Vranic M, et al. Insulin alone increases hypothalamo-pituitary-adrenal activity, and diabetes lowers peak stress responses. Endocrinology 2005;146:1382–1390.
140. Stewart PM, Shackleton CH, Beastall GH, Edwards CR. 5 alpha-reductase activity in polycystic ovary syndrome. Lancet 1990;335:431–433.
141. Fernandez-Real JM, Grasa M, Casamitjana R, Pugeat M, Barret C, Ricart W. Plasma total and glycosylated corticosteroid-binding globulin levels are associated with insulin secretion. J Clin Endocrinol Metab 1999;84:3192–3196.
142. Invitti C, Pecori Giraldi F, Dubini A, De Martin M, Cavagnini F. Increased urinary free cortisol and decreased serum corticosteroid-binding globulin in polycystic ovary syndrome. Acta Endocrinol (Copenh) 1991;125:28–32.
143. Pirich K, Vierhapper H. 24-hour serum concentration profile of cortisol in patients with Cushing's disease. Exp Clin Endocrinol 1988;92:275–279.
144. Corcuff JB, Tabarin A, Rashedi M, Duclos M, Roger P, Ducassou D. Overnight urinary free cortisol determination: a screening test for the diagnosis of Cushing's syndrome. Clin Endocrinol 1998;48:503–508.
145. Ness-Abramof R, Nabriski D, Apovian CM, Niven M, Weiss E, Shapito MS, et al. Overnight dexamethasone suppression test: a reliable screen for Cushing's syndrome in the obese. Obes Res 2002;10:1217–1221.
146. Crapo L. Cushing's syndrome: a review of diagnostic tests. Metabolism 1979;28:955–977.
147. Sahin M, Kebapcilar L, Taslipinar A, Azal O, Ozgurtas T, Corakci A, et al. Comparison of 1 mg and 2 mg overnight dexamethasone suppression tests for the screening of Cushing's syndrome in obese patients. Intern Med 2009;48:33–39.
148. Zoppini G, Targher G, Venturi C, Zamboni C, Muggeo M. Relationship of nonalcoholic hepatic steatosis to overnight low-dose dxamethasone suppression test in obese individuals. Clin Endocrinol 2004;61:711–715.
149. Ljung T, Andersson B, Bengtsson BA, Björntorp P, Mårin P. Inhibition of cortisol secretion by dexamethasone in relation to body fat distribution: a dose-response study. Obes Res 1996;4:277–282.
150. Fleseriu M, Ludlam WH, Teh SH, Yedinak CG, Deveney C, Sheppard BC. Cushing's syndrome might be underappreciated in patients seeking bariatric surgery: a plea for screening. Surg Obes Relat Dis 2009;5:116–122.
151. Taniguchi, T., Hamasaki, A., and Okamoto, M. (2008) Subclinical hypercortisolism in hospitalized patients with type 2 diabetes mellitus. Endocr J 55, 429–432.
152. Reimondo G, Pia A, Allasino B, Tassone F, Bovio S, Borretta G, et al. Screening of Cushing's syndrome in adult patients with newly diagnosed diabetes mellitus. Clin Endocrinol 2007;67:225–229.
153. Catargi B, Rigalleau V, Poussin A, Ronci-Chaix N, Bex V, Vergnot V, et al. Occult Cushing's syndrome in type-2 diabetes. J Clin Endocrinol Metab 2003;88:5808–5813.
154. Chiodini I, Torlontano M, Scillitani A, Arosio M, Bacci S, Di Lembo S, et al. Association of subclinical hypercortisolism with type 2 diabetes mellitus: a case-control study in hospitalized patients. Eur J Endocrinol 2005;153:837–844.

7 Laboratorial Diagnosis of Cushing's Syndrome: Differential Diagnosis Among the Different Causes of ACTH-Dependent and ACTH-Independent Cushing's Syndrome

Antonio M. Lerário and Marcello D. Bronstein

Contents

Summary

Once the diagnosis of Cushing's syndrome is established, it is imperative to differentiate among the various possible causes. The first step is to differentiate between adrenocorticotropic hormone (ACTH)-independent and ACTH-dependent causes. This is readily achieved by the determination of ACTH levels by an immunometric assay. Low ACTH levels are suggestive of an adrenal cause, which can be readily identified by abdominal imaging studies. On the other hand, the differential diagnosis of ACTH-dependent Cushing syndrome can be very challenging, as clinical and laboratorial manifestations of Cushing's disease (CD) and ectopic ACTH syndrome (EAS) are usually very similar. In order to differentiate between the two etiologies, many non-invasive dynamic tests have been proposed. Unfortunately, all these tests have limitations. The gold-standard in differentiating CD from EAS is the bilateral inferior petrosal sinus sampling, but this test is laborious and not readily available. The correct diagnosis is achieved by a composite of clinical, laboratorial and imaging studies allied to a precise clinical judgment. The following chapter describes how laboratorial tests can help in differentiating among the many etiologies of Cushing's syndrome. The most used laboratorial tools, its advantages and limitations are briefly presented.

Key Words: Cushing syndrome/diagnosis/etiology, adrenocorticotropic hormone, corticotropin-releasing hormone, deamino arginine vasopressin (desmopressin), dexamethasone suppression test, bilateral inferior petrosal sinus sampling, ectopic ACTH syndrome

From: *Contemporary Endocrinology: Cushing's Syndrome: Pathophysiology, Diagnosis and Treatment*
Edited by: M.D. Bronstein (ed.), DOI 10.1007/978-1-60327-449-4_7,

Table 1
Causes of Endogenous Cushing's syndrome. [Reproduced from *(53)*]

Cause of CS	*% of cases*	*Female-to-male rate*
ACTH-dependent	80%	
Cushing's disease (ACTH-secreting pituitary adenoma)	70%	3.5:1
Ectopic ACTH syndrome	10%	1:1
ACTH-independent (primary adrenal diseases)	20%	
Adrenocortical adenoma	10%	4:1
Adrenocortical carcinoma	5%	1:1
Macronodular hyperplasia (AIMAH)	<2%	1:1
Primary pigmented micronodular hyperplasia (PPNAD)	<2%	1:1
McCune–Albright syndrome	<2%	1:1

INTRODUCTION

Once the laboratorial diagnosis of Cushing's syndrome (CS) has been biochemically established as described on previous chapter, the following step is to differentiate among the various possible causes (Table 1). It should be remarked that all the tests described in this section must be performed only after hypercortisolism is clearly demonstrated. Endogenous CS is caused by an excessive cortisol production by the adrenal glands – either by a primary adrenal disease or secondary to an excessive ACTH stimulation. In the first case, the high levels of cortisol inhibit the corticotroph cells on the anterior lobe of the pituitary, resulting in low circulating levels of ACTH. As a result, CS caused by a primary adrenal disease can be classified as ACTH-independent. On the other hand, ACTH-dependent CS is caused by an abnormal production of ACTH – either "topically," by a pituitary tumor (Cushing's disease), or "ectopically," by a myriad of neuroendocrine tumors from many sites (the ectopic ACTH syndrome), as discussed below. Rarely, ACTH-dependent CS may be caused by eutopic (hypothalamic) or ectopic CRH-producing tumors. In these situations, plasma ACTH levels are either normal or elevated.

The first step in establishing the differential diagnosis of CS is determining whether the hypercortisolism is ACTH-dependent or independent. This is achieved simply by measuring plasma ACTH. The newer immunometric ACTH assays reliably detect concentrations as low as 5 pg/mL. On the contrary, the older radioimmunoassays were not reliable in such low concentrations and consequently, were not accurate enough to distinguish between ACTH dependent and independent causes *(1–3)*. If ACTH levels are consistently <5 pg/mL, the diagnosis of ACTH-independent CS is established. Conversely, ACTH levels >15 pg/mL are consistent with ACTH-dependent CS *(3, 4)*. Intermediate levels can be troublesome, but adrenal causes are easily identified by a CT scan in most of times, except in some rare forms of primary adrenal disease (primary pigmented nodular adrenal disease-PPNAD), in which adrenal glands are normal or only slightly enlarged, as discussed in Chapters 8 and 18. In this situation, other tests may be helpful. One of such tests is the CRH stimulation test. In ACTH-independent CS, normal corticotrophs are usually suppressed by excessive cortisol production. Thus, serum ACTH does not rise in response to exogenous CRH (see CRH test below in the section *dynamic tests*) *(3)*. On the other hand, a rise in ACTH levels in response to exogenous CRH

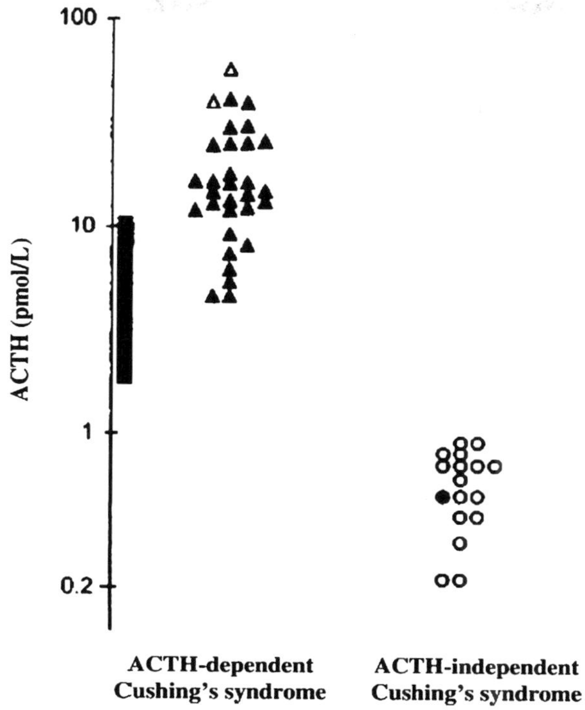

Fig. 1. High accuracy of basal morning plasma ACTH measured by an immunometric assay in distinguishing between ACTH-independent and ACTH-dependent CS. Black triangles: Cushing's disease. White triangle: ectopic ACTH syndrome. White circles: Adrenocortical Adenoma. Black circle: adrenocortical carcinoma. ACTH are plotted in pmol/L. Multiply by 4.5 to convert to pg/mL [reproduced from *(3)*].

is suggestive of an ACTH-dependent etiology. Some care should be taken in collecting blood samples destined to ACTH determination, as it is quickly degraded by plasma proteases. In order to keep the molecules intact until the assay is performed, blood samples should be collected in an EDTA-containing non-glass tube and immediately put on an ice water bath. The sample should be processed in not more than few hours after it is collected (or stored at -40°C for later processing). Otherwise, degradation by plasma proteases will lead lo false low results (Fig. 1).

ACTH-Independent CS

As stated above, if ACTH levels are below 5 pg/mL, the diagnosis of ACTH-independent CS is established. The causes of ACTH-independent CS are listed in Table 1 and discussed in detail elsewhere in other chapters of this book. The following step is to perform an imaging study of the adrenal glands. Either computed tomography or magnetic resonance are very sensitive in identifying adrenal lesions (for a complete discussion about radiologic features of adrenocortical imaging in ACTH-independent CS, see Chapter 8). The presence of high serum levels of androgenic precursors, such as DHEAS, is an important laboratorial tool to differentiate adrenocortical carcinoma from benign adrenal lesions causing CS (hyperplasias and adenomas), which usually are associated to low androgenic levels, although some adenomas may exhibit a mixed hormonal production *(5, 6)*.

ACTH-Dependent CS

In ACTH-dependent CS, the adrenal glands are overstimulated by abnormal amounts of ACTH, leading to cortisol overproduction. The source of ACTH is the pituitary gland in 85–90% of cases (CD) or neuroendocrine tumors elsewhere in the body (ectopic ACTH syndrome – EAS) in the remaining cases. Rarely, ACTH-dependent CS may be caused by CRH-producing tumors. It is imperative to differentiate among these causes, as the therapeutic approach is different. Since both pituitary adenomas and ectopic ACTH producing tumors are often small and difficult to visualize by imaging methods, and the results of such examinations are sometimes unspecific, localization of these tumors relies on biochemical testing to direct the imaging studies to the appropriate sites. A myriad of non-invasive dynamic tests have been developed. Since the pre-test probability for CD is 90%, neither of these tests alone is conclusive. The correct etiologic diagnosis of ACTH-dependent CS is achieved by a composite of biochemical tests and imaging studies, allied to precise clinical judgment. Preferably, this investigation process should be performed with the supervision of an experienced endocrinologist. In doubtful situations, the bilateral inferior petrous sinus sampling (IPSS), an invasive and laborious test, is required. The IPSS is considered the gold standard in the differential diagnosis of ACTH-dependent CS, as will be discussed below.

Although clinical and laboratorial manifestations of CD and EAS are indistinguishable from each other in the majority of cases, there are some clinical and laboratorial clues that make the diagnosis of EAS more likely. Generally, basal ACTH levels tend to be higher in ectopic ACTH syndrome as a group, but there is a considerable overlap between the two entities. One reason for this overlap is that many ectopic ACTH-producing tumors secrete an abnormally processed molecule of ACTH (so called *big ACTH*), due to a defective post-translational processing of proopiomelanocortin (POMC) caused by deficient expression levels of convertases enzymes *(7–10)*. As the primary antibodies of the newer two-site imunnometric assays for ACTH are monoclonal and design to detect specifically the mature molecule (ACTH 1–39), the higher molecular weight molecules associated to EAS may be poorly recognized by the assay, leading to falsely lower levels *(1)*. In this aspect, the older polyclonal assays had a better performance, as the abnormally processed POMC derivates were also detected by the assay *(1)*. Two-site immunometric assays to detect these abnormally processed POMC-derived peptides have been developed *(11)*. It was shown that serum levels of non-processed POMC derivates – POMC itself and pro-ACTH – were able to reliably differentiate CD caused by microadenomas from EAS *(7, 11)*. However, it was later demonstrated that pituitary macroadenomas also exhibited an abnormal processing of POMC and an overlap between CD caused by such tumors and EAS existed *(12, 13)*. Although determination of these peptides was proven to be helpful in the differential diagnosis between CD and EAS, these assays are not currently available in clinical practice.

As a consequence of the generally higher ACTH levels in EAS, hyperpigmentation, psychiatric manifestations, profound muscular weakness and metabolic disarrangements such as diabetes mellitus, hypertriglyceridemia and hypokalemia tend to be more prevalent in this condition. Hypokalemia is usually present in approximately 60% of EAS cases, but in only 10% of CD patients *(14, 15)*. It is present in virtually all patients with high urinary free cortisol levels (>6,000 mcg/24 h) *(15)*. An important characteristic of the neuroendocrine tumors associated to EAS is their ability to secrete various products and peptides, such as gastrin, vasoactive-intestinal peptide (VIP), CA19.9, calcitonin, alpha-fetoprotein, hCG and carcinoembryonic antigen, besides ACTH itself. In a recent series from the St. Bartholomew's Hospital of London, 22 out of 40 patients with hystologically-proven ectopic ACTH syndrome exhibited elevated serum levels of at least one of such peptides. The most commonly elevated tumor marker was calcitonin (3 MTC) and gastrin (1 pancreatic tumor), present in 50% of these patients. Other peptides such as glucagon, somatostatin and urinary 5-HIAA were present in sporadic cases *(16)*. In 25 cases of ectopic ACTH syndrome followed in our institution, elevated levels of gastrin were present in 7 cases, CEA in 6 cases, calcitonin in 3 cases and bHCG and alfa-fetoprotein in one case each *(17)*. Although only a subset of neuroendocrine tumors produces these substances, abnormal serum levels of these peptides make the diagnosis of ectopic ACTH syndrome very likely.

Dynamic Tests

As stated before, the differential diagnosis between CD and ectopic ACTH syndrome relies on a composite of dynamic tests, imaging studies and very often, the IPSS. The main objective of the dynamic tests is to address whether the presumed source of ACTH is the pituitary (Cushing's disease) or an ectopic tumor, and then, direct the efforts to localize such tumors by appropriate imaging methods. In the following section, the most commonly used dynamic tests as well as the rationale behind them will be briefly described (Table 2).

Non-invasive Tests

High-dose Dexamethasone Suppression Test

The high-dose dexamethasone suppression test has been used for many years in the differential diagnosis of ACTH-dependent CS. It was initially proposed to differentiate between ACTH dependent and independent CS, when reliable ACTH assays were not available *(18)*. Early observations suggested that this test had a role in the differential diagnosis of ACTH-dependent Cushing's syndrome, as corticotroph adenomas retained some responsiveness to negative feedback of dexamethasone, while ectopic ACTH-producing tumors did not. The original test is based on 24-h urine collections

Table 2
Dynamic Tests Proposed for Differentiating Between EAS and CD

Test	*Sensitivity*[a] *(%)*	*Specificity* [a] *(%)*	*Expected response in CD*	*Comments*
High-dose dexamethasone suppression test	80	70–90	A 50% fall in serum cortisol levels after oral dexamethasone	Does not improve the pre-test probability for CD
CRH stimulation test	85	94	An ACTH and/or cortisol rise after stimulation	CRH is expensive and unavailable in many countries
Desmopressin stimulation test	84	83	An ACTH and/or cortisol rise after stimulation	Desmopressin is cheap and widespread available; less discriminative than CRH; does not improve the pre-test probability for CD
IPSS	94	100	A central-to-periphery ACTH ratio >2 in basal conditions and >3 after stimulation	Considered the gold-standard; low complication rate; and technically difficult test

[a]For the diagnosis of CD

and determinations of cortisol metabolites (17-OHCS) or cortisol itself, before and after the oral administration of 2 mg dexamethasone each 6 h for 48 h *(18)*. Later on, it has been shown that urinary determinations could be substituted by a morning cortisol serum level, without impairing the test accuracy *(19)*. A simplification of the test consist in giving a single oral 8 mg dexamethasone dose at 11:00 – 12:00 p.m. and collecting a serum level of cortisol at 8:00 – 9:00 a.m. on the previous and following days. A 50% fall in cortisol level after dexamethasone is considered a positive response - suggestive of CD *(20)*. The original 48-h test has a better accuracy but is somewhat cumbersome *(21)*. So, the simplicity of the overnight test justifies its use. Considering the 50% cutoff for morning serum cortisol, the percentage of ectopic ACTH-producing tumors that exhibit a positive response varies from 10–30% (false-positives), and around 20% of corticotroph adenomas are nonresponsive to dexamethasone (false-negatives) *(19, 20, 22, 23)*. That makes the overall performance of the test below the pre-test probability for Cushing's disease. For this reason, the results of this test should be interpreted with care and a therapeutic decision should not be relied solely in its result.

CRH Stimulation Test

Corticotropin-releasing hormone (CRH) is a hormone produced by hypothalamic neurons of the paraventricular nucleus. Physiologically, it is released according to circadian rhythms and also in response to *stress*, such as cold exposure, pain, psychological stress and hypoglycemia. CRH stimulates the production and release of ACTH by the corticotroph cells of the anterior pituitary, through its actions on specific receptors, as discussed on previous chapters. The CRH test is based on the assumption that pituitary corticotroph tumors are responsive to CRH as most of them express CRH receptors, while ectopic ACTH-producing ectopic tumors are not, because they usually do not express CRH receptors. The test consists of giving an intravenous injection of 100 mcg (or 1 mcg/kg) of ovine or human CRH, and assaying ACTH and cortisol at standardized time points. There is no consensus in the literature regarding the time points or criterion for interpreting the results, and variations have been described among different centers. In a large series that included 100 patients with CD and 16 patients with EAS, a rise of 35% in ACTH levels (usually at 15 or 30 min after CRH injection) had a sensitivity and specificity of 93% and 100% for CD, which makes it a useful test in the differential diagnosis of ACTH-dependent CS *(24)*. The cortisol response was less discriminatory, with a sensitivity of 91% and a specificity of 88% for a 20% rise in serum levels after the stimulus *(24)*. However, this study performed the stimulation test with ovine CRH, whose molecule is slightly different from human CRH and leads to a more potent stimulus. Because of this fact, there was a concern about the performance of the test if human CRH were used. An Italian multicenter study addressed this issue by performing the same test with both human and ovine CRH, in 148 patients with CD and 12 with EAS. Adjusting the ACTH cutoff to a 50% rise, the sensitivity was 85% and 87% for ovine and human ACTH respectively. However, the performance of serum cortisol in discriminating CD from EAS was better when ovine CRH was injected (sensitivities of 67% for oCRH and 50% for hCRH) *(25)*. A variant of the CRH test consist of injecting the peptide 2 h following the completion of a low-dose dexamethasone suppression test (the dexamethasone-CRH test). This procedure is useful in differentiating mild cases of CD from pseudo-Cushing states *(26)*. In the original report, the dexamethasone-CRH test was more accurate in differentiating CS from pseudo-Cushing states than the low-dose dexamethasone test or the CRH test alone. A plasma cortisol concentration greater than 1.37 mcg/dL (38 nmol/L) measured 15 min after the administration of CRH correctly identified all cases of Cushing's syndrome and all cases of pseudo-Cushing's states (100% specificity, sensitivity and diagnostic accuracy) *(26)*.

As discussed above, the CRH test is a valuable tool in the differential diagnosis of ACTH-dependent CS. However, some points have to be taken into account. First, hCRH and oCRH are expensive and unavailable in many countries, including Brazil. For this reason, stimulation test with other peptides such as the more available and cheaper desmopressin, were proposed, as will be discussed on the following topic. Second, the sensitivity of the test is almost the same as the pre-test probability for CD, in spite of being rather specific, as shown above. Third, as the experience with the test increases worldwide, there are reports of ectopic ACTH syndrome that respond to CRH stimulation (false-positive cases) *(27)*. It should also be kept in mind that rarer cases of ACTH-dependent CS due to ectopic CRH production may also respond to CRH stimulation test.

Desmopressin Stimulation Test

Desmopressin (DDAVP) is a synthetic peptide, analogous to the natural- occurring vasopressin. It stimulates specifically the V2 and V3 (V1b) isoforms of vasopressin receptors, but does not activate the vascular isoform V1. The DDAVP stimulation test was proposed as an alternative to the CRH stimulation test, due to the availability in most centers and the lower cost of the peptide. The rationale behind this test is that pituitary ACTH producing adenomas overexpress the pituitary-specific V3 (V1b) and the V2 receptors *(28)* while most of the ACTH-producing ectopic tumors do not. The test consists in injecting 10 mcg of DDAVP intravenously and to determine serum ACTH and cortisol concentrations in basal conditions and standardized times. To avoid a possible water overload, the patients should be advised to reduce water intake at the day of the test. In the original report of Malerbi et al., a positive response was observed in 15 out of 16 patients with CD while 8 patients with adrenal tumors and a case of ectopic ACTH syndrome did not respond. The same patients were also stimulated with oCRH and a high degree of concordance was observed *(29)*. Among 15 normal individuals studied, 2 exhibited an ACTH response. These results suggested that DDAVP would be an attractive alternative to the CRH stimulation test, as their accuracy were quite similar *(29)*. However, later studies have shown that the precision of the test was not as good as the original report, as a considerable fraction of ectopic ACTH producing tumors may respond to DDAVP. Subsequently, it was demonstrated that these tumors, mainly lung carcinoids, may express the V2 and V3 receptors, which may cause them to respond to DDAVP *(30–32)*. The combined results from three previously published small series reveal an overall sensitivity and specificity of 84 and 83% for a cortisol rise of 20 and 77% and 73% for an ACTH rise of 35%, as proposed in the original study. In spite of the limited number of patients, these results suggest that the DDAVP stimulation test is less discriminative than the CRH stimulation test in differentiating CD from EAS. In a recent review from our institution, among 13 patients with EAS, a positive response to ACTH and cortisol was observed in 6 and 5 patients, respectively *(17)*. For this reason, the DDAVP stimulation test should be performed only if CRH is not available, keeping in mind all the limitations of the test.

Combined Non-invasive Strategies

As exposed above, all the non-invasive dynamic tests have limitations in discriminating CD from EAS. It has been proposed that combining the results of different tests could be more discriminative than each test alone. One of such proposed combinations is the classical (48 h) high-dose dexamethasone suppression test and the CRH stimulation test. A combined-test strategy requiring a negative cortisol response in the CRH stimulation test plus a cortisol suppression <50% in the dexamethasone test to exclude a diagnosis of Cushing's disease yielded a sensitivity of 98–100% and a specificity of 88–100% *(23, 33)*. Similar results have been obtained when the results of the classical 48 h low-dose dexamethasone suppression test and CRH-stimulation test were associated *(34)*. Thus, the combined-test strategy is thought to have a superior performance than the CRH stimulation test alone, although this observation should be confirmed in larger series. Discordant results between the two tests have been observed more often in CD caused by macroadenomas *(35)*. However, this situation is less problematic, as an image study of the sellar region will reinforce the diagnosis of CD.

To improve the sensitivity of the CRH test in diagnosing CD, a dual stimulation with both hCRH and DDAVP has been proposed. The initial results were promising, as a cutoff for cortisol rise could perfectly discriminate patients with CD and ectopic ACTH syndrome *(36)*. However, these data were not confirmed by other series, and an overlap response between the two conditions remained *(37)*

BILATERAL INFERIOR PETROSAL SINUS SAMPLING

This test is considered the gold-standard in the differential diagnosis of ACTH-dependent CS. The objective of the test is to assess whether or not the source of ACTH is the pituitary. This is achieved by positioning catheters in both inferior petrosal sinuses (which receive tributaries directly from the pituitary circulation) and simultaneously collecting blood samples for ACTH determination from the sinuses and from a peripheral vein. The technical aspects of the test are discussed in details in chapter 9. In order to enhance the sensitivity, blood samples are also collected 2, 5 and 10 min following an intravenous CRH injection *(38)*. A serum ACTH ratio between the petrosal sinuses/peripheral vein greater than 2 in basal condition or greater than 3 after CRH stimulation is consistent with CD. This test is very discriminative, with an overall sensitivity of 94% and a specificity approaching 100%. However, false-negative and false-positive tests have been reported *(39, 40)*. Recent publications have reported a false-negative ratio up to 10% in patients with proven CD *(39, 41–43)*. Failure in diagnosing CD by IPSS has been attributed to many factors, such as technical problems, anomalous venous drainage or bizarre localization of a corticotroph tumor *(43)*. It has been proposed that measures such as to biochemically reassure the hypercortisolemic state and documenting the correct localization of the catheters by a retrograde sinusography should be taken routinely *(40, 44)*. However, false-positive results have been observed even in cases in which these routine measures were performed *(45)*. For this reason, some authors recommend performing a normalization of the ACTH levels by the prolactin levels, in order to correct ACTH values for eventual non-uniform sinus drainage or sampling dilution *(45, 46)*. The IPSS may also be useful in defining the lateralization of a microadenoma within the pituitary. An ACTH gradient between both inferior petrosal sinus >1.4 suggests that the lesion is at the side of the higher value, with an accuracy of 59–83% *(38, 47)*. However, if the left-to-right gradient is reverted after the stimulus, lateralization prediction is not reliable *(48)*. It is important to assess the anatomy of the petrosal sinuses by performing a retrograde sinosography, as non-uniform drainage might lead to erroneous interpretation.

Desmopressin (DDAVP) is also an acceptable alternative in centers where CRH is not available. In a series of 56 patients with ACTH-dependent CS submitted to IPSS in our institution, a positive central-to-periphery gradient was found in 40 in basal conditions and in 47 after the DDAVP stimulation. The test accuracy after DDAVP stimulation was similar to that of CRH stimulation, with a sensitivity of 92.1% and a specificity of 100% *(49)*. In our experience, even in cases which presented no peripheral ACTH or cortisol response in a previous DDAVP test, an increment in ACTH secretion may be documented in the petrosal sinuses after stimulation.

The complication rate of the procedure is reported to be very low *(50, 51)*. The reported complications include transient ear discomfort or pain, groin hematoma, transient and permanent neurologic lesions and one case of pituitary apoplexy *(50–52)*.

Overall, the IPSS is the most accurate test for the differential diagnosis of ACTH-dependent CS, but the procedure is technically difficult and not universally available. Due to its complexity, in our opinion, this test should be reserved for situations in which the diagnosis could not be established based on non-invasive tests and imaging exams – i.e. discordant results of non-invasive dynamic tests and/or absent imaging findings.

FINAL CONSIDERATIONS

The differential diagnosis of endogenous CS can be very challenging, especially among the ACTH-dependent etiologies as no single test is totally reliable and the final diagnosis relies on a composite of many tests. In addition, atypical cases such as cyclic hypercortisolism, (see Chapter 23) bizarre localization of corticotroph tumors and CRH producing tumors, allied to frequently observed unspecific imaging findings can be very tricky. Defining a flowchart for the differential diagnosis of ACTH-dependent CS is not an easy task, and should be individualized not only according to each center expertise but also in an individual basis. For this reason, a correct clinical judgment is essential and these investigations should be performed with the supervision of an experienced endocrinologist whenever possible. In addition, once the diagnosis is established, treatment is also a challenging task, with high failure rates. A possibility for an unsuccessful treatment is an initial misdiagnosis, which is not uncommon even in specialized centers. For this reason, if failure occurs, it is always important to review the diagnosis, as many tests results require interpretation, sometimes based on individual experience.

REFERENCES

1. Raff H, Findling JW. A new immunoradiometric assay for corticotropin evaluated in normal subjects and patients with Cushing's syndrome. Clin Chem 1989;35:596–600.
2. Talbot JA, Kane JW, White A. Analytical and clinical aspects of adrenocorticotrophin determination. Ann Clin Biochem 2003;40:453–471.
3. Klose M, Kofoed-Enevoldsen A, Ostergaard Kristensen L. Single determination of plasma ACTH using an immunoradiometric assay with high detectability differentiates between ACTH-dependent and -independent Cushing's syndrome. Scand J Clin Lab Invest 2002;62:33–37.
4. Newell-Price J, Trainer P, Besser M, Grossman A. The diagnosis and differential diagnosis of Cushing's syndrome and pseudo-Cushing's states. Endocr Rev 1998;19:647–672.
5. Bertagna C, Orth DN. Clinical and laboratory findings and results of therapy in 58 patients with adrenocortical tumors admitted to a single medical center (1951 to 1978). Am J Med 1981;71:855–875.
6. Ng L, Libertino JM. Adrenocortical carcinoma: diagnosis, evaluation and treatment. J Urol 2003;169:5–11.
7. White A, Gibson S. ACTH precursors: biological significance and clinical relevance. Clin Endocrinol (Oxf) 1998;48: 251–255.
8. Stewart MF, Crosby SR, Gibson S, Twentyman PR, White A. Small cell lung cancer cell lines secrete predominantly ACTH precursor peptides not ACTH. Br J Cancer 1989;60:20–24.
9. Stewart PM, Gibson S, Crosby SR, et al. ACTH precursors characterize the ectopic ACTH syndrome. Clin Endocrinol (Oxf) 1994;40:199–204.
10. Crosby SR, Stewart MF, Farrell WE, Gibson S, White A. Comparison of ACTH and ACTH precursor peptides secreted by human pituitary and lung tumour cells in vitro. J Endocrinol 1990;125:147–152.
11. Crosby SR, Stewart MF, Ratcliffe JG, White A. Direct measurement of the precursors of adrenocorticotropin in human plasma by two-site immunoradiometric assay. J Clin Endocrinol Metab 1988;67:1272–1277.
12. Gibson S, Ray DW, Crosby SR, et al. Impaired processing of proopiomelanocortin in corticotroph macroadenomas. J Clin Endocrinol Metab 1996;81:497–502.
13. Raffin-Sanson ML, Massias JF, Dumont C, et al. High plasma proopiomelanocortin in aggressive adrenocorticotropin-secreting tumors. J Clin Endocrinol Metab 1996;81:4272–4277.
14. Howlett TA, Drury PL, Perry L, Doniach I, Rees LH, Besser GM. Diagnosis and management of ACTH-dependent Cushing's syndrome: comparison of the features in ectopic and pituitary ACTH production. Clin Endocrinol (Oxf) 1986;24:699–713.
15. Torpy DJ, Mullen N, Ilias I, Nieman LK. Association of hypertension and hypokalemia with Cushing's syndrome caused by ectopic ACTH secretion: a series of 58 cases. Ann N Y Acad Sci 2002;970:134–144.

16. Isidori AM, Kaltsas GA, Pozza C, et al. The ectopic adrenocorticotropin syndrome: clinical features, diagnosis, management, and long-term follow-up. J Clin Endocrinol Metab 2006;91:371–377.
17. Salgado LR, Fragoso MC, Knoepfelmacher M, et al. Ectopic ACTH syndrome: our experience with 25 cases. Eur J Endocrinol 2006;155:725–733.
18. Liddle GW. Tests of pituitary-adrenal suppressibility in the diagnosis of Cushing's syndrome. J Clin Endocrinol Metab 1960;20:1539–1560.
19. Dichek HL, Nieman LK, Oldfield EH, Pass HI, Malley JD, Cutler GB, Jr. A comparison of the standard high dose dexamethasone suppression test and the overnight 8-mg dexamethasone suppression test for the differential diagnosis of adrenocorticotropin-dependent Cushing's syndrome. J Clin Endocrinol Metab 1994;78:418–422.
20. Tyrrell JB, Findling JW, Aron DC, Fitzgerald PA, Forsham PH. An overnight high-dose dexamethasone suppression test for rapid differential diagnosis of Cushing's syndrome. Ann Intern Med 1986;104:180–186.
21. Bruno OD, Rossi MA, Contreras LN, et al. Nocturnal high-dose dexamethasone suppression test in the aetiological diagnosis of Cushing's syndrome. Acta Endocrinol (Copenh) 1985;109:158–162.
22. Howlett TA, Grossman A, Rees LH, Besser GM. Differential diagnosis of Cushing's syndrome. Lancet 1986;2:871.
23. Nieman LK, Chrousos GP, Oldfield EH, Avgerinos PC, Cutler GB, Jr., Loriaux DL. The ovine corticotropin-releasing hormone stimulation test and the dexamethasone suppression test in the differential diagnosis of Cushing's syndrome. Ann Intern Med 1986;105:862–867.
24. Nieman LK, Oldfield EH, Wesley R, Chrousos GP, Loriaux DL, Cutler GB, Jr. A simplified morning ovine corticotropin-releasing hormone stimulation test for the differential diagnosis of adrenocorticotropin-dependent Cushing's syndrome. J Clin Endocrinol Metab 1993;77:1308–1312.
25. Pecori Giraldi F, Invitti C, Cavagnini F. The corticotropin-releasing hormone test in the diagnosis of ACTH-dependent Cushing's syndrome: a reappraisal. Clin Endocrinol (Oxf) 2001;54:601–607.
26. Yanovski JA, Cutler GB, Jr., Chrousos GP, Nieman LK. Corticotropin-releasing hormone stimulation following low-dose dexamethasone administration. A new test to distinguish Cushing's syndrome from pseudo-Cushing's states. JAMA 1993;269:2232–2238.
27. Suda T, Kageyama K, Nigawara T, Sakihara S. Evaluation of Diagnostic Tests for ACTH-Dependent Cushing's Syndrome. Endocr J 2009;56:469–476.
28. Dahia PL, Grossman AB. The molecular pathogenesis of corticotroph tumors. Endocr Rev 1999;20:136–155.
29. Malerbi DA, Mendonca BB, Liberman B, et al. The desmopressin stimulation test in the differential diagnosis of Cushing's syndrome. Clin Endocrinol (Oxf). 1993;38:463–472.
30. Arlt W, Dahia PL, Callies F, et al. Ectopic ACTH production by a bronchial carcinoid tumour responsive to desmopressin in vivo and in vitro. Clin Endocrinol (Oxf). 1997;47:623–627.
31. Dahia PL, Ahmed-Shuaib A, Jacobs RA, et al. Vasopressin receptor expression and mutation analysis in corticotropin-secreting tumors. J Clin Endocrinol Metab. 1996;81:1768–1771.
32. de Keyzer Y, Lenne F, Auzan C, et al. The pituitary V3 vasopressin receptor and the corticotroph phenotype in ectopic ACTH syndrome. J Clin Invest. 1996;97:1311–1318.
33. Grossman AB, Howlett TA, Perry L, et al. CRF in the differential diagnosis of Cushing's syndrome: a comparison with the dexamethasone suppression test. Clin Endocrinol (Oxf). 1988;29:167–178.
34. Isidori AM, Kaltsas GA, Mohammed S, et al. Discriminatory value of the low-dose dexamethasone suppression test in establishing the diagnosis and differential diagnosis of Cushing's syndrome. J Clin Endocrinol Metab. 2003;88:5299–5306.
35. Woo YS, Isidori AM, Wat WZ, et al. Clinical and biochemical characteristics of adrenocorticotropin-secreting macroadenomas. J Clin Endocrinol Metab. 2005;90:4963–4969.
36. Newell-Price J, Perry L, Medbak S, et al. A combined test using desmopressin and corticotropin-releasing hormone in the differential diagnosis of Cushing's syndrome. J Clin Endocrinol Metab. 1997;82:176–181.
37. Tsagarakis S, Kaskarelis IS, Kokkoris P, Malagari C, Thalassinos N. The application of a combined stimulation with CRH and desmopressin during bilateral inferior petrosal sinus sampling in patients with Cushing's syndrome. Clin Endocrinol (Oxf). 2000;52:355–361.
38. Oldfield EH, Doppman JL, Nieman LK, et al. Petrosal sinus sampling with and without corticotropin-releasing hormone for the differential diagnosis of Cushing's syndrome. N Engl J Med. 1991;325:897–905.
39. Swearingen B, Katznelson L, Miller K, et al. Diagnostic errors after inferior petrosal sinus sampling. J Clin Endocrinol Metab. 2004;89:3752–3763.
40. Yamamoto Y, Davis DH, Nippoldt TB, Young WF, Jr., Huston J, 3rd, Parisi JE. False-positive inferior petrosal sinus sampling in the diagnosis of Cushing's disease. Report of two cases. J Neurosurg. 1995;83:1087–1091.

41. Bonelli FS, Huston J, 3rd, Carpenter PC, Erickson D, Young WF, Jr., Meyer FB. Adrenocorticotropic hormone-dependent Cushing's syndrome: sensitivity and specificity of inferior petrosal sinus sampling. AJNR Am J Neuroradiol. 2000;21:690–696.
42. Lopez J, Barcelo B, Lucas T, et al. Petrosal sinus sampling for diagnosis of Cushing's disease: evidence of false negative results. Clin Endocrinol (Oxf). 1996;45:147–156.
43. Doppman JL, Chang R, Oldfield EH, Chrousos G, Stratakis CA, Nieman LK. The hypoplastic inferior petrosal sinus: a potential source of false-negative results in petrosal sampling for Cushing's disease. J Clin Endocrinol Metab. 1999;84:533–540.
44. McCance DR, McIlrath E, McNeill A, et al. Bilateral inferior petrosal sinus sampling as a routine procedure in ACTH-dependent Cushing's syndrome. Clin Endocrinol (Oxf). 1989;30:157–166.
45. Findling JW, Kehoe ME, Raff H. Identification of patients with Cushing's disease with negative pituitary adrenocorticotropin gradients during inferior petrosal sinus sampling: prolactin as an index of pituitary venous effluent. J Clin Endocrinol Metab. 2004;89:6005–6009.
46. McNally PG, Bolia A, Absalom SR, Falconer-Smith J, Howlett TA. Preliminary observations using endocrine markers of pituitary venous dilution during bilateral simultaneous inferior petrosal sinus catheterization in Cushing's syndrome: is combined CRF and TRH stimulation of value? Clin Endocrinol (Oxf). 1993;39: 681–686.
47. Kaltsas GA, Giannulis MG, Newell-Price JD, et al. A critical analysis of the value of simultaneous inferior petrosal sinus sampling in Cushing's disease and the occult ectopic adrenocorticotropin syndrome. J Clin Endocrinol Metab. 1999;84: 487–492.
48. Miller DL, Doppman JL, Nieman LK, et al. Petrosal sinus sampling: discordant lateralization of ACTH-secreting pituitary microadenomas before and after stimulation with corticotropin-releasing hormone. Radiology. 1990;176: 429–431.
49. Machado MC, de Sa SV, Domenice S, et al. The role of desmopressin in bilateral and simultaneous inferior petrosal sinus sampling for differential diagnosis of ACTH-dependent Cushing's syndrome. Clin Endocrinol (Oxf). 2007;66: 136–142.
50. Miller DL, Doppman JL, Peterman SB, Nieman LK, Oldfield EH, Chang R. Neurologic complications of petrosal sinus sampling. Radiology 1992;185: 143–147.
51. Lefournier V, Gatta B, Martinie M, et al. One transient neurological complication (sixth nerve palsy) in 166 consecutive inferior petrosal sinus samplings for the etiological diagnosis of Cushing's syndrome. J Clin Endocrinol Metab 1999;84:3401–3402.
52. Rotman-Pikielny P, Patronas N, Papanicolaou DA. Pituitary apoplexy induced by corticotrophin-releasing hormone in a patient with Cushing's disease. Clin Endocrinol (Oxf) 2003;58:545–549.
53. Newell-Price J, Bertagna X, Grossman AB, Nieman LK. Cushing's syndrome. Lancet 2006;367:1605–1617.

8 Imaging for the Differential Diagnosis of Cushing's Syndrome: MRI, CT, and Isotopic Scanning

Wouter W. de Herder and Richard A. Feelders

Contents

Summary

In this chapter, the current available radiological (and scintigraphic) techniques used for intra-pituitary tumor localization in the ACTH-dependent CS will be discussed. In general this involves dedicated MRI protocols and sometimes sampling procedures are required. Adrenal imaging in CS can involve CT, MRI and scintigraphic procedures. Several radiological techniques such as CT, MRI, and sampling procedures, but also scintigraphic procedures are useful for localizing the extra-pituitary source of ACTH overproduction in the ectopic ACTH syndrome. Still the (occult) ACTH-producing tumor may sometimes not be revealed.

Key Words: Adrenal, pituitary, MRI, CT, ultrasound, scintigraphy, sampling, Cushing pituitary imaging in the ACTH-dependent Cushing's syndrome

RADIOLOGY IN THE ACTH-DEPENDENT CUSHING'S SYNDROME

MRI

Patients with the adrenocorticotropin (ACTH)-dependent Cushing's syndrome (CS) should eventually all undergo dedicated pituitary magnetic resonance imaging (MRI) *(1–3)*. Corticotroph pituitary adenomas are characteristically hypointense on MRI (Fig. 2a) and fail to enhance following administration

From: *Contemporary Endocrinology: Cushing's Syndrome: Pathophysiology, Diagnosis and Treatment*
Edited by: M.D. Bronstein (ed.), DOI 10.1007/978-1-60327-449-4_8,

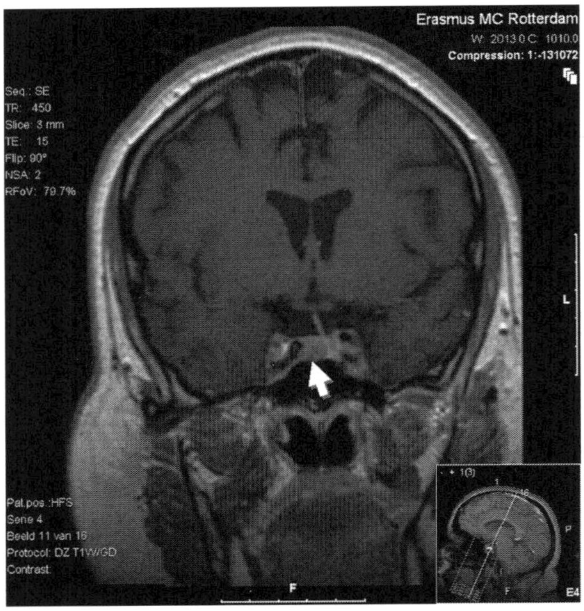

Fig. 1. T1-weighted Gd-DTPA-enhanced image in the coronal plane of a corticotroph pituitary microadenoma (*arrow*) located in the proximity of the internal carotid artery and showing as a hypointense area in a contrast-enhanced pituitary. Also note the deviation of the pituitary stalk to the contralateral (*left*) side.

of gadopentetate dimeglumine (Gd-DPTA) contrast (Figs.1 and 2b). Precontrast scans and Gd-DPTA-enhanced studies always should be performed in conjunction to improve diagnostic accuracy (Fig. 2a, b). The sensitivity of T1-weighted spin echo (SE) pituitary MRI is between 50 and 60% *(4–6)*. False-negative pituitary MRIs may result from small tumor size (picoadenomas – small microadenomas) or signal characteristics and contrast enhancement characteristics of the ACTH-secreting tumor that are similar to normal, surrounding pituitary tissue *(5, 7–11)*. In addition, the specificity of T1-weighted SE MRI is limited, as incidental pituitary lesions (incidentalomas) are present in up to 10% of the normal population *(3, 12–17)*. Therefore, most experts require an inferior petrosal sinus sampling for ACTH for differentiating pituitary from ectopic sources of ACTH (Fig. 7c). It was stated at a recent consensus meeting that pituitary MRI may provide a definitive diagnosis without the need for further invasive testing in the setting of a greater than 6-mm pituitary adenoma with classic clinical and dynamic biochemical results *(1)*.

A recent series evaluated the possibility for improved tumor detection using MRI with 1-mm spoiled gradient recalled acquisition in the steady-state (SPGR) sequences compared with T1-weighted SE MRI *(9)*. This technique has potential benefits, such as faster acquisition, provision of thinner slices, and better soft tissue enhancement *(9, 18)*. Compared with T1-weighted SE MRI for the detection of tumor, SPGR had superior sensitivity (80% versus 49%) but a higher false-positive rate (2% versus 4%). The authors recommend the addition of coronal post-contrast SPGR to conventional SE pituitary imaging protocols to improve MRI detection of ACTH-secreting pituitary tumors. This technique should be used in combination, not alone, however, to minimize false positives *(9)*. In individual cases, T2-weighted MRI images may provide superior results when compared to per- and post-contrast T1-weighted imaging *(3)* (Fig. 2c).

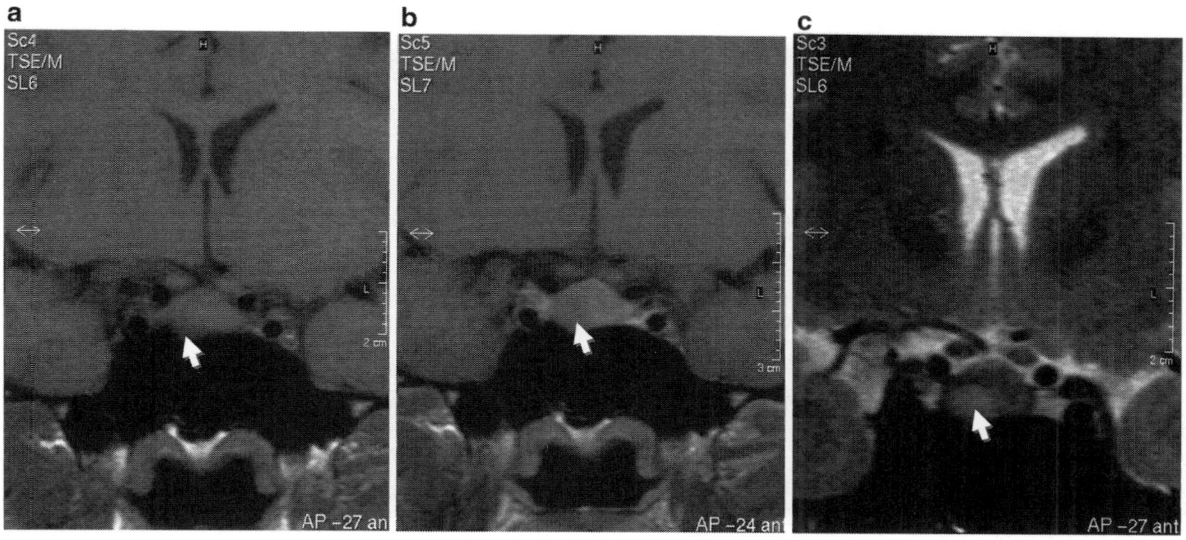

Fig. 2. (**a**) T1-weighted non-enhanced MR image in the coronal plane of a corticotroph pituitary microadenoma (*arrow*) showing as a hypointense area at the right side. (**b**) T1-weighted Gd-DTPA-enhanced MR image in the coronal plane of a corticotroph pituitary microadenoma (*arrow*) showing as a hypointense area at the right side. (same patients as in (**a**)). Visualization is slightly improved as compared to (**a**). (**c**) T2-weighted MR image in the coronal plane of a corticotroph pituitary microadenoma (*arrow*) showing as a hyperintense area at the right side. (same patients as in (**a**) and –(**b**)). Visualization is improved as compared to (**a**) and –(**b**).

SCINTIGRAPHY IN THE ACTH-DEPENDENT CS

Somatostatin Receptor Scintigraphy in Cushing's Disease

^{111}In-pentetreotide SPECT was negative in patients with ACTH-secreting pituitary microadenomas *(19)*. ^{111}In-pentetreotide scintigraphy was positive in patients with ACTH-secreting macroadenomas *(19–21)*. Generally, the somatostatin receptor subtype 2 (sst_2) number is low in corticotroph adenomas because of suppressive effects of high circulating cortisol levels on sst_2 expression, which limits binding of a preferential sst_2 binding radioligand such as ^{111}In-pentetreotide *(22, 23)*.

ADRENAL IMAGING IN CS

On computed tomography (CT) and MRI, the maximum width of the right adrenal limb is 2.8mm and the left adrenal limb is 3.3mm *(24)*. In 15–25% of cases of CS, the cause is a primary adrenocortical neoplasm, usually a benign adenoma *(2)*.

ADRENAL RADIOLOGY IN CS

CT

Thin-section CT or MRI of the adrenal glands is often the final diagnostic test in patients who have ACTH-independent causes of CS *(25, 26)*. Adrenocortical adenomas causing CS are usually larger than 2.0cm in diameter. CT can detect adrenal masses with a diameter more than 5mm. Adrenocortical adenomas in the ACTH-independent CS should, therefore, be easily visualized using CT. However, CT is known to underestimate the size of adrenal tumors *(27)*.

Most adrenocortical adenomas in patients with ACTH-independent CS are rich in lipid content and thus have an attenuation less than 10 Hounsfield units (HU) at non-enhanced CT *(26, 28–34)* (Fig. 3). However, lipid-poor adenomas might have unenhanced CT attenuation values more than 10 HU *(35, 36)*.

Cortisol-producing carcinomas tend to be larger than adenomas at the time of discovery. Usually their diameter is larger than 4cm *(29, 37–41)*. The majority of these carcinomas have irregular margins and contain inhomogeneous areas of necrosis, hemorrhage and calcifications *(34, 37, 42)* (Fig. 4).

In the presence of heterogeneous masses, or a mass of >10 HU, contrast-enhanced CT should be performed. Adenomas may show the same density as normal adrenal tissue on unenhanced CT. On contrast-enhanced CT, they enhance rapidly with intravenous contrast agent and wash it out rapidly *(35, 43–47)*. The absolute contrast washout can be used to distinguish between adenomas (>60% contrast washout) and carcinomas (<40% contrast washout) *(42, 44, 48–52)*. The pattern of enhancement of carcinomas can be inhomogeneous in the presence of central necrosis or hemorrhage *(34, 42, 44, 48–51, 53)*.

Features compatible with an autonomously functioning adrenocortical adenoma include atrophy of the contralateral adrenal gland. In the absence of atrophy of the contralateral adrenal gland or the remaining involved gland, the diagnosis should be reconsidered. If the diagnosis is biochemically affirmed, ACTH-dependent micronodular or macronodular adrenocortical hyperplasia should be considered (Fig. 5). Bilateral micronodular disease, with or without Carney's complex, is suggested by classic clinical and biochemical features *(54)*. In these patients, imaging of the adrenal glands may reveal slightly enlarged glands with or without discernable nodules, but a proportion will have normal-size adrenal glands *(54)*.

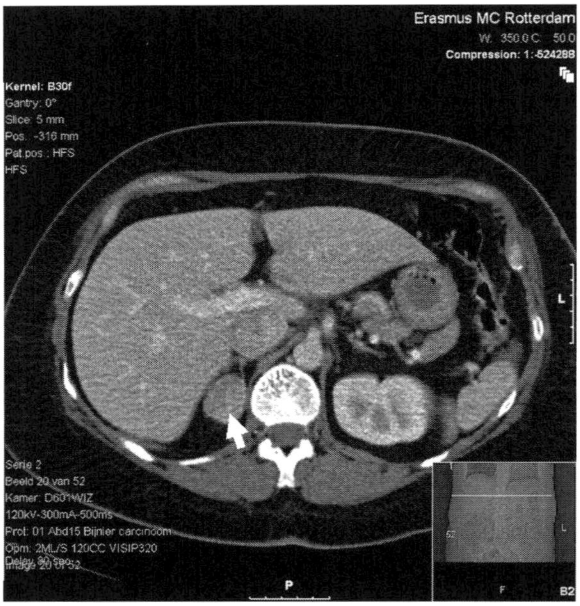

Fig. 3. CT in the transversal plane showing a right-sided adrenal adenoma (diameter: 3 × 4 × 2 cm) causing Cushing's syndrome.

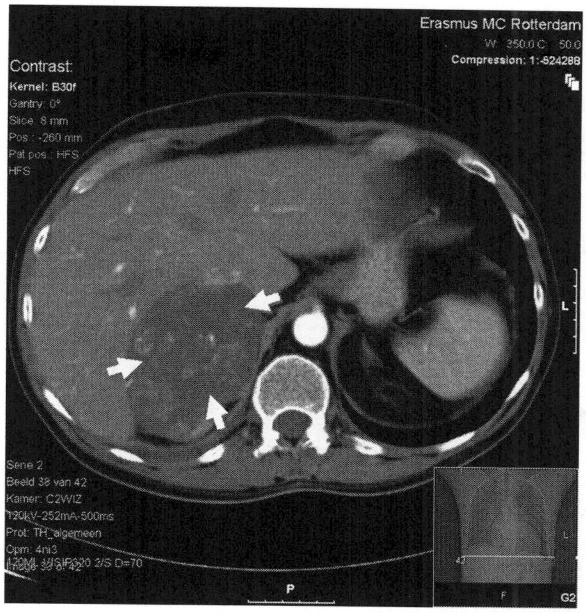

Fig. 4. CT in the transversal plane after the administration of contrast agent showing a right-sided adrenal carcinoma (diameter: 8.5 × 6 × 9 cm) causing Cushing's syndrome. Please note the inhomogeneous aspect at CT.

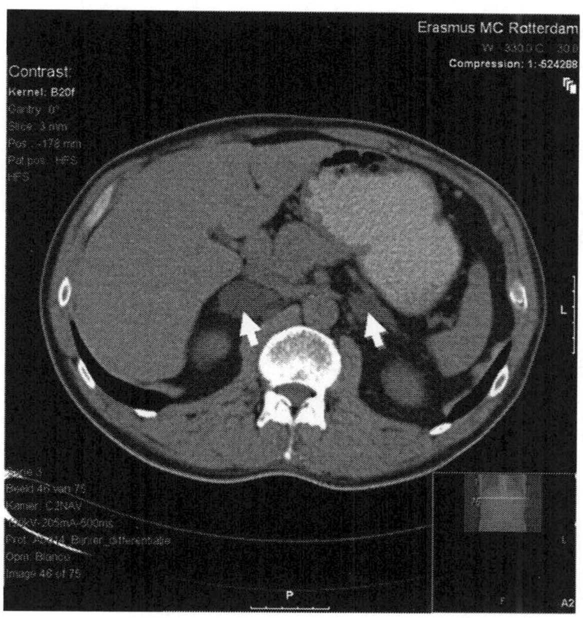

Fig. 5. Non-contrast-enhanced CT in the transversal plane showing bilateral nodular adrenal hyperplasia (*arrows*) in a patient with food-dependent Cushing's syndrome.

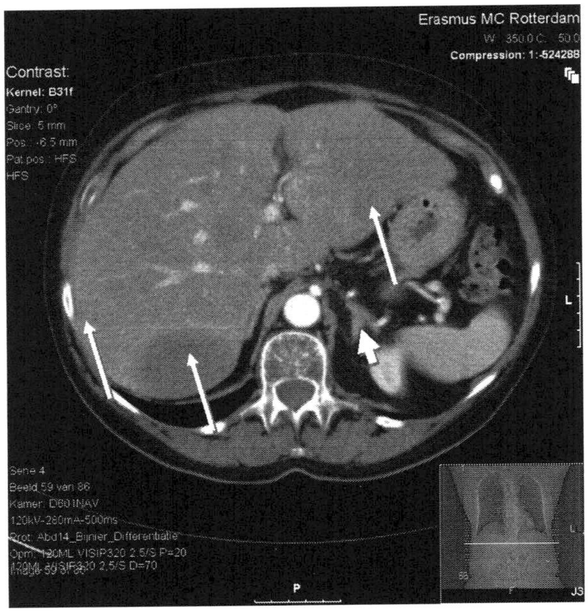

Fig. 6. CT in the transversal plane after the administration of contrast agent showing a left-sided adrenal hyperplasia (*thick arrow*) in a patient with a metastatic neuroendocrine tumor of the lung with liver metastases (*small arrows*) and the ectopic ACTH syndrome.

The adrenal glands are often symmetrically enlarged in patients with ACTH-dependent Cushing syndrome; however, up to 30% of patients will have normal-size adrenal glands *(55)* (Fig. 6).

MRI

Various MR imaging parameters can be used to characterize adrenocortical masses, including T1 and T2 characteristics, enhancement patterns, and chemical shift characteristics *(47, 56–64)*.

On MRI, adenomas appear homogeneous on all sequences. Adenomas have low or equal signal intensity to the liver on T2-weighted images and may appear of lower signal intensity than the rest of the adrenal gland *(29, 34, 42)*. Because of their lipid content, adenomas lose signal on the out-of-phase images with chemical shift imaging. In general, carcinomas contain larger amounts of fluid than adenomas and thus appear bright on T2-weighted images. Heterogeneity is also noted on T2-weighted images because of hemorrhage and/or necrosis. They show intermediate to high signal intensity on T1-weighted images. Adrenocortical carcinomas seem to have no or only partial loss of signal intensity on out-of-phase images with chemical shift imaging *(34, 42, 48, 65–67)*.

Contrast-enhanced CT and MRI studies further enable the assessment of retroperitoneal lymph nodes, vascular extension and thrombosis, and encroachment of adrenal and renal veins, or the inferior vena cava *(42, 48, 65)*.

ADRENAL SCINTIGRAPHY IN CS

Functional Imaging Modalities Specific for Adrenocortical Tumors

[^{131}I]-6-Iodomethyl norcholesterol (NP-59) is a radio-pharmaceutical which is stored in the adrenocortical intracellular lipid droplets after receptor-mediated uptake. Conventional NP-59 examinations are planar, although recently single photon emission computed tomography (SPECT) with NP-59 has been assessed *(68, 69)*. Normal adrenals are visualized at 5 days after injection of NP-59 *(51)*. Unilateral adrenal uptake seen before day 5 suggests a functioning steroid-synthesizing adenoma *(51, 65, 69)*. The minimum size of the adrenocortical mass to be evaluated with NP-59 is more than 2cm. Its practical use is further hampered by limited availability *(51, 65, 69)*.

[^{11}C]-Metomidate is a positron emission tomography (PET) ligand that inhibits the synthesis of adrenocortical steroids via binding with steroidogenic enzymes. It has been assessed in small series of adrenocortical masses, showing indiscriminately high (sometimes irregular) uptake in adenomas and carcinomas and may thus indicate whether an adrenal mass is of adrenocortical or non-adrenocortical (pheochromocytoma, adrenal metastasis) origin *(70–74)*.

Non-specific Functional Imaging Modalities for Adrenocortical Tumors

Fluorine-18 [^{18}F]-deoxyglucose (FDG) PET has been predominantly suggested as a useful tool in the evaluation of non-hyperfunctioning adrenocortical masses. In general, malignant adrenocortical masses show increased uptake of [^{18}F]-FDG because of increased glucose utilization, but benign lesions show no evidence of increased [^{18}F]-FDG uptake *(70, 72, 75–79)*.

IMAGING IN THE ECTOPIC ACTH SYNDROME

Localization of ectopic ACTH-secreting tumors is challenging and primarily relies on CT, MRI, and nuclear medicine imaging. The ectopic ACTH syndrome can develop in patients with already diagnosed, mostly metastatic, mostly neuroendocrine tumors, such as small cell lung cancer, carcinoids of the bronchi and thymus, pancreatic, endocrine tumors (islet cell tumors), medullary thyroid carcinoma, pheochromocytoma, gastrinoma, and prostate cancer with endocrine differentiation *(80–83)*. However, sometimes these tumors cause a diagnostic challenge with regard to their localization and remain occult because of their small size during follow-up. Many of these tumors express somatostatin receptors, and specifically sst_2 on their cell surface, thereby facilitating localization using somatostatin receptor scintigraphy (SRS) *(84)*.

SCINTIGRAPHY IN THE ECTOPIC ACTH SYNDROME

Somatostatin Receptor Scintigraphy and PET

^{111}In-pentetreotide scintigraphy has been successful for the localization of extra-pituitary ACTH- and CRH-secreting tumors and their metastases, especially in those difficult cases in which conventional radiological studies had initially failed to localize the tumors. (Fig. 7a) *(19, 85–98)*. The imaging protocol requires the administration of laxatives from –24h. throughout imaging period, an recommended injected dose of 222MBq (6mCi) and planar imaging and SPECT at 24h p.i. and 48h p.i. and sometimes after 72h *(99)*. Results heavily depend on the imaging protocol. An analysis of recent studies examining the usefulness of SRS in the ectopic ACTH syndrome demonstrated diagnostic sensitivity ranging from 33% to 80% for tumor localization *(92, 95, 100)*. Comparison of these series is not straightforward given variable study design and whether outcomes were based on single or multiple imaging procedures or even on final histological diagnosis *(87, 92, 93, 95, 100, 101)*. Using a range of dosing regimens (6–18mCi), the smallest tumor size detected using SRS was 0.6cm *(87, 95)*. SRS always should be correlated with conventional imaging because of false-positive results observed with thyroid nodes and nodules, inflammation, radiation fibrosis, and accessory spleen *(93, 100)*. There have been a few reports of negative SRS becoming positive, and repeat SRS every 6–12 months should be considered during long-term follow-up in persistent occult disease *(92)*.

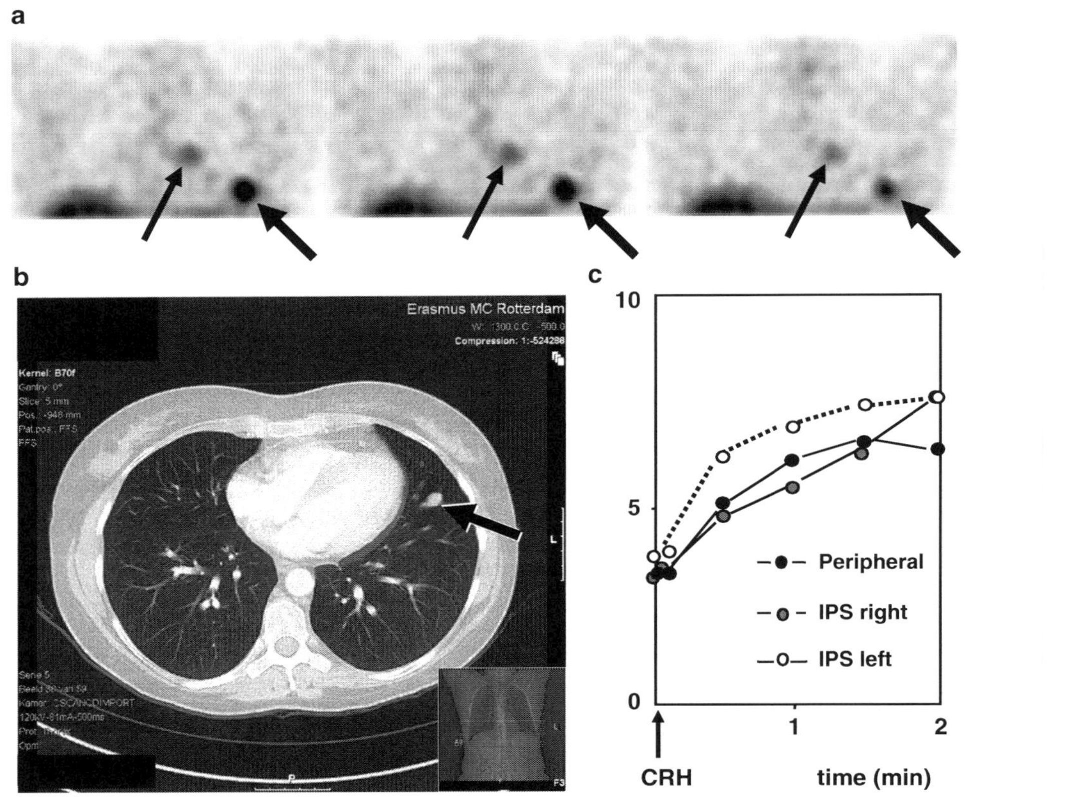

Fig. 7. (**a**) ^{111}In-pentetreotide SPECT in the coronal plane in a patient with the ectopic ACTH syndrome showing an area of intense uptake in the left lung (*thick arrow*) corresponding to a bronchial carcinoid and a central lymph node metastasis (*small arrow*). (**b**) CT scan of the chest in the transversal plane showing the primary bronchial carcinoid in the left lung. (**c**) Results of bilateral inferior petrosal sinus (IPS) sampling for ACTH before and after the administration of CRH, pointing to an ectopic ACTH source. Note the absence of a gradient between central IPS and peripheral ACTH levels and the ACTH response to CRH, which erroneously points to a pituitary source.

In the near future, somatostatin receptor SPECT with ^{111}In-pentetreotide will probably be replaced by PET using ^{68}Ga-labelled tracers, like ^{68}Ga-labelled 1,4,7,10-tetraazacyclododecane-*N*,*N*',*N*'',*N*'''-tetraacetic acid-d-Phe(1)-Tyr(3)-octreotide (^{68}Ga-DOTA-TOC) *(98, 102–104)*. The fast pharmacokinetics and rapid tumor accumulation of this peptide allow for PET studies approximately less than 1 h. after tracer administration. ^{68}Ga is a positron emitter which is easily available and does not need to be produced by an on-site cyclotron. As compared to SPECT, PET produces images with a better spatial resolution and preliminary data show that smaller lesions might be detected with this technique *(104)*.

Currently, the combination of SRS, or PET using ^{68}Ga-labelled somatostatin analogs and conventional CT/MRI probably facilitates the best overall localization in these difficult cases (Fig. 7a–c).

^{18}F-FDG PET

[^{18}F]-FDG PET has been shown to localize ectopic ACTH-secreting tumors in 35% of cases, but failed to identify tumors that were occult on CT/MRI *(95)*. In this series, the sensitivity of CT and combined SRS was higher than that of MRI or [^{18}F]-FDG–PET. This suggests that [^{18}F]-FDG–PET confers no additional benefit for detection of ectopic ACTH-secreting tumors beyond existing modalities *(95, 98, 105)*.

^{18}F-L-DOPA PET and /^{11}C-5-HT PET

Studies with whole-body ^{11}C-5-hydroxy-l-tryptophan (^{11}C-5-HT) PET and ^{18}F-l-dihydroxophenylalanine (^{18}F-l-DOPA) PET show potential additional usefulness for the improved localization of neuroendocrine tumors *(98, 102, 103, 106–108)*. However, the experience with these techniques in the ectopic ACTH syndrome is very limited and until now these techniques were only available in a few centers worldwide.

CONCLUSIONS

Various radiological and scintigraphic techniques for pituitary, adrenal or whole body imaging have also been applied for the localization of pituitary, adrenal or other pathologies in CS.

REFERENCES

1. Arnaldi G, Angeli A, Atkinson AB, Bertagna X, Cavagnini F, Chrousos GP, et al. Diagnosis and complications of Cushing's syndrome: a consensus statement. J Clin Endocrinol Metab 2003;88(12):5593–5602.
2. Kaye TB, Crapo L. The Cushing syndrome: an update on diagnostic tests. Ann Intern Med 1990;112(6):434–444.
3. Bonneville JF, Bonneville F, Barrali E, Jacquet G, Cattin F. Magnetic resonance imaging of the pituitary area: pathologic aspects. In: de Herder WW, editor. Functional and morphological imaging of the endocrine system. Boston: Kluwer Academic Publishers, 2000: 3–34.
4. Boscaro M, Barzon L, Fallo F, Sonino N. Cushing's syndrome. Lancet 2001;357(9258):783–791.
5. Dwyer AJ, Frank JA, Doppman JL, Oldfield EH, Hickey AM, Cutler GB, et al. Pituitary adenomas in patients with Cushing disease: initial experience with Gd-DTPA-enhanced MR imaging. Radiology 1987;163(2):421–426.
6. Doppman JL, Frank JA, Dwyer AJ, Oldfield EH, Miller DL, Nieman LK, et al. Gadolinium DTPA enhanced MR imaging of ACTH-secreting microadenomas of the pituitary gland. J Comput Assist Tomogr 1988;12(5):728–735.
7. Lienhardt A, Grossman AB, Dacie JE, Evanson J, Huebner A, Afshar F, et al. Relative contributions of inferior petrosal sinus sampling and pituitary imaging in the investigation of children and adolescents with ACTH-dependent Cushing's syndrome. J Clin Endocrinol Metab 2001;86(12):5711–5714.
8. Tabarin A, Laurent F, Catargi B, Olivier-Puel F, Lescene R, Berge J, et al. Comparative evaluation of conventional and dynamic magnetic resonance imaging of the pituitary gland for the diagnosis of Cushing's disease. Clin Endocrinol (Oxf) 1998;49(3):293–300.
9. Patronas N, Bulakbasi N, Stratakis CA, Lafferty A, Oldfield EH, Doppman J, et al. Spoiled gradient recalled acquisition in the steady state technique is superior to conventional postcontrast spin echo technique for magnetic resonance imaging detection of adrenocorticotropin-secreting pituitary tumors. J Clin Endocrinol Metab 2003;88(4):1565–1569.
10. Colombo N, Loli P, Vignati F, Scialfa G. MR of corticotropin-secreting pituitary microadenomas. AJNR Am J Neuroradiol 1994;15(8):1591–1595.
11. de Herder WW, Uitterlinden P, Pieterman H, Tanghe HL, Kwekkeboom DJ, Pols HA, et al. Pituitary tumour localization in patients with Cushing's disease by magnetic resonance imaging. Is there a place for petrosal sinus sampling? Clin Endocrinol (Oxf) 1994;40(1):87–92.
12. Elster AD. Imaging of the sella: anatomy and pathology. Semin Ultrasound CT MR 1993;14(3):182–194.
13. Elster AD. Modern imaging of the pituitary. Radiology 1993;187(1):1–14.
14. Elster AD. Sellar susceptibility artifacts: theory and implications. AJNR Am J Neuroradiol 1993;14(1):129–136.
15. Hall WA, Luciano MG, Doppman JL, Patronas NJ, Oldfield EH. Pituitary magnetic resonance imaging in normal human volunteers: occult adenomas in the general population. Ann Intern Med 1994;120(10):817–820.
16. Arnaldi G, Mancini T, Kola B, Appolloni G, Freddi S, Concettoni C, et al. Cyclical Cushing's syndrome in a patient with a bronchial neuroendocrine tumor (typical carcinoid) expressing ghrelin and growth hormone secretagogue receptors. J Clin Endocrinol Metab 2003;88(12):5834–5840.
17. Friedman TC, Zuckerbraun E, Lee ML, Kabil MS, Shahinian H. Dynamic pituitary MRI has high sensitivity and specificity for the diagnosis of mild Cushing's syndrome and should be part of the initial workup. Horm Metab Res 2007; 39(6):451–456.
18. Stadnik T, Stevenaert A, Beckers A, Luypaert R, Buisseret T, Osteaux M. Pituitary microadenomas: diagnosis with two- and three-dimensional MR imaging at 1.5 T before and after injection of gadolinium. Radiology 1990;176(2):419–428.

19. de Herder WW, Kwekkeboom DJ, Reijs AEM, Kooy PPM, Hofland LJ, Krenning EP, et al. Receptor scintigraphy with somatostatin analogues and dopamine antagonists of pituitary tumours. In: Von Werder K, Fahlbusch R, editors. Pituitary adenomas. From basic research to diagnosis and therapy. Amsterdam: Elsevier Science BV, 1996: 93–104.
20. de Herder WW, Lamberts SW. Somatostatin analogs as radiodiagnostic tools. Rev Endocr Metab Disord 2005;6(1): 23–27.
21. de Herder WW, Ferone D, Kwekkeboom DJ, Lamberts SWJ. Scintigraphy of pituitary tumors. In: de Herder WW, editor. Functional and morphological imaging of the endocrine system. Boston: Kluwer Academic Publishers, 2000: 47–58.
22. de Bruin C, Feelders RA, Waaijers AM, van Koetsveld PM, Sprij-Mooij DM, Lamberts SW, et al. Differential regulation of human dopamine D2 and somatostatin receptor subtype expression by glucocorticoids in vitro. J Mol Endocrinol 2009;42(1):47–56.
23. de Bruin C, Pereira AM, Feelders RA, Romijn JA, Roelfsema F, Sprij-Mooij DM, et al. Co-expression of dopamine and somatostatin receptor subtypes in corticotroph adenomas. J Clin Endocrinol Metab 2009;94(4):1118–24.
24. Vincent JM, Morrison ID, Armstrong P, Reznek RH. The size of normal adrenal glands on computed tomography. Clin Radiol 1994;49(7):453–455.
25. Perry RR, Nieman LK, Cutler GB, Jr., Chrousos GP, Loriaux DL, Doppman JL, et al. Primary adrenal causes of Cushing's syndrome. Diagnosis and surgical management. Ann Surg 1989;210(1):59–68.
26. NIH state-of-the-science statement on management of the clinically inapparent adrenal mass ("incidentaloma"). NIH Consens State Sci Statements 2002;19(2):1–25.
27. Fajardo R, Montalvo J, Velazquez D, Arch J, Bezaury P, Gamino R, et al. Correlation between radiologic and pathologic dimensions of adrenal masses. World J Surg 2004;28(5):494–497.
28. Mansmann G, Lau J, Balk E, Rothberg M, Miyachi Y, Bornstein SR. The clinically inapparent adrenal mass: update in diagnosis and management. Endocr Rev 2004;25(2):309–340.
29. Thompson GB, Young WF, Jr. Adrenal incidentaloma. Curr Opin Oncol 2003;15(1):84–90.
30. Korobkin M, Francis IR. Imaging of adrenal masses. Urol Clin North Am 1997;24(3):603–622.
31. Korobkin M. CT characterization of adrenal masses: the time has come. Radiology 2000;217(3):629–632.
32. Hamrahian AH, Ioachimescu AG, Remer EM, Motta-Ramirez G, Bogabathina H, Levin HS, et al. Clinical utility of noncontrast computed tomography attenuation value (hounsfield units) to differentiate adrenal adenomas/hyperplasias from nonadenomas: Cleveland Clinic experience. J Clin Endocrinol Metab 2005;90(2):871–877.
33. Korobkin M, Giordano TJ, Brodeur FJ, Francis IR, Siegelman ES, Quint LE, et al. Adrenal adenomas: relationship between histologic lipid and CT and MR findings. Radiology 1996;200(3):743–747.
34. van Dijk LC, Krestin GP. Imaging of the adrenal glands. In: de Herder WW, editor. Functional and morphological imaging of the endocrine system. Boston: Kluwer Academic Publishers, 2000: 145–162.
35. Korobkin M, Brodeur FJ, Yutzy GG, Francis IR, Quint LE, Dunnick NR, et al. Differentiation of adrenal adenomas from nonadenomas using CT attenuation values. AJR Am J Roentgenol 1996;166(3):531–536.
36. Caoili EM, Korobkin M, Francis IR, Cohan RH, Dunnick NR. Delayed enhanced CT of lipid-poor adrenal adenomas. AJR Am J Roentgenol 2000;175(5):1411–1415.
37. Lockhart ME, Smith JK, Kenney PJ. Imaging of adrenal masses. Eur J Radiol 2002;41(2):95–112.
38. Mantero F, Terzolo M, Arnaldi G, Osella G, Masini AM, Ali A, et al. A survey on adrenal incidentaloma in Italy. Study Group on Adrenal Tumors of the Italian Society of Endocrinology. J Clin Endocrinol Metab 2000;85(2):637–644.
39. Rockall AG, Babar SA, Sohaib SA, Isidori AM, Diaz-Cano S, Monson JP, et al. CT and MR imaging of the adrenal glands in ACTH-independent cushing syndrome. Radiographics 2004;24(2):435–452.
40. Dunnick NR, Korobkin M, Francis I. Adrenal radiology: distinguishing benign from malignant adrenal masses. AJR Am J Roentgenol 1996;167(4):861–867.
41. Lee MJ, Hahn PF, Papanicolaou N, Egglin TK, Saini S, Mueller PR, et al. Benign and malignant adrenal masses: CT distinction with attenuation coefficients, size, and observer analysis. Radiology 1991;179(2):415–418.
42. Ilias I, Sahdev A, Reznek RH, Grossman AB, Pacak K. The optimal imaging of adrenal tumours: a comparison of different methods. Endocr Relat Cancer 2007;14(3):587–599.
43. Dunnick NR, Korobkin M. Imaging of adrenal incidentalomas: current status. AJR Am J Roentgenol 2002;179(3): 559–568.
44. Boland GW, Hahn PF, Pena C, Mueller PR. Adrenal masses: characterization with delayed contrast-enhanced CT. Radiology 1997;202(3):693–696.
45. Boland GW, Lee MJ, Gazelle GS, Halpern EF, McNicholas MM, Mueller PR. Characterization of adrenal masses using unenhanced CT: an analysis of the CT literature. AJR Am J Roentgenol 1998;171(1):201–204.
46. Caoili EM, Korobkin M, Francis IR, Cohan RH, Platt JF, Dunnick NR, et al. Adrenal masses: characterization with combined unenhanced and delayed enhanced CT. Radiology 2002;222(3):629–633.

47. Outwater EK, Siegelman ES, Huang AB, Birnbaum BA. Adrenal masses: correlation between CT attenuation value and chemical shift ratio at MR imaging with in-phase and opposed-phase sequences. Radiology 1996;200(3):749–752.
48. Dunnick NR. CT and MRI of adrenal lesions. Urol Radiol 1988;10(1):12–16.
49. Szolar DH, Schmidt-Kloiber C, Preidler KW. Computed tomography evaluation of adrenal masses. Curr Opin Urol 1999;9(2):143–151.
50. Szolar DH, Korobkin M, Reittner P, Berghold A, Bauernhofer T, Trummer H, et al. Adrenocortical carcinomas and adrenal pheochromocytomas: mass and enhancement loss evaluation at delayed contrast-enhanced CT. Radiology 2005;234(2):479–485.
51. Mayo-Smith WW, Boland GW, Noto RB, Lee MJ. State-of-the-art adrenal imaging. Radiographics 2001;21(4):995–1012.
52. Korobkin M, Brodeur FJ, Francis IR, Quint LE, Dunnick NR, Londy F. CT time-attenuation washout curves of adrenal adenomas and nonadenomas. AJR Am J Roentgenol 1998;170(3):747–752.
53. Slattery JM, Blake MA, Kalra MK, Misdraji J, Sweeney AT, Copeland PM, et al. Adrenocortical carcinoma: contrast washout characteristics on CT. AJR Am J Roentgenol 2006;187(1):W21–W24.
54. Doppman JL, Travis WD, Nieman L, Miller DL, Chrousos GP, Gomez MT, et al. Cushing syndrome due to primary pigmented nodular adrenocortical disease: findings at CT and MR imaging. Radiology 1989;172(2):415–420.
55. Sohaib SA, Hanson JA, Newell-Price JD, Trainer PJ, Monson JP, Grossman AB, et al. CT appearance of the adrenal glands in adrenocorticotrophic hormone-dependent Cushing's syndrome. AJR Am J Roentgenol 1999;172(4): 997–1002.
56. Mayo-Smith WW, Lee MJ, McNicholas MM, Hahn PF, Boland GW, Saini S. Characterization of adrenal masses (< 5 cm) by use of chemical shift MR imaging: observer performance versus quantitative measures. AJR Am J Roentgenol 1995;165(1):91–95.
57. Bilbey JH, McLoughlin RF, Kurkjian PS, Wilkins GE, Chan NH, Schmidt N, et al. MR imaging of adrenal masses: value of chemical-shift imaging for distinguishing adenomas from other tumors. AJR Am J Roentgenol 1995;164(3):637–642.
58. Korobkin M, Lombardi TJ, Aisen AM, Francis IR, Quint LE, Dunnick NR, et al. Characterization of adrenal masses with chemical shift and gadolinium-enhanced MR imaging. Radiology 1995;197(2):411–418.
59. Tsushima Y, Ishizaka H, Matsumoto M. Adrenal masses: differentiation with chemical shift, fast low-angle shot MR imaging. Radiology 1993;186(3):705–709.
60. Mitchell DG, Crovello M, Matteucci T, Petersen RO, Miettinen MM. Benign adrenocortical masses: diagnosis with chemical shift MR imaging. Radiology 1992;185(2):345–351.
61. Reinig JW, Stutley JE, Leonhardt CM, Spicer KM, Margolis M, Caldwell CB. Differentiation of adrenal masses with MR imaging: comparison of techniques. Radiology 1994;192(1):41–46.
62. Ichikawa T, Ohtomo K, Uchiyama G, Fujimoto H, Nasu K. Contrast-enhanced dynamic MRI of adrenal masses: classification of characteristic enhancement patterns. Clin Radiol 1995;50(5):295–300.
63. Lee MJ, Mayo-Smith WW, Hahn PF, Goldberg MA, Boland GW, Saini S, et al. State-of-the-art MR imaging of the adrenal gland. Radiographics 1994;14(5):1015–1029.
64. Semelka RC, Shoenut JP, Lawrence PH, Greenberg HM, Maycher B, Madden TP, et al. Evaluation of adrenal masses with gadolinium enhancement and fat-suppressed MR imaging. J Magn Reson Imaging 1993;3(2):337–343.
65. Lumachi F, Zucchetta P, Marzola MC, Bui F, Casarrubea G, Angelini F, et al. Usefulness of CT scan, MRI and radiocholesterol scintigraphy for adrenal imaging in Cushing's syndrome. Nucl Med Commun 2002;23(5):469–473.
66. Chezmar JL, Robbins SM, Nelson RC, Steinberg HV, Torres WE, Bernardino ME. Adrenal masses: characterization with T1-weighted MR imaging. Radiology 1988;166(2):357–359.
67. Heinz-Peer G, Honigschnabl S, Schneider B, Niederle B, Kaserer K, Lechner G. Characterization of adrenal masses using MR imaging with histopathologic correlation. AJR Am J Roentgenol 1999;173(1):15–22.
68. Imperiale A, Olianti C, Mannelli M, La Cava G, Pupi A. Tomographic evaluation of [131I] 6beta-iodomethyl-norcholesterol standardised uptake trend in clinically silent monolateral and bilateral adrenocortical incidentalomas. Q J Nucl Med Mol Imaging 2005;49(3):287–296.
69. Gross MD, Shapiro B, Shreve P, Shulkin BI. Scintigraphy of adrenal disorders. In: de Herder WW, editor. Functional and morphological imaging of the endocrine system. Boston: Kluwer Academic Publishers, 2000: 163–190.
70. Zettinig G, Mitterhauser M, Wadsak W, Becherer A, Pirich C, Vierhapper H, et al. Positron emission tomography imaging of adrenal masses: (18)F-fluorodeoxyglucose and the 11beta-hydroxylase tracer (11)C-metomidate. Eur J Nucl Med Mol Imaging 2004;31(9):1224–1230.
71. Eriksson B, Orlefors H, Oberg K, Sundin A, Bergstrom M, Langstrom B. Developments in PET for the detection of endocrine tumours. Best Pract Res Clin Endocrinol Metab 2005;19(2):311–324.
72. Gross MD, Avram A, Fig LM, Fanti S, Al Nahhas A, Rubello D. PET in the diagnostic evaluation of adrenal tumors. Q J Nucl Med Mol Imaging 2007;51(3):272–283.

73. Hennings J, Lindhe O, Bergstrom M, Langstrom B, Sundin A, Hellman P. [11C]metomidate positron emission tomography of adrenocortical tumors in correlation with histopathological findings. J Clin Endocrinol Metab 2006;91(4): 1410–1414.
74. Mitterhauser M, Dobrozemsky G, Zettinig G, Wadsak W, Vierhapper H, Dudczak R, et al. Imaging of adrenocortical metastases with [11C]metomidate. Eur J Nucl Med Mol Imaging 2006;33(8):974.
75. Blake MA, Slattery JM, Kalra MK, Halpern EF, Fischman AJ, Mueller PR, et al. Adrenal lesions: characterization with fused PET/CT image in patients with proved or suspected malignancy-initial experience. Radiology 2006;238(3): 970–977.
76. Tenenbaum F, Groussin L, Foehrenbach H, Tissier F, Gouya H, Bertherat J, et al. 18F-fluorodeoxyglucose positron emission tomography as a diagnostic tool for malignancy of adrenocortical tumours? Preliminary results in 13 consecutive patients. Eur J Endocrinol 2004;150(6):789–792.
77. Mackie GC, Shulkin BL, Ribeiro RC, Worden FP, Gauger PG, Mody RJ, et al. Use of [18F]fluorodeoxyglucose positron emission tomography in evaluating locally recurrent and metastatic adrenocortical carcinoma. J Clin Endocrinol Metab 2006;91(7):2665–2671.
78. Leboulleux S, Dromain C, Bonniaud G, Auperin A, Caillou B, Lumbroso J, et al. Diagnostic and prognostic value of 18-fluorodeoxyglucose positron emission tomography in adrenocortical carcinoma: a prospective comparison with computed tomography. J Clin Endocrinol Metab 2006;91(3):920–925.
79. Maurea S, Mainolfi C, Bazzicalupo L, Panico MR, Imparato C, Alfano B, et al. Imaging of adrenal tumors using FDG PET: comparison of benign and malignant lesions. AJR Am J Roentgenol 1999;173(1):25–29.
80. Isidori AM, Kaltsas GA, Grossman AB. Ectopic ACTH syndrome. Front Horm Res 2006;35:143–156.
81. Isidori AM, Kaltsas GA, Pozza C, Frajese V, Newell-Price J, Reznek RH, et al. The ectopic ACTH syndrome: Clinical features, diagnosis, management and long-term follow-up. J Clin Endocrinol Metab 2006;91(2):371–7.
82. Beuschlein F, Hammer GD. Ectopic pro-opiomelanocortin syndrome. Endocrinol Metab Clin North Am 2002;31(1): 191–234.
83. Wajchenberg BL, Mendonca BB, Liberman B, Pereira MA, Carneiro PC, Wakamatsu A, et al. Ectopic adrenocorticotropic hormone syndrome. Endocr Rev 1994;15(6):752–787.
84. Doppman JL, Nieman L, Miller DL, Pass HI, Chang R, Cutler GB, Jret al.., Ectopic adrenocorticotropic hormone syndrome: localization studies in 28 patients. Radiology 1989;172(1):115–124.
85. de Herder WW, Krenning EP, Malchoff CD, Hofland LJ, Reubi JC, Kwekkeboom DJ, et al. Somatostatin receptor scintigraphy: its value in tumor localization in patients with Cushing's syndrome caused by ectopic corticotropin or corticotropin-releasing hormone secretion. Am J Med 1994;96(4):305–312.
86. Weiss M, Yellin A, Husza'r M, Eisenstein Z, Bar-Ziv J, Krausz Y. Localization of adrenocorticotropic hormone-secreting bronchial carcinoid tumor by somatostatin-receptor scintigraphy. Ann Intern Med 1994;121(3):198–199.
87. Phlipponneau M, Nocaudie M, Epelbaum J, de Keyzer Y, Lalau JD, Marchandise X et al. Somatostatin analogs for the localization and preoperative treatment of an adrenocorticotropin-secreting bronchial carcinoid tumor. J Clin Endocrinol Metab 1994;78(1):20–24.
88. Lefebvre H, Jegou S, Leroux P, Dero M, Vaudry H, Kuhn JM. Characterization of the somatostatin receptor subtype in a bronchial carcinoid tumor responsible for Cushing's syndrome. J Clin Endocrinol Metab 1995;80(4):1423–1428
89. Matte J, Roufosse F, Rocmans P, Schoutens A, Jacobovitz D, Mockel J. Ectopic Cushing's syndrome and pulmonary carcinoid tumour identified by [^{111}In-DTPA-D-Phe^{1}]octreotide. Postgrad Med J 1998;74(868):108–110.
90. Tremble JM, Buxton-Thomas M, Hopkins D, Kane P, Bailey D, Harris PE. Cushing's syndrome associated with a chemodectoma and a carcinoid tumour. Clin Endocrinol (Oxf) 2000;52(6):789–793.
91. Bakalakos EA, Cawley K, O'Dorisio TM, Heck C, Schirmer WJ. Localization of ectopic corticotropin-producing carcinoid tumor with use of indium-111 pentetreotide scintigraphy. Endocr Pract 1998;4(6):378–381.
92. Tsagarakis S, Christoforaki M, Giannopoulou H, Rondogianni F, Housianakou I, Malagari C, et al. A reappraisal of the utility of somatostatin receptor scintigraphy in patients with ectopic adrenocorticotropin Cushing's syndrome. J Clin Endocrinol Metab 2003;88(10):4754–4758.
93. Tabarin A, Valli N, Chanson P, Bachelot Y, Rohmer V, Bex-Bachellerie V, et al. Usefulness of somatostatin receptor scintigraphy in patients with occult ectopic adrenocorticotropin syndrome. J Clin Endocrinol Metab 1999;84(4):1193–1202.
94. de Herder WW, Lamberts SW. Octapeptide somatostatin-analogue therapy of Cushing's syndrome. Postgrad Med J 1999;75(880):65–66.
95. Pacak K, Ilias I, Chen CC, Carrasquillo JA, Whatley M, Nieman LK. The role of [(18)F]fluorodeoxyglucose positron emission tomography and [(111)In]-diethylenetriaminepentaacetate-D-Phe-pentetreotide scintigraphy in the localization of ectopic adrenocorticotropin-secreting tumors causing Cushing's syndrome. J Clin Endocrinol Metab 2004;89(5):2214–2221.

96. de Herder WW, Lamberts SW. Is there a role for somatostatin and its analogs in Cushing's syndrome? Metabolism 1996;45(8 Suppl 1):83–85.
97. de Herder WW, Lamberts SW. Tumor localization-the ectopic ACTH syndrome. J Clin Endocrinol Metab 1999;84(4): 1184–1185.
98. Sundin A, Garske U, Orlefors H. Nuclear imaging of neuroendocrine tumours. Best Pract Res Clin Endocrinol Metab 2007;21(1):69–85.
99. Balon HR, Goldsmith SJ, Siegel BA, Silberstein EB, Krenning EP, Lang O, et al. Procedure guideline for somatostatin receptor scintigraphy with (111)In-pentetreotide. J Nucl Med 2001;42(7):1134–1138.
100. Torpy DJ, Chen CC, Mullen N, Doppman JL, Carrasquillo JA, Chrousos GP, et al. Lack of utility of (111)In-pentetreotide scintigraphy in localizing ectopic ACTH producing tumors: follow-up of 18 patients [see comments]. J Clin Endocrinol Metab 1999;84(4):1186–1192.
101. Granberg D, Sundin A, Janson ET, Oberg K, Skogseid B, Westlin JE. Octreoscan in patients with bronchial carcinoid tumours. Clin Endocrinol (Oxf) 2003;59(6):793–799.
102. Haug A, Auernhammer CJ, Wangler B, Tiling R, Schmidt G, Goke B, et al. Intraindividual comparison of (68) Ga-DOTA-TATE and (18)F-DOPA PET in patients with well-differentiated metastatic neuroendocrine tumours. Eur J Nucl Med Mol Imaging, 2009;36(5):765–70.
103. Ambrosini V, Tomassetti P, Castellucci P, Campana D, Montini G, Rubello D, et al. Comparison between 68Ga-DOTA-NOC and 18F-DOPA PET for the detection of gastro-entero-pancreatic and lung neuro-endocrine tumours. Eur J Nucl Med Mol Imaging 2008;35(8):1431–1438.
104. Buchmann I, Henze M, Engelbrecht S, Eisenhut M, Runz A, Schafer M, et al. Comparison of 68Ga-DOTATOC PET and 111In-DTPAOC (Octreoscan) SPECT in patients with neuroendocrine tumours. Eur J Nucl Med Mol Imaging 2007;34(10):1617–1626.
105. Kumar J, Spring M, Carroll PV, Barrington SF, Powrie JK. 18Flurodeoxyglucose positron emission tomography in the localization of ectopic ACTH-secreting neuroendocrine tumours. Clin Endocrinol (Oxf) 2006;64(4):371–374.
106. Orlefors H, Sundin A, Garske U, Juhlin C, Oberg K, Langstrom B, et al. Whole-body ^{11}C-5-hydroxytryptophan positron emission tomography as a universal imaging technique for neuroendocrine tumors - comparison with somatostatin receptor scintigraphy and computed tomography. J Clin Endocrinol Metab 2005;90:3392–3400.
107. Koopmans KP, de Vries EG, Kema IP, Elsinga PH, Neels OC, Sluiter WJ, et al. Staging of carcinoid tumours with 18F-DOPA PET: a prospective, diagnostic accuracy study. Lancet Oncol 2006;7(9):728–734.
108. Koopmans KP, Neels OC, Kema IP, Elsinga PH, Sluiter WJ, Vanghillewe K, et al. Improved staging of patients with carcinoid and islet cell tumors with 18F-dihydroxy-phenyl-alanine and 11C-5-hydroxy-tryptophan positron emission tomography. J Clin Oncol 2008;;26(9):1489–1495.

9 Inferior Petrosal Sampling for the Differential Diagnosis of ACTH-Dependent Cushing's Syndrome

Bradley R. Javorsky, MD and James W. Findling, MD

CONTENTS

SUMMARY

Despite the high pretest probability of a pituitary adenoma in patients with adrenocorticotropic hormone (ACTH)-dependent Cushing's syndrome, a definitive diagnosis is elusive for many patients. Pituitary imaging and biochemical testing have limited diagnostic accuracy. Bilateral simultaneous inferior petrosal sinus ACTH sampling (IPSS) has become the test of choice in the differential evaluation of ACTH-dependent Cushing's syndrome. Administration of corticotropin-releasing hormone further enhances the sensitivity of this test. The use of IPSS for lateralization of corticotroph microadenomas is controversial and has not yet replaced the thorough examination of the pituitary gland by an experienced neurosurgeon after the diagnosis of Cushing's disease has been made. IPSS is feasible and safe in most individuals. It is not, however, without significant risks, costs, and limitations. IPSS should be incorporated into clinical practice in a logical manner to minimize risks and maximize diagnostic utility.

Key Words: Cushing's syndrome, Cushing's disease, adrenocorticotropic hormone, ectopic ACTH syndrome, inferior petrosal sinus sampling, cavernous sinus sampling

From: *Contemporary Endocrinology: Cushing's Syndrome: Pathophysiology, Diagnosis and Treatment*
Edited by: M.D. Bronstein (ed.), DOI 10.1007/978-1-60327-449-4_9,

INTRODUCTION

Since its initial description in 1932, Cushing's syndrome has been plagued by diagnostic uncertainty *(1)*. The protean effects of cortisol excess are commonly the result of neoplasms only a few millimeters in size. These tumors continue to evade even the most sensitive modern imaging tests. Additional diagnostic modalities have therefore been studied. Vascular sampling has long been utilized in the diagnostic evaluation of endocrine syndromes of excess hormone production (e.g. aldosterone secreting adrenal tumors, insulinomas, and parathyroid tumors). Over the past 30 years, bilateral simultaneous inferior petrosal sinus adrenocorticotropic hormone (ACTH) sampling (IPSS) has emerged as the gold standard for the differentiation of pituitary-dependent from non-pituitary ACTH-dependent hypercortisolism.

In the 1970s, the introduction of pituitary microsurgery as a treatment choice for patients with ACTH-secreting pituitary adenomas (Cushing's disease), as well as the recognition that some non-pituitary ACTH-secreting tumors (ectopic ACTH syndrome) were not radiographically identifiable for years after the clinical presentation of hypercortisolism, mandated a precise differential diagnostic test. Historically, clinicians had relied on dexamethasone suppression testing to distinguish these two forms of ACTH-dependent Cushing's syndrome. However, biochemical studies such as high-dose dexamethasone suppression testing and eventually corticotropin-releasing hormone (CRH) stimulation were associated with limited diagnostic accuracy *(2, 3)*.

Since the majority of patients with ACTH-dependent Cushing's syndrome harbor a corticotroph microadenoma (80–90%), radiologic imaging of the pituitary gland has always been an important part of the differential diagnostic investigation. Despite dramatic improvements in the quality of pituitary imaging, from sella polytomography to computed tomography (CT) to magnetic resonance imaging (MRI), approximately 20–50% of patients with pathologically confirmed Cushing's disease do not have tumors seen on even the most sensitive studies *(4)*. Furthermore, non-functioning tumors are visualized on MRI in as many as 10% of the normal population making false-positive results a concern *(5)*.

In light of the high pretest probability of Cushing's disease in patients with ACTH-dependent Cushing's syndrome, and the poor performance of biochemical testing and radiologic imaging, IPSS emerged as the differential diagnostic test of choice. This chapter will highlight the history, technical aspects, interpretation, clinical data, and the potential risks and limitations of this procedure. Recommendations on how and when IPSS should be incorporated into clinical practice will also be made.

HISTORY OF INFERIOR PETROSAL SINUS SAMPLING

The hypothalamic–pituitary–adrenal axis is a tightly regulated and highly conserved system that is essential for normal functioning. Dysregulation of this system with excessive amounts of the end product, the glucocorticoid cortisol, results in the clinical disorder known as Cushing's syndrome. Endogenous hypercortisolism may be the result of excessive production of cortisol from an adrenal neoplasm, or from excessive production of ACTH from the pituitary or ectopic source. Inappropriate or ectopic secretion of CRH as a cause of hypercortisolism is uncommon, but has been described in case reports *(6–8)*.

A case report in 1977 by Corrigan et al. described the use of selective catheterization of bilateral petrosal sinuses to successfully differentiate ectopic ACTH secretion from Cushing's disease *(9)*. In 1981, Findling et al. published a case series of 10 patients who underwent IPSS *(10)*. This study demonstrated the importance of sampling from the petrosal sinus (as opposed to other vascular sites) for the differential diagnosis of ACTH-dependent Cushing's syndrome. It also showed that IPSS was safe and reliable in patients with inconclusive biochemical studies. Many studies have been performed since that time confirming and expanding these findings *(11–23)*.

The addition of CRH stimulation during IPSS has increased the sensitivity and specificity of the test. CRH was isolated and sequenced in 1981 by Vale et al. *(24)*. Orth et al. demonstrated that administration of CRH potently stimulates release of ACTH in normal subjects and patients with Cushing's disease *(25)*. Other factors such as vasopressin, oxytocin, prolactin, GH, TSH, and alpha-subunit are also released *(26–28)*. Muller et al. *(29)* first used CRH administration in the differential diagnosis of Cushing's disease, while Landolt et al. combined CRH with IPSS *(30)*. ACTH is intermittently secreted in Cushing's disease, and in contrast to pituitary adenomas, non-pituitary ACTH-producing tumors respond poorly to CRH administration. For these reasons, ACTH is now sampled several times before and after CRH administration during IPSS.

ANATOMY AND TECHNICAL DETAILS

IPSS should be performed at centers with considerable experience and a dedicated team to ensure proper and safe execution of the study. Diagnostic accuracy is high, and complications are uncommon, in institutions that perform IPSS regularly *(11, 31–34)*.

The anatomy of venous drainage from the human pituitary has been previously described in detail *(35–39)*. Hypophyseal veins exit from the anterior pituitary lobe into the ipsilateral cavernous sinus. The pituitary fossa is surrounded laterally by venous channels known as the cavernous sinuses that drain into the inferior petrosal sinuses (which then drain into the jugular veins) (Fig. 1). The carotid arteries and cranial nerves (III, IV, V1, V2, and VI) course through the cavernous sinuses. Given the drainage patterns of the hypophyseal veins, lateralization of a pituitary adenoma should theoretically be achieved based on measurements of hormone secretion within the inferior petrosal sinuses. However, venous drainage patterns can vary from individual to individual. In one series, 39% of subjects had asymmetric venous drainage *(40)*. Some authors therefore recommend routine venous angiography to help interpret lateralization data *(40)*.

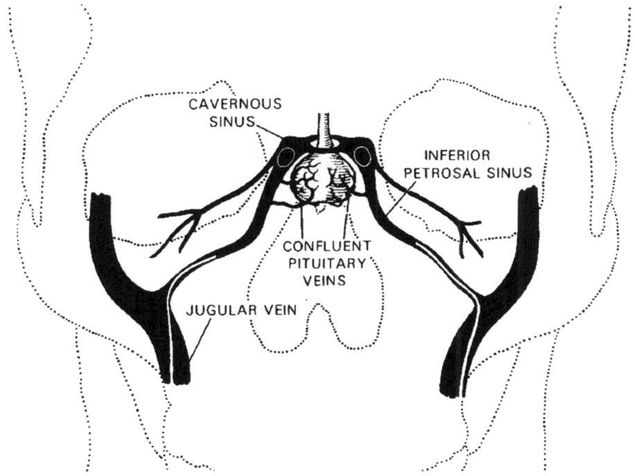

Fig. 1. Catheter placement for bilateral simultaneous blood sampling of the inferior petrosal sinuses. Confluent pituitary veins empty laterally into the cavernous sinuses, which drain into the inferior petrosal sinuses. Used with permission from Ref. *(49)*, Copyright 1985, Massachusetts Medical Society, all rights reserved.

A percutaneous bilateral femoral approach is used. To sample the inferior petrosal sinuses, a pre-shaped 5-French catheter is directed anteromedially in the internal jugular vein. To prevent the risk of cavernous sinus thrombosis, the catheter should not be advanced too deeply into the petrosal sinus. In addition, patients should be routinely heparinized prior to the procedure. Conscious sedation should be used (rather than general anesthesia) so that symptoms can be monitored to avoid adverse effects. Digital subtraction angiography should be performed to establish correct catheter positioning and assess for abnormal venous anatomy. Blood is withdrawn simultaneously from both catheters and a peripheral vein (superior vena cava) for hormonal assays. Bilateral sampling should be performed since small pituitary adenomas may drain unilaterally into the cavernous sinus. Thus, false-negative studies are possible when done unilaterally. Although controversial, bilateral sampling may also provide a modest improvement in the ability to predict lateralization of the tumor.

Samples are collected for ACTH and prolactin at two baseline time points (–5 and 0 min) and then at 3, 5, and 10 min after intravenous administration of 1 μg/kg or 100 μg CRH. A final peripheral venous blood sample is also obtained at 30 min. Proper collection of ACTH is essential. It should be collected in chilled tubes containing EDTA, centrifuged to separate plasma within 45 min, and stored at –20°C until the assay is performed. Prolactin samples are stored and measured when results are equivocal or there is a question of atypical venous anatomy. Contrast medium is administered again at the end of the study to confirm stable and appropriate positioning of the catheters throughout the sampling procedure. A retrograde flux of contrast to the contralateral cavernous sinus should be seen. The length of the procedure is generally 1–2 h and the patient is discharged the same day. In our institution, patients are asked to collect a midnight salivary cortisol sample the night prior to IPSS. This can be used to confirm periprocedural hypercortisolism should the results be perplexing.

INTERPRETATION OF IPSS DATA

Petrosal sinus to peripheral (IPS:P) ACTH ratios ≥2.0 at baseline *or* a peak ≥3.0 after CRH administration (at any of the time points) are diagnostic of Cushing's disease (Table 1). By convention, tests that meet these criteria are called positive tests.

The false-negative rate for IPSS is 1–10% *(13, 15, 23, 41)*. Anomalous venous drainage may be responsible for these diagnostic errors *(13, 40)*. For these patients, it may take years before the diagnosis of Cushing's disease is made, resulting in unnecessary morbidity *(41, 42)*. In situations where

Table 1
Interpretation of IPSS Results for the Differential Diagnosis of Cushing's Syndrome. Inferior Petrosal Sinus to Peripheral Ratio (IPS:P)

Cushing's disease is confirmed if:
Baseline IPS:P ACTH ratio (any baseline value, either side) ≥2
OR
CRH stimulated IPS:P ACTH ratio (any post administration value, either side) ≥3
If results suggest ectopic ACTH syndrome, evaluate for false negative by normalizing IPS:P ACTH ratio to IPS:P prolactin ratio:
Normalized ACTH/prolactin IPS:P ratio= (Dominant peak post-CRH IPS:P ACTH ratio)/(Ipsilateral basal IPS:P prolactin ratio)
>0.8 → indicative of Cushing's disease
<0.6 → indicative of ectopic ACTH syndrome

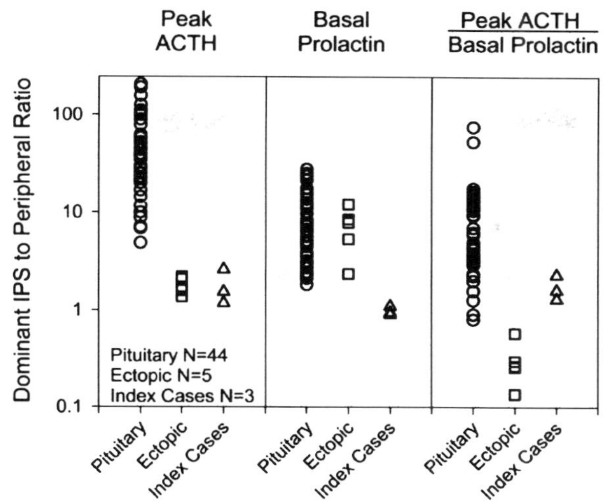

Fig. 2. IPS:P ratios for patients with proven Cushing's disease (pituitary; circles), ectopic ACTH syndrome (ectopic; squares), and the three index cases (triangles). The left panel is the post-CRH IPS to peripheral ACTH ratio. The middle panel is the basal (pre-CRH) IPS to peripheral prolactin ratio from the same sites as the ACTH ratios. The right panel is the left panel divided by the middle panel giving IPS:P ratios normalized to the ipsilateral prolactin ratio. Notice the overlap of the IPS–peripheral ACTH ratio for the ectopic ACTH and index cases, that the index cases had IPS–peripheral prolactin ratios that were lower than in pituitary and ectopic ACTH, and that normalizing the peak ACTH IPS:P ratio to the ipsilateral prolactin ratio led to results in index cases (with subsequently proven Cushing's disease) similar to prospectively proven pituitary Cushing's disease. Used with permission from Ref. *(42)*, Copyright 2004, The Endocrine Society.

the IPSS results suggest ectopic ACTH syndrome, normalization of the IPS:P ACTH ratio to the IPS:P prolactin ratio can increase the diagnostic accuracy of this test (Fig. 2) *(42)*. This is possible since the IPS:P prolactin ratio is an effective index of pituitary venous effluent. Normalized ratios greater than 0.8 are indicative of Cushing's disease, while ratios less than 0.6 are seen in patients with ectopic ACTH syndrome (Table 1) *(42)*. Thus, prolactin samples should be collected at the time of IPSS and stored until the time of measurement, should they be needed.

TRIAL RESULTS: SENSITIVITY AND SPECIFICITY

Differential Diagnosis

Cushing's disease and ectopic ACTH syndrome may be clinically indistinguishable. Radiological studies and dynamic tests of steroid secretion are also often inconclusive in separating these disease entities *(2, 12, 17, 43)*. The inability to correctly diagnose the etiology of hypercortisolism puts patients at risk of additional and unnecessary morbidity. Similarly, transphenoidal surgical exploration carries with it significant risks and should be avoided if less invasive testing can demonstrate that it is unnecessary. Since ~90% of patients with Cushing's syndrome have an ACTH-secreting pituitary adenoma, it is essential that further diagnostic testing have an even greater diagnostic accuracy.

In the first large series of IPSS, Oldfield et al. prospectively studied 281 patients with Cushing's syndrome *(11)*. IPSS was successfully performed in 278 patients (99%) and 262 also received CRH during the procedure. With the exception of groin hematomas, no major complications were reported.

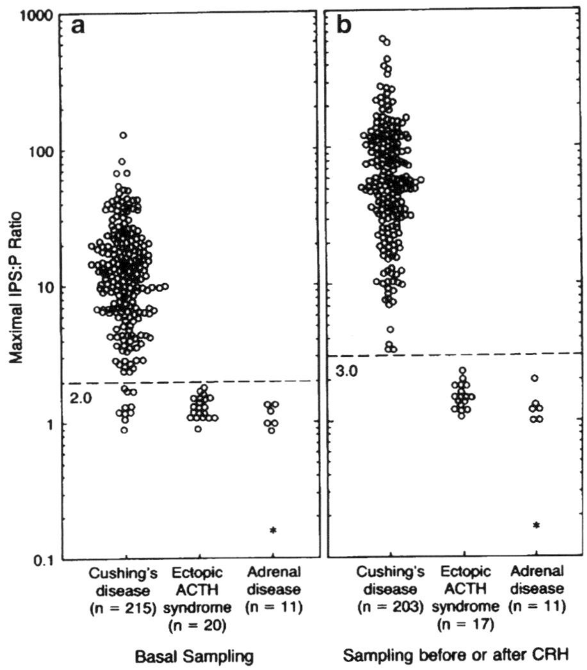

Fig. 3. Maximal IPS:P ACTH ratio in patients with Cushing's syndrome. During basal sampling (panel a), the maximal ratio was ≥2.0 in 205 of 215 patients with confirmed Cushing's disease but below 2.0 in all patients with ectopic ACTH syndrome or primary adrenal disease. Panel b shows that all patients with Cushing's disease who received CRH had maximal ratios of ≥3.0, whereas all patients with ectopic ACTH syndrome had ratios of <3.0. The asterisks represent five patients with primary adrenal disease in whom ACTH was undetectable in peripheral-blood plasma before and after CRH administration. Used with permission from Ref. *(11)*, Copyright 1991, Massachusetts Medical Society, all rights reserved.

Sensitivity of a central-to-peripheral (IPS:P) ACTH ratio ≥2.0 for Cushing's disease was 95% with a specificity of 100%. After CRH administration, both sensitivity and specificity of a peak IPS:P ACTH ratio ≥3.0 was 100%. It should be noted, however, that 32 patients whose diagnosis could not be confirmed were excluded from their analysis (Fig. 3).

In a subsequent report by Findling et al., 29 patients with ACTH-dependent hypercortisolism were prospectively studied by means of IPSS with CRH stimulation *(12)*. In all patients confirmed to have Cushing's disease (n = 20), IPS:P ACTH ratios were >2.0. In contrast, the nine patients with occult ectopic ACTH-secreting adenomas had IPS:P ACTH ratios <2.0. The authors also demonstrated that CRH administration was necessary to correctly classify all patients since rare patients may have a baseline IPS:P ACTH ratio <2.0. Furthermore, bilateral sampling was essential since the non-dominant IPS:P ACTH ratio was less than 2.0 in 33% of patients with Cushing's disease even after CRH administration. Finally, high-dose dexamethasone testing incorrectly diagnosed 24% of patients in this report.

Subsequent studies have largely replicated these findings, reporting sensitivities ranging from 85 to 100% with specificities of 90–100% *(12–23)*. A 1998 review by Newell-Price et al. of 21 studies found an overall sensitivity and specificity of 96 and 100%, respectively *(44)*.

Lateralization

Given the hypophyseal venous anatomy in most individuals, lateralization of a pituitary adenoma should theoretically be possible using IPSS. Early studies in monkeys demonstrated minimal mixture of blood between the cavernous sinuses and inferior petrosal sinuses *(45)*. However, as noted previously, venous drainage patterns can vary significantly between individuals and therefore may preclude accurate lateralization if not accounted for. Furthermore, multi-focal ACTH-secreting pituitary adenomas have been described *(46)*. These observations have led some pituitary specialists to conclude that lateralization using IPSS is "no better than the flip of a coin." Indeed, at least one study reported correct lateralization only 50% of the time using IPSS *(14)*. Liu et al. found that hemihypophysectomy based on lateralization data was successful only ~50% of the time in patients with suspected Cushing's disease based on central venous sampling and no tumor visualized by MRI or the surgeon intraoperatively *(47)*. However, other studies have generally reported lateralization rates of 58–100% and the review by Newell-Price et al. found an overall diagnostic accuracy of 78% *(44)*.

The first report of lateralization by Manni et al. described three Cushing's disease patients with peripherally located intra-pituitary tumors. All three had lateralizing ratios >2 *(48)*. Oldfield et al. subsequently reported that 10 out of 10 patients were cured of Cushing's disease when a lateralizing ratio of ≥1.4 was used to localize the adenoma *(49)*. Seven of eight patients in a series by Vignati et al. showed lateralization of ACTH at baseline and after CRH administration *(50)*. Lefournier et al. demonstrated that diagnostic accuracy of IPSS in predicting lateralization increased from 57 to 71% when both venous flow anatomy and catheter positions were symmetric *(51)*. Miller et al. reported on seven patients that had conflicting basal and post-CRH lateralization results, suggesting that neither can be relied on uniformly *(52)*. In the large series of 281 patients by Oldfield et al., an inter-petrosal ACTH gradient of ≥1.4 correctly predicted the microadenoma location in 71% of patients after CRH administration *(11)*. Clearly, while lateralization data should not be taken without some skepticism (and should not obviate the need for a thorough surgical exploration of the entire pituitary gland) it may provide a starting point for neurosurgeons, especially when adenomas are not seen on imaging studies.

Comparison with Other Tests

High-dose dexamethasone suppression (HDD), CRH stimulation testing, and imaging studies have traditionally been used to distinguish between excessive pituitary-dependent and pituitary-independent ACTH secretion. The sensitivity, specificity, and diagnostic accuracy of these tests are reviewed in detail in other chapters of this text. Here, we will comment on several reports comparing these modalities to IPSS.

The pretest probability of pituitary adenomas in patients with ACTH-dependent Cushing's syndrome is approximately 90%. Furthermore, a regression analysis using easily obtained clinical data such as the patient's gender, age, duration of symptoms, urinary-free cortisol, plasma potassium, and plasma ACTH yields a diagnostic sensitivity greater than 92% *(2)*. A successful diagnostic study must therefore have a sensitivity and specificity greater than these figures.

Using IPSS as a gold standard, Aron et al. reported a sensitivity and specificity of HDD (using the standard criterion of ≥50% cortisol suppression) for the diagnosis of Cushing's syndrome to be 81 and 66.7%, respectively *(2)*. HDD misclassified 24% of patients in another report *(12)*. In a NIH series of 90 patients with ectopic ACTH syndrome, 86% had no suppression of urinary-free cortisol after 2-day HDD, 90% had no suppression of plasma cortisol after overnight HDD, and 92% had no rise in plasma cortisol in response to CRH administration. In contrast, 66 of 67 (98%) patients failed to have significant central to peripheral ACTH gradients with IPSS *(53)*. Wiggam et al. compared IPSS (without CRH administration) to HDD and CRH testing in 44 patients with confirmed Cushing's disease and 1 patient with confirmed ectopic ACTH syndrome *(43)*. Stringent response criteria were used (>90% suppression with HDD and >50% rise in serum cortisol with CRH for the diagnosis of Cushing's disease) to maximize specificity. They showed that in patients with proven pituitary disease, only 48% met the criteria for HDD and 70% met the criteria for CRH testing (only 35% had a correct response to both tests). In contrast, IPSS successfully indicated Cushing's disease in 82% of cases (had CRH been administered during IPSS, the sensitivity would have presumably been even higher).

In a study comparing the ability of MRI and IPSS to determine the cause of Cushing's syndrome, Kaskarelis et al. showed that the accuracy for detecting a pituitary source of ACTH was 50% for MRI and 88% for successful IPSS *(54)*. Of the 54 patients with confirmed final diagnoses, MRI resulted in 25 false negatives and 2 false positives, while IPSS had 2 false negatives and 3 false positives.

A number of studies have also compared IPSS to imaging with CT and MRI for the localization of tumors within the pituitary. In 38 patients with Cushing's disease, Landolt et al. found that pituitary adenomas were correctly localized in 6 of 20 (30%) patients by CT, 11 of 29 (38%) patients by MRI, and 29 of 38 (76%) patients by CRH-stimulated IPSS *(55)*. Booth et al. also found that IPSS was more likely than imaging studies to localize an adenoma (70% vs. 49%, $p < 0.06$) and agree with final pathology (63% vs. 13%, $p < 0.10$) *(56)*. However, a study by de Herder et al. showed that MRI, when positive for an adenoma, was a superior localizing technique as compared to IPSS *(57)*.

Cavernous Sinus and Jugular Vein Sampling

Since IPSS is not always technically successful even at centers with experienced interventional radiologists, and has been associated with rare but significant complications, other less technically demanding procedures have been investigated. In Corrigan's initial 1977 report, jugular bulb ACTH levels were 1.6 times higher than peripheral levels, while the IPS:P ACTH ratio was 2.1 *(9)*. In other studies, however, jugular bulb and jugular vein sampling were non-diagnostic *(10, 58)*. Doppman et al. directly compared IPSS with internal jugular vein sampling (before and after CRH stimulation) in 20 patients with Cushing's disease and 1 patient with the ectopic ACTH syndrome *(59)*. Sensitivity for the diagnosis of Cushing's disease with internal jugular vein sampling and IPSS were 80 and 95%, respectively. They concluded that since jugular vein sampling is less invasive than IPSS, negative results with the former procedure should be confirmed with the latter. Similar findings were reported by Erickson et al. in a group of 35 patients showing a sensitivity of 81.3% for internal jugular vein sampling and 93.8% for IPSS *(60)*. In a larger group of patients reported by the investigators at the NIH (65 with Cushing's disease and 13 with ectopic ACTH secretion), IPSS had a sensitivity of 94% while jugular vein sampling had a sensitivity of 83% (100% specificity for both tests) *(61)*.

Results for cavernous sinus sampling have been mixed. Teramoto et al. reported on seven patients with Cushing's disease that had more reliable and significantly greater central to peripheral ACTH gradients with cavernous sinus sampling than with IPSS *(58)*. Though CRH was not administered in this study, the authors concluded that it was unnecessary. Lateralization could be predicted in all but one subject based on intercavernous gradients. A subsequent report by Teramoto et al. on 44 patients with ACTH-dependent Cushing's syndrome supported these findings *(62)*. Oliverio et al. demonstrated that cavernous sinus sampling with and without CRH stimulation had a sensitivity of 94 and 71%, respectively (using a central to peripheral ratio of ≥3.0) *(63)*. Lateralization was correct in all patients with intercavernous gradients ≥1.4. Graham et al. reported a 100% sensitivity and specificity for CRH-stimulated cavernous sinus sampling in 90 patients with ACTH-dependent Cushing's syndrome, though these calculations were based on only 70 patients that had a proven source of ACTH *(64)*.

A subsequent study by Doppman et al. decreased enthusiasm for this procedure. They compared cavernous sinus ACTH levels to inferior petrosal sinus ACTH levels before and after CRH stimulation in patients with surgically proven Cushing's disease *(65)*. Using a central to peripheral ACTH ratio of >2.0, sensitivity for the diagnosis of Cushing's disease was 80% for the unstimulated cavernous sinus samples, while the sensitivity for unstimulated and CRH stimulated inferior petrosal sinus samples was 87 and 100%, respectively. Lateralization of the pituitary adenoma was correct in only 40% of patients using cavernous sinus samples and 60% of patients using inferior petrosal sinus samples (defined as interpetrosal and intercavernous ACTH ratios of ≥1.4). Lefournier et al. did not see an improvement in lateralization using cavernous sinus sampling compared to IPSS *(51)*. Furthermore, two transient sixth nerve palsies occurred during cavernous sinus catheterization. In a study of 95 patients with ACTH-dependent Cushing's syndrome by Liu et al., cavernous sinus sampling without CRH was not superior to IPSS for tumor localization or sensitivity for the detection of Cushing's disease *(47)*.

Taken together, these studies underscore several important points. First, IPSS is more sensitive than jugular vein sampling, and possibly cavernous sinus sampling, for the diagnosis of Cushing's disease. Second, to achieve the highest possible diagnostic accuracy, CRH is an essential component of IPSS. Third, lateralization of adenomas using jugular vein sampling is not better than IPSS. Finally, these procedures are technically successful in most patients and complications are rare. Of note, many studies exclude suspected, but unproven, cases of Cushing's disease or ectopic ACTH syndrome in their analysis, necessitating caution in interpretation of sensitivity and specificity data. Nevertheless, these observations suggest that IPSS with CRH stimulation should be the differential diagnostic test of choice in centers with experienced radiologists.

IPSS with Desmopressin

The posterior pituitary hormone vasopressin has long been known to be a potent stimulus for the secretion of ACTH. Since vasopressin receptors are present on corticotroph adenoma cells and only rarely on ectopic tumors producing ACTH, and CRH is not available in all centers, desmopressin (a synthetic analog of vasopressin) administration during IPSS has been investigated in several studies. Castinetti et al. reported on 43 patients with Cushing's syndrome *(66)*. Using an IPS:P ACTH ratio >2 after desmopressin administration, sensitivity and specificity were 95 and 100%, respectively. This technique was not effective for localization of the tumor in this study. Machado et al. found a sensitivity of 92.1% and specificity of 100% using an IPS:P ACTH ≥3 after desmopressin stimulation *(67)*. In that study, lateralization of the pituitary tumor was surgically confirmed in 78.7%. Tsagarakis et al. used a combination of CRH with desmopressin during IPSS *(68, 69)*. In their report of 30 patients with Cushing's disease, 15 patients received desmopressin plus CRH during IPSS, while 15 received only CRH. Using an IPS:P ACTH ratio >2, they found a sensitivity of 100% for the combined approach, but only 87% for CRH alone. A subsequent study of 47 patients with Cushing's disease and 7 patients with the ectopic ACTH syndrome found a sensitivity and specificity of 97.9 and 100%, respectively, using the combined desmopressin and CRH approach. In summary, desmopressin administration during IPSS, either in combination with CRH or alone, appears to be a safe and effective diagnostic strategy. These results need to be confirmed in larger studies before this practice is adopted on a widespread basis.

LIMITATIONS AND COMPLICATIONS

In experienced hands, IPSS has been shown to be a safe and reliable procedure *(11, 31–34)*. There are, however, important risks and limitations. The decision to use IPSS as a diagnostic tool, therefore, must be made with considerable care and thought.

IPSS Cannot Diagnose Cushing's Syndrome

It must be stressed that IPSS cannot be used to establish the diagnosis of hypercortisolism or Cushing's syndrome, and should not be used when other tests to diagnose Cushing's syndrome are confusing or contradictory. Normal individuals and patients with "pseudo-Cushing" states have IPSS results that overlap with patients shown to have pathology confirmed pituitary adenomas *(70)*. In a study of 40 individuals with mild to moderate Cushing's disease, 8 with pseudo-Cushing states, and 7 normal volunteers, Yanovski et al. demonstrated that basal ACTH levels, ACTH after CRH stimulation, or central to peripheral ACTH ratios had, at best, a diagnostic accuracy of 81% *(70)*. Thus, IPSS offers no diagnostic improvement over other less invasive tests. IPSS, therefore, should only be considered after hypercortisolism has been firmly established and imaging studies are inconclusive or negative for a pituitary adenoma.

Pituitary Venous Drainage Variability

Variation in pituitary venous drainage has been well described *(13, 40)*. These anatomical differences may be a significant source of false-negative or false-lateralization IPSS results. In a series of 501 patients reported by Doppman et al., 4 patients had false-negative IPSS results. All four patients were found to have a hypoplastic or plexiform inferior petrosal sinus ipsilateral to an ACTH-secreting tumor *(13)*. For this reason, attempts have been made to correct for this variation or minimize error. This includes routine venography and prolactin measurements *(40, 42)*.

Episodic Hypercortisolism

Several reports in the literature describe a subset of patients with episodic hypercortisolemia *(71)*. These patients pose a problem when trying to interpret IPSS results. Since eucortisolemic individuals have IPSS results that overlap with Cushing's disease, false-positive results may be reported in patients with episodic hypercortisolemia secondary to ectopic ACTH secretion if patients happen to be eucortisolemic during the IPSS study. Indeed, Yamamoto et al. reported two such cases *(72)*. It is for this reason that we recommend assessing cortisol levels periprocedurally. We measure late-night salivary cortisol levels the evening prior to IPSS.

Ectopic CRH

Ectopic production of CRH as a cause of Cushing's syndrome is rare, but has been reported *(6–8)*. Sources of the ectopic CRH include neuroendocrine pancreatic tumors, pheochromocytoma, and bronchial carcinoid tumors. These patients may have false-positive central-to-peripheral ACTH gradients during IPSS. Production of CRH by the tumor likely prevents the suppression of the pituitary–adrenal axis usually seen with ectopic ACTH secretion.

Complications

Minor groin hematomas are the most common complication of IPSS, occurring at a frequency of 3–4% *(31)*. Major neurological complications are rare, occurring in only 0.2% of procedures at one center *(32)*. In that report, brain stem injury was felt to be due to variant anatomy and catheter type causing localized venous hypertension. The authors concluded that both catheters should be removed, or the entire IPSS procedure should be terminated, at the first sign of unusual symptoms or signs. These include paresthesias, difficulty with speech, arterial hypertension, or vomiting. In a series reported by Lefournier et al., neurological complications occurred in 1 of 166 patients undergoing IPSS (transient sixth nerve palsy) *(34)*.

Thromboembolic complications have also been reported *(73, 74)*. Blevins et al. reported 2 of 34 patients who had developed deep venous thromboses after the procedure. Of note, heparin was not routinely administered during IPSS at that institution. Factors that promote thrombotic complications in patients with Cushing's syndrome include the hypercoaguable state of hypercortisolism, immobilization, obesity, hypertension, surgery, and vessel trauma during the procedure. Venous subarachnoid hemorrhage with subsequent acute obstructive hydrocephalus has also been reported, occurring in 1 of 94 patients *(75)*. This complication was associated with anomalous venous anatomy and arterial hypertension.

ROLE OF IPSS IN THE EVALUATION OF CUSHING'S SYNDROME

The role of IPSS in clinical practice varies considerably from institution to institution. No formal societal guidelines address how or when it should be utilized in the evaluation of Cushing's syndrome. Some investigators advocate that IPSS be used routinely in all patients with ACTH-dependent Cushing's syndrome *(19)*. In centers where IPSS is not available, other diagnostic modalities are relied upon including imaging studies, HDD, and CRH stimulation testing.

Most authorities agree that because of the costs and potential risks, IPSS should be reserved for cases that have negative imaging studies or equivocal biochemical test results. A recent study tested this approach *(33)*. This report described the experience of one neurosurgeon on 193 patients referred for surgical treatment of presumed Cushing's disease. IPSS was performed in 105 of these patients who did not have an identifiable lesion on pituitary imaging and/or biochemical testing or clinical features were not consistent with Cushing's disease (IPSS was not performed in the other 88 patients). There was no statistical difference between these groups in the remission rate after first transsphenoidal surgery, recurrence rate, and long-term remission rate. Cushing's disease was confirmed in all patients except one in each group. This report suggests that Cushing's disease can be successfully diagnosed and treated using this algorithm for selective use of IPSS.

Further refinements in imaging capabilities, or new imaging techniques, may ultimately reduce the number of IPSS procedures that are performed. Indeed, the spoiled gradient recalled acquisition in the steady-state MRI sequence, a relatively new MRI technique, was shown to have a higher sensitivity for the detection of pituitary adenomas in patients with Cushing's disease as compared to standard T1-weighted spin echo MRI (80% vs. 49%), though the false-positive rate also increased (4% vs. 2%) *(4)*.

While the diagnostic accuracy is superior to other modalities for the differential diagnosis of Cushing's syndrome, its cost-effectiveness compared to imaging studies and biochemical tests remains unclear as few studies have addressed this question. A 1995 decision analysis by Midgette and Aron comparing IPSS and HDD testing concluded that selective use of IPSS after a negative HDD test was the most cost-effective approach, assuming a diagnostic accuracy of 100% for IPSS and sensitivity and specificity of 81 and 79%, respectively, for HDD *(76)*. However, it was noted that the IPSS strategy saves lives whenever HDD specificity is less than 100%. The incremental benefit of IPSS was $1,000,000 per life saved.

SUMMARY AND CONCLUSIONS

Elucidating the cause of ACTH-dependent Cushing's syndrome remains a challenging diagnostic exercise for clinicians. The introduction of effective surgical techniques several decades ago necessitated the development of more precise diagnostic techniques. Imaging studies and traditional biochemical provocative tests lack the sensitivity and specificity required to surpass the 90% pretest probability of pituitary adenomas in patients with ACTH-dependent Cushing's syndrome. Bilateral simultaneous IPSS has the high sensitivity and specificity required of a test to distinguish between Cushing's disease and ectopic ACTH syndrome. As a result, IPSS has become the gold standard for the differential diagnosis of ACTH-dependent Cushing's syndrome.

REFERENCES

1. Cushing H. The basophil adenomas of the pituitary body and their clinical manifestations (pituitary basophilism). Bulletin of the Johns Hopkins Hospital 1932;50:137–195.
2. Aron DC, Raff H, Findling JW. Effectiveness versus efficacy: the limited value in clinical practice of high dose dexamethasone suppression testing in the differential diagnosis of adrenocorticotropin-dependent Cushing's syndrome. J Clin Endocrinol Metab 1997;82:1780–1785.
3. Kaye TB, Crapo L. The Cushing syndrome: an update on diagnostic tests. Ann Intern Med 1990;112:434–444.
4. Patronas N, Bulakbasi N, Stratakis CA, et al. Spoiled gradient recalled acquisition in the steady state technique is superior to conventional postcontrast spin echo technique for magnetic resonance imaging detection of adrenocorticotropin-secreting pituitary tumors. J Clin Endocrinol Metab 2003;88:1565–1569.
5. Hall WA, Luciano MG, Doppman JL, Patronas NJ, Oldfield EH. Pituitary magnetic resonance imaging in normal human volunteers: occult adenomas in the general population. Ann Intern Med 1994;120:817–820.
6. Case records of the Massachusetts General Hospital. Weekly clinicopathological exercises. Case 52–1987. A 20-year-old woman with Cushing's disease and a pulmonary nodule. N Engl J Med 1987;317:1648–1658.
7. O'Brien T, Young WF, Jr, Davila DG, et al. Cushing's syndrome associated with ectopic production of corticotrophin-releasing hormone, corticotrophin and vasopressin by a phaeochromocytoma. Clin Endocrinol (Oxf) 1992;37:460–467.
8. Young J, Deneux C, Grino M, Oliver C, Chanson P, Schaison G. Pitfall of petrosal sinus sampling in a Cushing's syndrome secondary to ectopic adrenocorticotropin-corticotropin releasing hormone (ACTH-CRH) secretion. J Clin Endocrinol Metab 1998;83:305–308.
9. Corrigan DF, Schaaf M, Whaley RA, Czerwinski CL, Earll JM. Selective venous sampling to differentiate ectopic ACTH secretion from pituitary Cushing's syndrome. N Engl J Med 1977;296:861–862.
10. Findling JW, Aron DC, Tyrrell JB, et al. Selective venous sampling for ACTH in Cushing's syndrome: differentiation between Cushing disease and the ectopic ACTH syndrome. Ann Intern Med 1981;94:647–652.
11. Oldfield EH, Doppman JL, Nieman LK, et al. Petrosal sinus sampling with and without corticotropin-releasing hormone for the differential diagnosis of Cushing's syndrome. N Engl J Med 1991;325:897–905.
12. Findling JW, Kehoe ME, Shaker JL, Raff H. Routine inferior petrosal sinus sampling in the differential diagnosis of adrenocorticotropin (ACTH)-dependent Cushing's syndrome: early recognition of the occult ectopic ACTH syndrome. J Clin Endocrinol Metab 1991;73:408–413.
13. Doppman JL, Chang R, Oldfield EH, Chrousos G, Stratakis CA, Nieman LK. The hypoplastic inferior petrosal sinus: a potential source of false-negative results in petrosal sampling for Cushing's disease. J Clin Endocrinol Metab 1999;84:533–540.
14. McCance DR, McIlrath E, McNeill A, et al. Bilateral inferior petrosal sinus sampling as a routine procedure in ACTH-dependent Cushing's syndrome. Clin Endocrinol (Oxf) 1989;30:157–166.
15. Bonelli FS, Huston J, 3rd, Carpenter PC, Erickson D, Young WF, Jr, Meyer FB. Adrenocorticotropic hormone-dependent Cushing's syndrome: sensitivity and specificity of inferior petrosal sinus sampling. AJNR Am J Neuroradiol 2000;21:690–696.
16. Colao A, Faggiano A, Pivonello R, et al. Inferior petrosal sinus sampling in the differential diagnosis of Cushing's syndrome: results of an Italian multicenter study. Eur J Endocrinol 2001;144:499–507.
17. Ilias I, Torpy DJ, Pacak K, Mullen N, Wesley RA, Nieman LK. Cushing's syndrome due to ectopic corticotropin secretion: twenty years' experience at the National Institutes of Health. J Clin Endocrinol Metab 2005;90:4955–4962.
18. Invitti C, Pecori Giraldi F, Cavagnini F. Inferior petrosal sinus sampling in patients with Cushing's syndrome and contradictory responses to dynamic testing. Clin Endocrinol (Oxf) 1999;51:255–257.
19. Kaltsas GA, Giannulis MG, Newell-Price JD, et al. A critical analysis of the value of simultaneous inferior petrosal sinus sampling in Cushing's disease and the occult ectopic adrenocorticotropin syndrome. J Clin Endocrinol Metab 1999;84:487–492.

20. Tabarin A, Greselle JF, San-Galli F, et al. Usefulness of the corticotropin-releasing hormone test during bilateral inferior petrosal sinus sampling for the diagnosis of Cushing's disease. J Clin Endocrinol Metab 1991;73:53–59.
21. Bessac L, Bachelot I, Vasdev A, et al. Catheterization of the inferior petrosal sinus. Its role in the diagnosis of Cushing's syndrome. Experience with 23 explorations. Ann Endocrinol (Paris) 1992;53:16–27.
22. Colao A, Merola B, Tripodi FS, et al. Simultaneous and bilateral inferior petrosal sinus sampling for the diagnosis of Cushing's syndrome: comparison of multihormonal assay, baseline multiple sampling and ACTH-releasing hormone test. Horm Res 1993;40:209–216.
23. Lopez J, Barcelo B, Lucas T, et al. Petrosal sinus sampling for diagnosis of Cushing's disease: evidence of false negative results. Clin Endocrinol (Oxf) 1996;45:147–156.
24. Vale W, Spiess J, Rivier C, Rivier J. Characterization of a 41-residue ovine hypothalamic peptide that stimulates secretion of corticotropin and beta-endorphin. Science 1981;213:1394–1397.
25. Orth DN, DeBold CR, DeCherney GS, et al. Pituitary microadenomas causing Cushing's disease respond to corticotropin-releasing factor. J Clin Endocrinol Metab 1982;55:1017–1019.
26. Nussey SS, Page SR, Peterson DB, et al. Corticotrophin releasing hormone (CRH1–41) stimulates the secretion of adrenocorticotrophin, vasopressin and oxytocin but not adrenocorticotrophin precursors: evidence from petrosal sinus sampling in man. Clin Endocrinol (Oxf) 1991;34:51–56.
27. Vignati F, Berselli ME, Boccardi E, Branca V, Loli P. Stimulatory effect of oCRH on alpha-subunit secretion during petrosal sinus sampling in patients with Cushing's disease. Horm Metab Res 1992;24:524–527.
28. Tabarin A, Corcuff JB, Rashedi M, et al. Multihormonal response to corticotropin-releasing hormone in inferior petrosal sinus blood of one patient with Cushing's disease: comparison with in vitro secretion of the tumoral corticotropes. Acta Endocrinol (Copenh) 1992;127:284–288.
29. Muller OA, Stalla GK, von Werder K. Corticotropin releasing factor: a new tool for the differential diagnosis of Cushing's syndrome. J Clin Endocrinol Metab 1983;57:227–229.
30. Landolt AM, Valavanis A, Girard J, Eberle AN. Corticotrophin-releasing factor-test used with bilateral, simultaneous inferior petrosal sinus blood-sampling for the diagnosis of pituitary-dependent Cushing's disease. Clin Endocrinol (Oxf) 1986;25:687–696.
31. Miller DL, Doppman JL. Petrosal sinus sampling: technique and rationale. Radiology 1991;178:37–47.
32. Miller DL, Doppman JL, Peterman SB, Nieman LK, Oldfield EH, Chang R. Neurologic complications of petrosal sinus sampling. Radiology 1992;185:143–147.
33. Jehle S, Walsh JE, Freda PU, Post KD. Selective use of bilateral inferior petrosal sinus sampling in patients with adrenocorticotropin-dependent Cushing's syndrome prior to transsphenoidal surgery. J Clin Endocrinol Metab 2008;93:4624–4632.
34. Lefournier V, Gatta B, Martinie M, et al. One transient neurological complication (sixth nerve palsy) in 166 consecutive inferior petrosal sinus samplings for the etiological diagnosis of Cushing's syndrome. J Clin Endocrinol Metab 1999;84:3401–3402.
35. Green HT. The venous drainage of the human hypophysis cerebri. Am J Anat 1957;100:435–469.
36. Xuereb GP, Prichard MM, Daniel PM. The arterial supply and venous drainage of the human hypophysis cerebri. Q J Exp Physiol Cogn Med Sci 1954;39:199–217.
37. Shiu PC, Hanafee WN, Wilson GH, Rand RW. Cavernous sinus venography. Am J Roentgenol Radium Ther Nucl Med 1968;104:57–62.
38. Doppman JL, Oldfield E, Krudy AG, et al. Petrosal sinus sampling for Cushing syndrome: anatomical and technical considerations. Work in progress. Radiology 1984;150:99–103.
39. Miller DL, Doppman JL, Chang R. Anatomy of the junction of the inferior petrosal sinus and the internal jugular vein. AJNR Am J Neuroradiol 1993;14:1075–1083.
40. Mamelak AN, Dowd CF, Tyrrell JB, McDonald JF, Wilson CB. Venous angiography is needed to interpret inferior petrosal sinus and cavernous sinus sampling data for lateralizing adrenocorticotropin-secreting adenomas. J Clin Endocrinol Metab 1996;81:475–481.
41. Swearingen B, Katznelson L, Miller K, et al. Diagnostic errors after inferior petrosal sinus sampling. J Clin Endocrinol Metab 2004;89:3752–3763.
42. Findling JW, Kehoe ME, Raff H. Identification of patients with Cushing's disease with negative pituitary adrenocorticotropin gradients during inferior petrosal sinus sampling: prolactin as an index of pituitary venous effluent. J Clin Endocrinol Metab 2004;89:6005–6009.
43. Wiggam MI, Heaney AP, McIlrath EM, et al. Bilateral inferior petrosal sinus sampling in the differential diagnosis of adrenocorticotropin-dependent Cushing's syndrome: a comparison with other diagnostic tests. J Clin Endocrinol Metab 2000;85:1525–1532.

44. Newell-Price J, Trainer P, Besser M, Grossman A. The diagnosis and differential diagnosis of Cushing's syndrome and pseudo-Cushing's states. Endocr Rev 1998;19:647–672.
45. Oldfield EH, Girton ME, Doppman JL. Absence of intercavernous venous mixing: evidence supporting lateralization of pituitary microadenomas by venous sampling. J Clin Endocrinol Metab 1985;61:644–647.
46. Laws ER, Jr. Multiple pituitary adenomas. J Neurosurg 2000;93:909–911.
47. Liu C, Lo JC, Dowd CF, et al. Cavernous and inferior petrosal sinus sampling in the evaluation of ACTH-dependent Cushing's syndrome. Clin Endocrinol (Oxf) 2004;61:478–486.
48. Manni A, Latshaw RF, Page R, Santen RJ. Simultaneous bilateral venous sampling for adrenocorticotropin in pituitary-dependent Cushing's disease: evidence for lateralization of pituitary venous drainage. J Clin Endocrinol Metab 1983;57:1070–1073.
49. Oldfield EH, Chrousos GP, Schulte HM, et al. Preoperative lateralization of ACTH-secreting pituitary microadenomas by bilateral and simultaneous inferior petrosal venous sinus sampling. N Engl J Med 1985;312:100–103.
50. Vignati F, Berselli ME, Scialfa G, Boccardi E, Loli P. Bilateral and simultaneous venous sampling of inferior petrosal sinuses for ACTH and PRL determination: preoperative localization of ACTH-secreting microadenomas. J Endocrinol Invest 1989;12:235–238.
51. Lefournier V, Martinie M, Vasdev A, et al. Accuracy of bilateral inferior petrosal or cavernous sinuses sampling in predicting the lateralization of Cushing's disease pituitary microadenoma: influence of catheter position and anatomy of venous drainage. J Clin Endocrinol Metab 2003;88:196–203.
52. Miller DL, Doppman JL, Nieman LK, et al. Petrosal sinus sampling: discordant lateralization of ACTH-secreting pituitary microadenomas before and after stimulation with corticotropin-releasing hormone. Radiology 1990;176:429–431.
53. Ilias I, Torpy DJ, Pacak K, Mullen N, Wesley RA, Nieman LK. Cushing's syndrome due to ectopic corticotropin secretion: twenty years' experience at the National Institutes of Health. J Clin Endocrinol Metab 2005;90:4955–4962.
54. Kaskarelis IS, Tsatalou EG, Benakis SV, et al. Bilateral inferior petrosal sinuses sampling in the routine investigation of Cushing's syndrome: a comparison with MRI. AJR Am J Roentgenol 2006;187:562–570.
55. Landolt AM, Schubiger O, Maurer R, Girard J. The value of inferior petrosal sinus sampling in diagnosis and treatment of Cushing's disease. Clin Endocrinol (Oxf) 1994;40:485–492.
56. Booth GL, Redelmeier DA, Grosman H, Kovacs K, Smyth HS, Ezzat S. Improved diagnostic accuracy of inferior petrosal sinus sampling over imaging for localizing pituitary pathology in patients with Cushing's disease. J Clin Endocrinol Metab 1998;83:2291–2295.
57. de Herder WW, Uitterlinden P, Pieterman H, et al. Pituitary tumour localization in patients with Cushing's disease by magnetic resonance imaging. Is there a place for petrosal sinus sampling? Clin Endocrinol (Oxf) 1994;40:87–92.
58. Teramoto A, Nemoto S, Takakura K, Sasaki Y, Machida T. Selective venous sampling directly from cavernous sinus in Cushing's syndrome. J Clin Endocrinol Metab 1993;76:637–641.
59. Doppman JL, Oldfield EH, Nieman LK. Bilateral sampling of the internal jugular vein to distinguish between mechanisms of adrenocorticotropic hormone-dependent Cushing syndrome. Ann Intern Med 1998;128:33–36.
60. Erickson D, Huston J, 3rd, Young WF, Jr, et al. Internal jugular vein sampling in adrenocorticotropic hormone-dependent Cushing's syndrome: a comparison with inferior petrosal sinus sampling. Clin Endocrinol (Oxf) 2004;60:413–419.
61. Ilias I, Chang R, Pacak K, et al. Jugular venous sampling: an alternative to petrosal sinus sampling for the diagnostic evaluation of adrenocorticotropic hormone-dependent Cushing's syndrome. J Clin Endocrinol Metab 2004;89:3795–3800.
62. Teramoto A, Yoshida Y, Sanno N, Nemoto S. Cavernous sinus sampling in patients with adrenocorticotrophic hormone-dependent Cushing's syndrome with emphasis on inter- and intracavernous adrenocorticotrophic hormone gradients. J Neurosurg 1998;89:762–768.
63. Oliverio PJ, Monsein LH, Wand GS, Debrun GM. Bilateral simultaneous cavernous sinus sampling using corticotropin-releasing hormone in the evaluation of Cushing disease. AJNR Am J Neuroradiol 1996;17:1669–1674.
64. Graham KE, Samuels MH, Nesbit GM, et al. Cavernous sinus sampling is highly accurate in distinguishing Cushing's disease from the ectopic adrenocorticotropin syndrome and in predicting intrapituitary tumor location. J Clin Endocrinol Metab 1999;84:1602–1610.
65. Doppman JL, Nieman LK, Chang R, et al. Selective venous sampling from the cavernous sinuses is not a more reliable technique than sampling from the inferior petrosal sinuses in Cushing's syndrome. J Clin Endocrinol Metab 1995;80:2485–2489.
66. Castinetti F, Morange I, Dufour H, et al. Desmopressin test during petrosal sinus sampling: a valuable tool to discriminate pituitary or ectopic ACTH-dependent Cushing's syndrome. Eur J Endocrinol 2007;157:271–277.
67. Machado MC, de Sa SV, Domenice S, et al. The role of desmopressin in bilateral and simultaneous inferior petrosal sinus sampling for differential diagnosis of ACTH-dependent Cushing's syndrome. Clin Endocrinol (Oxf) 2007;66:136–142.

68. Tsagarakis S, Kaskarelis IS, Kokkoris P, Malagari C, Thalassinos N. The application of a combined stimulation with CRH and desmopressin during bilateral inferior petrosal sinus sampling in patients with Cushing's syndrome. Clin Endocrinol (Oxf) 2000;52:355–361.
69. Tsagarakis S, Vassiliadi D, Kaskarelis IS, Komninos J, Souvatzoglou E, Thalassinos N. The application of the combined corticotropin-releasing hormone plus desmopressin stimulation during petrosal sinus sampling is both sensitive and specific in differentiating patients with Cushing's disease from patients with the occult ectopic adrenocorticotropin syndrome. J Clin Endocrinol Metab 2007;92:2080–2086.
70. Yanovski JA, Cutler GB, Jr, Doppman JL, et al. The limited ability of inferior petrosal sinus sampling with corticotropin-releasing hormone to distinguish Cushing's disease from pseudo-Cushing states or normal physiology. J Clin Endocrinol Metab 1993;77:503–509.
71. Atkinson AB, Kennedy AL, Carson DJ, Hadden DR, Weaver JA, Sheridan B. Five cases of cyclical Cushing's syndrome. Br Med J (Clin Res Ed) 1985;291:1453–1457.
72. Yamamoto Y, Davis DH, Nippoldt TB, Young WF, Jr, Huston J, 3rd, Parisi JE. False-positive inferior petrosal sinus sampling in the diagnosis of Cushing's disease. Report of two cases. J Neurosurg 1995;83:1087–1091.
73. Blevins LS, Jr, Clark RV, Owens DS. Thromboembolic complications after inferior petrosal sinus sampling in patients with Cushing's syndrome. Endocr Pract 1998;4:365–367.
74. Obuobie K, Davies JS, Ogunko A, Scanlon MF. Venous thrombo-embolism following inferior petrosal sinus sampling in Cushing's disease. J Endocrinol Invest 2000;23:542–544.
75. Bonelli FS, Huston J, 3rd, Meyer FB, Carpenter PC. Venous subarachnoid hemorrhage after inferior petrosal sinus sampling for adrenocorticotropic hormone. AJNR Am J Neuroradiol 1999;20:306–307.
76. Midgette AS, Aron DC. High-dose dexamethasone suppression testing versus inferior petrosal sinus sampling in the differential diagnosis of adrenocorticotropin-dependent Cushing's syndrome: a decision analysis. Am J Med Sci 1995;309:162–170.

10 The Surgical Management of Cushing's Disease

Ian F. Dunn and Edward R. Laws, Jr

Contents

Abstract

The prompt and effective lowering of increased cortisol becomes essential for the well-being of patient's with Cushing's disease. As 80% of patients with the clinical signs and symptoms of Cushing's disease have a pituitary source of excessive and uncontrolled adrenocorticotropic hormone (ACTH) secretion, well-trained pituitary surgeons are required to deal with this complex disease. At present, surgical removal of a pituitary adenoma which is the source of excessive ACTH provides the most reliable method of reducing cortisol, with the potential for "cure" of the tumor and immediate remission of disease. The most popular methods are endonasal microsurgical or endoscopic approaches, which have become increasingly safe and effective. The goals of surgery are to reverse the endocrinopathy and restore normal pituitary function; eliminate mass effect and restore normal neurological function; eliminate or minimize the possibility of tumor recurrence; and obtain a definitive histologic diagnosis. Reported long-term recurrence rates mandate close monitoring in this patient population.

Key Words: Surgical management, Cushing's disease, ACTH adenoma, transsphenoidal surgery, cortisol, endoscopy

From: *Contemporary Endocrinology: Cushing's Syndrome: Pathophysiology, Diagnosis and Treatment*
Edited by: M.D. Bronstein (ed.), DOI 10.1007/978-1-60327-449-4_10,

INTRODUCTION

Once the diagnosis of Cushing's disease is made, prompt and effective lowering of increased cortisol becomes essential for the well-being of the patient. It has been demonstrated that 80% of patients with the clinical signs and symptoms of Cushing's disease have a pituitary source of excessive and uncontrolled adrenocorticotropic hormone (ACTH) secretion *(29)*, underscoring the need for focused and well-trained pituitary surgeons to deal with this complex and debilitating disease first recognized by Harvey Cushing *(25)*.

At present, surgical removal of a pituitary adenoma which is the source of excessive ACTH provides the most reliable method of reducing cortisol, with the potential for "cure" of the tumor and immediate remission of disease. The initial selective transsphenoidal microadenomectomy was first performed by Hardy in the 1960s *(3, 13, 14)* and soon thereafter by Salassa and Laws *(30, 45, 46)*; since then, several large surgical series have been published, validating this approach in the management of Cushing's disease (Table 1). The goals of surgery today are the same as they were in Hardy's day: reverse the endocrinopathy and restore normal pituitary function; eliminate mass effect and restore normal neurological function; eliminate or minimize the possibility of tumor recurrence; and obtain a definitive histologic diagnosis.

Table 1
Surgical Series of Cushing's Disease After 1999[a]

Author and Year	*Patients*	*Follow-up in months, mean (range)*	*% Remission*[b]	*Criteria for remission*	*% Recurrence*
Invitti et al., 1999 *(17)*	288	27 (6–115)	69	Variable	17
Swearingen et al., 1999 *(53)*	161	96 (12–240)	85	Low morning cortisol/ low urine-free cortisol	7
Chee et al., 2001 *(5)*	61	88 (7–211)	78	Low-dose dexamethasone suppression normal	14.6
Rees et al., 2002 *(43)*	54	72 (6–252)	77	Low morning serum cortisol level	5
Shimon et al., 2002 *(50)*	82	50 (no range given)	78	24 h urinary cortisol normal	5
Yap et al., 2002 *(54)*	97	92 (6–348)	69	Low morning serum cortisol level	11.5
Chen et al., 2003 *(6)*	174	At least 60	73	24 h urinary cortisol normal	7
Flitsch et al., 2003 *(10)*	147	61 (14–123)	98	Low morning serum cortisol level	5.5
Pereira et al. 2003 *(40)*	78	84 (12–288)	65	Low morning serum cortisol level	17

(continued)

Table 1 (continued)

Author and Year	*Patients*	*Follow-up in months, mean (range)*	*% Remission*[b]	*Criteria for remission*	*% Recurrence*
Hammer et al., 2004 *(12)*	289	133 (12–288)	82	Low-dose dexamethasone suppression normal	6
Rollin et al., 2004 *(44)*	41	58 (4–170)	88	Low-dose dexamethasone suppression normal	5
Atkinson et al., 2005 *(1)*	63	115 (12–252)	71	Low-dose dexamethasone suppression normal	22
Esposito et al., 2006 *(9)*	40	33 (14–65)	93	Subnormal morning cortisol level	3
Hofmann et al., 2008 *(16)*	426	72 (3–300)	76	2 mg dexamethasone suppression normal	15
Patil et al., 2008 *(38)*	215	45 (6–166)	86	24 h urinary cortisol normal	17
Fomekong et al., 2009 *(11)*	40	87 (20–152)	80	24 h urinary cortisol normal	9.4

[a]Listed are those with at least 40 patients included
[b]After initial surgery

MAKING THE DIAGNOSIS

In the evaluation of the patient with Cushing's syndrome and characteristic features of excess cortisol secretion, it is essential to prove that increased levels of circulating cortisol actually exist. This is done by measuring fasting cortisol and ACTH levels in the serum, 24-h urinary excretion of cortisol, as well as salivary cortisol. The goal is to demonstrate significantly elevated cortisol, moderately elevated ACTH, and a loss of the normal diurnal variation in cortisol secretion. If the clinical symptoms and laboratory findings are not classical, it is essential to rule out extra-pituitary sources. Ordinarily this would involve imaging of the adrenal glands, and efforts to rule out an ectopic source of excess ACTH or corticotropin-releasing hormone (CRH). Imaging of the chest and abdomen can detect carcinoid and other tumors that may be ectopic sources of ACTH or CRH. In the face of demonstrated excess levels of circulating cortisol, bilateral inferior petrosal sinus sampling is the best method currently available to rule out such an ectopic source and help lateralize a pituitary source *(2, 31, 35)*.

Careful and comprehensive pituitary imaging studies are essential. New methods that take advantage of 3T MR imaging *(23)*, dynamic postcontrast sequences *(7)*, and methionine PET/3T fusion have promise in improving the detection of small intrasellar ACTH-secreting tumors (Fig. 1). In evaluating the imaging studies, careful attention must be paid to the cavernous sinuses and the supra-diaphragmatic area where ectopic pituitary adenoma tissue may be present.

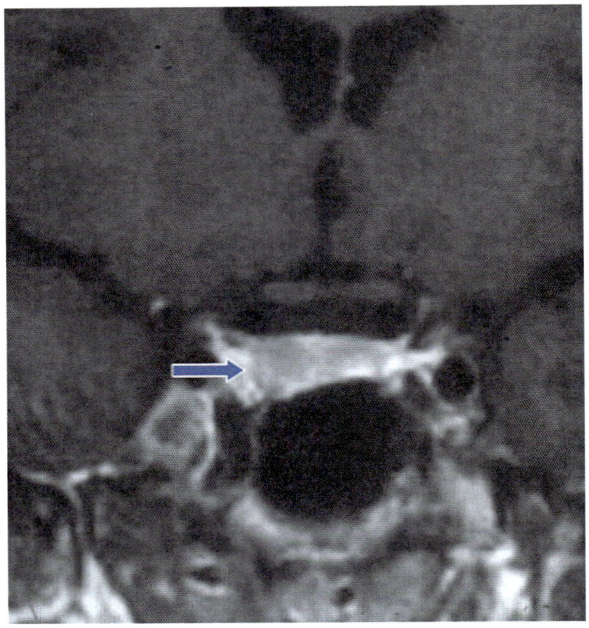

Fig. 1. T1 coronal MRI showing an ACTH-secreting microadenoma (blue arrow). Note the cortical atrophy in this young patient, a recently recognized phenomenon in Cushing's disease *(37, 52)*.

SURGICAL PRINCIPLES

With the confirmation of a pituitary source for Cushing's disease, exploration of the pituitary is indicated. Currently, this is almost always done using one or another variant of the transsphenoidal approach. The most popular methods are endonasal microsurgical or endoscopic approaches, which have become increasingly safe and effective.

Anatomic aspects in patients with Cushing's disease complicate the operation. The sella turcica itself is often quite small. The lack of sellar enlargement and increased intra-sellar pressure from a large lesion predisposes the patient to venous bleeding from the channels between the leaves of the sellar dura. Because the sella is small, manipulations within it can cause inadvertent trauma and damage to the posterior pituitary, making diabetes insipidus riskier in these patients as compared to other pituitary tumor patients.

Another anatomic feature of the typical patient with Cushing's disease is centripetal obesity, often producing increased intra-abdominal and intrathoracic venous pressure. Recognizing this, we are diligent in positioning the patient for surgery, being certain that the head and thorax are elevated 20–30 degrees above the horizontal.

It is our practice in operating for Cushing's disease not to administer perioperative corticosteroids, as these patients already have high circulating levels of cortisol. This policy allows for prompt postoperative assessment of the lowering of cortisol following excision of the pituitary tumor. In these patients we also tend to avoid the routine use of an abdominal fat graft, which is employed only when an intraoperative spinal fluid leak is present. Similarly, we avoid the routine use of a lumbar intrathecal catheter and postoperative spinal drainage.

Because patients with Cushing's disease are at a higher than normal risk for the development of deep venous thromboses, it is our practice to institute low-dose aspirin therapy immediately following surgery, and to use sequential lower limb compression devices until the patient is ambulatory. Occasionally, in high-risk patients subcutaneous heparin is utilized during the hospitalization.

TECHNICAL ASPECTS OF THE SURGERY FOR CUSHING'S DISEASE

Once the sella is exposed through an endonasal endoscopic or microscopic approach, the following steps have been useful:

1. Wide exposure of the dura, from one cavernous sinus to the other
2. Wide opening of the dura, usually with an "X-shaped" incision and cauterization of the dural leaves
3. Broad subdural exposure of the face of the pituitary gland
4. Explore for and remove obvious tumor detected visually, as directed by imaging studies, or by softness upon palpation
5. With appropriate incision of the gland, attempt to define and resect the pseudocapsule *(27)* around the tumor, removing all tumor and the adjacent margin of normal gland.

If no tumor is readily detected, we systematically incise the gland and explore within it. If there are no anatomic clues from the imaging studies, the initial exploration is an excisional biopsy of the central mucoid wedge of the pituitary gland where the highest concentrations of ACTH cells are present. This includes the pars intermedia just anterior to the posterior pituitary. If tumor is still undetected, a subdural exploration and delivery to the center of the exposure of the lateral lobes of the pituitary is carried out, searching for tumor. A thin rim of normal gland is preserved superiorly to protect the pituitary stalk, unless a total hypophysectomy is planned. Any manipulation or stretching of the pituitary stalk is assiduously avoided in an attempt to avoid postoperative diabetes insipidus. Finally, one may carefully biopsy the posterior pituitary. During exploration, one must also consider the possibility that more than one adenoma may be present *(26, 34)*. It is our practice to explore carefully with the angled endoscopes the cavernous sinus walls, and to remove intracavernous extensions when possible; we have not routinely attempted to resect invaded dura of the cavernous sinus.

After a brief trial of using intraoperative ultrasound for the detection of microadenomas we have not persisted in using this modality, although others have found it useful.

In accordance with the advice of experienced pituitary pathologists, it is our practice not to use intraoperative smears, touch preparations or frozen sections in an attempt to confirm the presence of tumor. This is a difficult challenge for most surgical pathologists and we prefer to have the maximum amount of tissue available for permanent study. When no gross tumor has been detected, the entire surgical specimen is embedded and serially sectioned in the search for a small tumor or other ACTH staining tissue.

The method of closure of the sella depends upon whether or not a spinal fluid leak is present. If there is no leak, it is our practice to fill the tumor cavity with Gelfoam and to reconstruct the floor of the sella with bone or an artificial material such as Porex. If a spinal fluid leak has occurred, an abdominal fat graft is obtained, usually from a sub-umbilical incision, is placed in the sella to occlude the leak, and is buttressed by the reconstruction of the sellar floor. Ordinarily the sphenoid sinus is not packed, nor are the nostrils.

POSTOPERATIVE MANAGEMENT

Patients are managed in a systematic manner to maximize safe and efficient patient care *(28)*. If the surgery has been uncomplicated, we do not routinely utilize the intensive care unit. Serum cortisol is measured every 6 h, with the anticipation that it will be essentially undetectable within about 18 h of surgery if the operation is successful *(51)*.

Careful management of intake and output with measurement of serum sodium is undertaken, and diabetes insipidus is managed appropriately with DDAVP.

Every effort is made to mobilize the patient as rapidly as possible, and routine nasal care is provided with saline irrigation and decongestants as indicated.

Patients who become clinically adrenally insufficient, or who have extremely low cortisol measurements are given replacement hydrocortisone, initially at a dose of 40 mg upon awakening in the morning, and 20 mg at 5–6 p.m. This is tapered to routine replacement doses after several days, according to the patient's condition.

COMPLICATIONS OF SURGERY

The complication rate of this operation has been carefully studied *(47)*. Fortunately, major complications are rare and occur in less than 2% of patients *(20)*. The most common and worrisome complication is a postoperative spinal fluid leak that potentially can lead to meningitis. Our strategy with his problem is to perform immediate reexploration and repair of the spinal fluid leak with a new abdominal fat graft.

Patients with Cushing's disease have fragile tissues and are prone to bleeding, so that careful hemostasis is important. Occasionally, postoperative nasal bleeding may occur. The complication that is more frequent after using the endoscopic approach is delayed epistaxis from unrecognized damage to the sphenopalatine artery. This bleeding requires prompt attention and is often best handled with endovascular occlusion of the main trunk of the bleeding artery.

Deep venous thrombosis and pulmonary embolus can occur in these patients. Appropriate precautions should be taken and prompt therapy initiated when such complications occur.

Diabetes insipidus and delayed hyponatremia from SIADH can occur as complications of the procedure. Diabetes insipidus is controlled with appropriate medical therapy using desmopressin. Hyponatremia is usually related to inappropriate ADH secretion and ordinarily responds well to aggressive fluid restriction.

Postoperative sinus complaints may occur. They include congestion, mucocele formation, infection, and inflammatory disease. Appropriate therapy is usually effective but may involve referral to an otorhinolaryngologist. Symptomatic nasal septal perforations have become extremely uncommon with improvements in technique. On rare occasions there can be alterations or loss of the sense of taste or smell.

RESULTS OF SURGERY

Recent series of surgery for Cushing's disease have reported remission rates of between 65% and 93% after initial surgery, though the series vary in length of follow-up and remission criteria *(1, 4, 5, 8–12, 16, 17, 20, 38, 40, 42–44, 50, 53, 54)*. Our overall series of surgery for Cushing's disease incorporates 672 patients operated upon between 1972 and 2009. The series has been reviewed a number of times with the goal of focusing on specific aspects of the management of this difficult disease entity *(20, 33, 37, 38, 39, 41, 42)*. In the optimal situation where a pituitary microadenoma is detected on MRI and removed, the initial remission rate has been 88% *(42)*; even in cases where a tumor is not identified on MR, initial remission rates are similar in experienced surgical hands *(48)*. Expectedly, remission rates are lower (50%) in cases without pathological confirmation of tumor *(41)*.

With macroadenomas, which are often invasive, the initial remission rate ranges from 55 *(20)* to 80% *(11)*.

In patients who do not achieve remission after the initial operation, assuming that the localization of the source of excess ACTH in the pituitary is correct, it is our practice to recommend immediate reexploration *(33)*, except for patients who have very mild disease or preferred to be followed. This strategy of immediate reexploration has yielded a 55% remission rate. In patients who have not achieved remission and who have major morbidity associated with their Cushing's disease, the reexploration is done with the intent of performing a total hypophysectomy.

When these strategies are unsuccessful, focused radiosurgery becomes an important adjunct in the management of persistent Cushing's disease *(18, 19, 29, 49)*.

POSTOPERATIVE RECURRENCE OF CUSHING'S DISEASE

With a sizable number of patients followed for more than 10 years, it has become evident that the recurrence rate inexorably increases with the passage of time *(38)*. Although it is true that most recurrences occur within the first 5 years, and that most are located in the same part of the sella as the original tumor, the recurrence rate after 20 years exceeds 20%. Moreover, the remission rates after surgery for recurrent Cushing's disease are lower than those reported after initial surgery *(15, 24, 39)*, further emphasizing the importance of as complete an extirpation as possible during the first operation. The reported long-term recurrence rates demand that these patients are closely monitored for recurrence; this is particularly true in the pediatric population *(21, 22, 30, 32, 36)*. Often, the patients can tell us that they are experiencing a recurrence even before the laboratory data are conclusive.

CONCLUSION

Cushing's disease remains a challenging diagnostic and therapeutic problem. With a systematic approach, most patients can achieve satisfactory control of this debilitating disease. At present, successful surgery remains the most effective management of achieving this goal.

REFERENCES

1. Atkinson AB, Kennedy A, Wiggam MI, McCance DR, Sheridan B. Long-term remission rates after pituitary surgery for Cushing's disease: the need for long-term surveillance. Clin Endocrinol (Oxf) 2005;63:549–559.
2. Batista D, Gennari M, Riar J, Chang R, Keil MF, Oldfield EH, Stratakis CA. An assessment of petrosal sinus sampling for localization of pituitary microadenomas in children with Cushing disease. J Clin Endocrinol Metab 2006;91:221–224.
3. Bigos ST, Robert F, Pelletier G, Hardy J. Cure of Cushing's disease by transsphenoidal removal of a microadenoma from a pituitary gland despite a radiographically normal sella turcica. J Clin Endocrinol Metab 1977;45:1251–1260.
4. Cavagnini F, Pecori Giraldi F. Epidemiology and follow-up of Cushing's disease. Ann Endocrinol (Paris) 2001;62:168–172.
5. Chee GH, Mathias DB, James RA, Kendall-Taylor P. Transsphenoidal pituitary surgery in Cushing's disease: can we predict outcome? Clin Endocrinol (Oxf) 2001;54:617–626.
6. Chen JC, Amar AP, Choi S, Singer P, Couldwell WT, Weiss MH. Transsphenoidal microsurgical treatment of Cushing disease: postoperative assessment of surgical efficacy by application of an overnight low-dose dexamethasone suppression test. J Neurosurg 2003;98:967–973.
7. Davis WL, Lee JN, King BD, Harnsberger HR. Dynamic contrast-enhanced MR imaging of the pituitary gland with fast spin-echo technique. J Magn Reson Imaging 1994;4:509–511.
8. De Tommasi C, Vance ML, Okonkwo DO, Diallo A, Laws ER, Jr. Surgical management of adrenocorticotropic hormone-secreting macroadenomas: outcome and challenges in patients with Cushing's disease or Nelson's syndrome. J Neurosurg 2005;103:825–830.
9. Esposito F, Dusick JR, Cohan P, Moftakhar P, McArthur D, Wang C, Swerdloff RS, Kelly DF. Clinical review: early morning cortisol levels as a predictor of remission after transsphenoidal surgery for Cushing's disease. J Clin Endocrinol Metab 2006;91:7–13.
10. Flitsch J, Knappe UJ, Ludecke DK. The use of postoperative ACTH levels as a marker for successful transsphenoidal microsurgery in Cushing's disease. Zentralbl Neurochir 2003;64:6–11.

11. Fomekong E, Maiter D, Grandin C, Raftopoulos C. Outcome of transsphenoidal surgery for Cushing's disease: a high remission rate in ACTH-secreting macroadenomas. Clin Neurol Neurosurg 2009;111:442–9.
12. Hammer GD, Tyrrell JB, Lamborn KR, Applebury CB, Hannegan ET, Bell S, Rahl R, Lu A, Wilson CB. Transsphenoidal microsurgery for Cushing's disease: initial outcome and long-term results. J Clin Endocrinol Metab 2004;89:6348–6357.
13. Hardy J. Transsphenoidal microsurgery for selective removal of functional pituitary microadenomas. Invited commentary. World J Surg 1977;1:84.
14. Hardy J. Presidential address: XVII Canadian Congress of Neurological Sciences. Cushing's disease: 50 years later. Can J Neurol Sci 1982;9:375–380.
15. Hofmann BM, Hlavac M, Kreutzer J, Grabenbauer G, Fahlbusch R. Surgical treatment of recurrent Cushing's disease. Neurosurgery 2006;58:1108–1118; discussion 1117–8.
16. Hofmann BM, Hlavac M, Martinez R, Buchfelder M, Muller OA, Fahlbusch R. Long-term results after microsurgery for Cushing disease: experience with 426 primary operations over 35 years. J Neurosurg 2008;108:9–18.
17. Invitti C, Pecori Giraldi F, de Martin M, Cavagnini F. Diagnosis and management of Cushing's syndrome: results of an Italian multicentre study. Study Group of the Italian Society of Endocrinology on the Pathophysiology of the Hypothalamic-Pituitary-Adrenal Axis. J Clin Endocrinol Metab 1999;84:440–448.
18. Jagannathan J, Kanter AS, Olson C, Sherman JH, Laws ER, Jr, Sheehan JP. Applications of radiotherapy and radiosurgery in the management of pediatric Cushing's disease: a review of the literature and our experience. J Neurooncol 2008;90:117–124.
19. Jagannathan J, Sheehan JP, Pouratian N, Laws ER, Steiner L, Vance ML. Gamma Knife surgery for Cushing's disease. J Neurosurg 2007;106:980–987.
20. Jane JA, Jr., Laws ER, Jr. The surgical management of pituitary adenomas in a series of 3,093 patients. J Am Coll Surg 2001;193:651–659.
21. Kane LA, Leinung MC, Scheithauer BW, Bergstralh EJ, Laws ER, Jr., Groover RV, Kovacs K, Horvath E, Zimmerman D. Pituitary adenomas in childhood and adolescence. J Clin Endocrinol Metab 1994;79:1135–1140.
22. Kanter AS, Diallo AO, Jane JA, Jr., Sheehan JP, Asthagiri AR, Oskouian RJ, Okonkwo DO, Sansur CA, Vance ML, Rogol AD, Laws ER, Jr. Single-center experience with pediatric Cushing's disease. J Neurosurg 2005;103:413–420.
23. Kim LJ, Lekovic GP, White WL, Karis J. Preliminary experience with 3-Tesla MRI and Cushing's disease. Skull Base 2007;17:273–277.
24. Knappe UJ, Ludecke DK. Persistent and recurrent hypercortisolism after transsphenoidal surgery for Cushing's disease. Acta Neurochir Suppl 1996;65:31–34.
25. Lanzino G, Maartens NF, Laws ER, Jr. Cushing's case XLV: Minnie G. J Neurosurg 2002;97:231–234.
26. Laws ER, Jr. Multiple pituitary adenomas. J Neurosurg 2000;93:909–911.
27. Laws ER, Jr. Pituitary pseudocapsule. J Neurosurg 2006;104:1–2; discussion 2–3.
28. Laws ER, Jr, Abboud CF, Kern EB. Perioperative management of patients with pituitary microadenoma. Neurosurgery 1980;7:566–570.
29. Laws ER, Reitmeyer M, Thapar K, Vance ML. Cushing's disease resulting from pituitary corticotrophic microadenoma. Treatment results from transsphenoidal microsurgery and gamma knife radiosurgery. Neurochirurgie 2002;48:294–299.
30. Laws ER, Scheithauer BW, Groover RV. Pituitary adenomas in childhood and adolescence. Prog Exp Tumor Res 1987;30:359–361.
31. Lefournier V, Martinie M, Vasdev A, Bessou P, Passagia JG, Labat-Moleur F, Sturm N, Bosson JL, Bachelot I, Chabre O. Accuracy of bilateral inferior petrosal or cavernous sinuses sampling in predicting the lateralization of Cushing's disease pituitary microadenoma: influence of catheter position and anatomy of venous drainage. J Clin Endocrinol Metab 2003;88:196–203.
32. Leinung MC, Kane LA, Scheithauer BW, Carpenter PC, Laws ER, Jr, Zimmerman D. Long term follow-up of transsphenoidal surgery for the treatment of Cushing's disease in childhood. J Clin Endocrinol Metab 1995;80:2475–2479.
33. Locatelli M, Vance ML, Laws ER. Clinical review: the strategy of immediate reoperation for transsphenoidal surgery for Cushing's disease. J Clin Endocrinol Metab 2005;90:5478–5482.
34. Meij BP, Lopes MB, Vance ML, Thorner MO, Laws ER, Jr. Double pituitary lesions in three patients with Cushing's disease. Pituitary 2000;3:159–168.
35. Oldfield EH, Doppman JL, Nieman LK, Chrousos GP, Miller DL, Katz DA, Cutler GB, Jr, Loriaux DL. Petrosal sinus sampling with and without corticotropin-releasing hormone for the differential diagnosis of Cushing's syndrome. N Engl J Med 1991;325:897–905.
36. Partington MD, Davis DH, Laws ER, Jr, Scheithauer BW. Pituitary adenomas in childhood and adolescence. Results of transsphenoidal surgery. J Neurosurg 1994;80:209–216.

37. Patil CG, Lad SP, Katznelson L, Laws ER, Jr. Brain atrophy and cognitive deficits in Cushing's disease. Neurosurg Focus 2007;23:E11.
38. Patil CG, Prevedello DM, Lad SP, Vance ML, Thorner MO, Katznelson L, Laws ER, Jr. Late recurrences of Cushing's disease after initial successful transsphenoidal surgery. J Clin Endocrinol Metab 2008;93:358–362.
39. Patil CG, Veeravagu A, Prevedello DM, Katznelson L, Vance ML, Laws ER, Jr. Outcomes after repeat transsphenoidal surgery for recurrent Cushing's disease. Neurosurgery 2008;63:266–270; discussion 270–1.
40. Pereira AM, van Aken MO, van Dulken H, Schutte PJ, Biermasz NR, Smit JW, Roelfsema F, Romijn JA. Long-term predictive value of postsurgical cortisol concentrations for cure and risk of recurrence in Cushing's disease. J Clin Endocrinol Metab 2003;88:5858–5864.
41. Pouratian N, Prevedello DM, Jagannathan J, Lopes MB, Vance ML, Laws ER, Jr. Outcomes and management of patients with Cushing's disease without pathological confirmation of tumor resection after transsphenoidal surgery. J Clin Endocrinol Metab 2007;92:3383–3388.
42. Prevedello DM, Pouratian N, Sherman J, Jane JA, Jr, Vance ML, Lopes MB, Laws ER, Jr. Management of Cushing's disease: outcome in patients with microadenoma detected on pituitary magnetic resonance imaging. J Neurosurg 2008;109:751–759.
43. Rees DA, Hanna FW, Davies JS, Mills RG, Vafidis J, Scanlon MF. Long-term follow-up results of transsphenoidal surgery for Cushing's disease in a single centre using strict criteria for remission. Clin Endocrinol (Oxf) 2002;56:541–551.
44. Rollin GA, Ferreira NP, Junges M, Gross JL, Czepielewski MA. Dynamics of serum cortisol levels after transsphenoidal surgery in a cohort of patients with Cushing's disease. J Clin Endocrinol Metab 2004;89:1131–1139.
45. Salassa RM, Laws ER, Carpenter PC, Northcutt RC. Cushing's disease-50 years later. Trans Am Clin Climatol Assoc 1983;94:122–129.
46. Salassa RM, Laws ER, Jr., Carpenter PC, Northcutt RC. Transsphenoidal removal of pituitary microadenoma in Cushing's disease. Mayo Clin Proc 1978;53:24–28.
47. Semple PL, Laws ER, Jr. Complications in a contemporary series of patients who underwent transsphenoidal surgery for Cushing's disease. J Neurosurg 1999;91:175–179.
48. Semple PL, Vance ML, Findling J, Laws ER. Transsphenoidal surgery for Cushing's disease: outcome in patients with a normal MRI scan. Neurosurgery 2000;46:553–559.
49. Sheehan JM, Vance ML, Sheehan JP, Ellegala DB, Laws ER, Jr. Radiosurgery for Cushing's disease after failed transsphenoidal surgery. J Neurosurg 2000;93:738–742.
50. Shimon I, Ram Z, Cohen ZR, Hadani M. Transsphenoidal surgery for Cushing's disease: endocrinological follow-up monitoring of 82 patients. Neurosurgery 2002;51:57–61; discussion 61–2.
51. Simmons NE, Alden TD, Thorner MO, Laws ER, Jr. Serum cortisol response to transsphenoidal surgery for Cushing disease. J Neurosurg 2001;95:1–8.
52. Simmons NE, Do HM, Lipper MH, Laws ER, Jr. Cerebral atrophy in Cushing's disease. Surg Neurol 2000;53:72–76.
53. Swearingen B, Biller BM, Barker FG, 2nd, Katznelson L, Grinspoon S, Klibanski A, Zervas NT. Long-term mortality after transsphenoidal surgery for Cushing disease. Ann Intern Med 1999;130:821–824.
54. Yap LB, Turner HE, Adams CB, Wass JA. Undetectable postoperative cortisol does not always predict long-term remission in Cushing's disease: a single centre audit. Clin Endocrinol (Oxf) 2002;56:25–31.

11 Adrenal-Directed Treatment Options for Cushing's Disease

William F. Young Jr. and Geoffrey B. Thompson

CONTENTS

SUMMARY

Adrenal-directed treatment for Cushing's disease should be considered when pituitary-directed treatment has not been successful. Bilateral adrenalectomy in this setting, although a secondary option, is a good treatment to decrease morbidity and mortality. Laparoscopic adrenalectomy is one of the most clinically important advances in the past two decades for the treatment of adrenal disorders. When compared to open adrenalectomy, laparoscopic adrenalectomy is equally safe, effective, and curative; it is more successful in shortening hospitalization and convalescence and has less long-term morbidity. The keys to successful laparoscopic adrenalectomy are appropriate patient selection, knowledge of anatomy, delicate tissue handling, meticulous hemostasis, and experience with the technique of laparoscopic adrenalectomy.

Key Words: Adrenalectomy, Cushing's syndrome, laparoscopic surgeries

INTRODUCTION AND BACKGROUND

The laparoscopic approach to removing the adrenal gland was first reported in 1992 *(1, 2)* and it has rapidly become the procedure of choice for unilateral adrenalectomy when the adrenal mass is less than 10 cm in size and there are no imaging findings to suggest malignancy (e.g., invasion of contiguous

From: *Contemporary Endocrinology: Cushing's Syndrome: Pathophysiology, Diagnosis and Treatment*
Edited by: M.D. Bronstein (ed.), DOI 10.1007/978-1-60327-449-4_11,

Table 1
Types of Cushing's Syndrome that may be Treated Laparoscopically

Unilateral adrenalectomy
Cortisol-producing adenoma
Asymmetric ACTH-independent macronodular adrenal hyperplasia (AIMAH)
Bilateral partial adrenalectomy
Bilateral cortisol-secreting adenomas
Bilateral adrenalectomy
ACTH-independent Cushing's syndrome caused by primary pigmented nodular adrenal disease (PPNAD) or AIMAH
ACTH-dependent Cushing's syndrome that failed attempts at removal of ACTH-secreting tumor (pituitary or ectopic)

ACTH corticotropin, *AIMAH* ACTH-independent macronodular adrenal hyperplasia, *PPNAD* primary pigmented nodular adrenal disease

structures, nodal or distant metastases) *(3)*. When compared to open adrenalectomy, the laparoscopic approach is associated with shorter postoperative recovery time and less long-term morbidity *(3)*.

In a review of 2,550 laparoscopic adrenalectomy procedures reported in the literature, the most frequent adrenal disorder operated laparoscopically was aldosterone-producing adenoma (36%) followed by cortisol-producing adenoma (19%), apparent nonfunctioning cortical adenoma (18%), and pheochromocytoma (18%) *(3)*. However, patients with corticotropin (ACTH)-dependent Cushing's syndrome who have experienced failed attempts to remove the ACTH-secreting neoplasm – whether pituitary or ectopic – are also ideal candidates for one-stage bilateral laparoscopic adrenalectomy *(4–6)*. The types of Cushing's syndrome that can be treated with laparoscopic unilateral or bilateral adrenalectomy are summarized in Table 1.

ADVANTAGES OF THE LAPAROSCOPIC APPROACH

The surgical approach to adrenal was revolutionized with the introduction of the laparoscope. Although laparoscopic adrenalectomy is technically more demanding to perform than conventional open anterior or posterior adrenalectomy, it is associated with shorter hospitalization, less morbidity, and earlier return to daily activities *(3, 6–12)*. Conventional open adrenalectomy – by the anterior or posterior approach – requires a large incision to gain access to a relatively small gland. In addition, the incision used for posterior adrenalectomy, with its associated 12th rib resection and subcostal nerve retraction, has been associated with incisional and musculoskeletal problems that may persist long after the operation *(6, 13)*. These incisional problems are especially pronounced and severe in patients with Cushing's syndrome because of poor wound healing, laxity of the abdominal wall, and glucocorticoid-associated obesity *(14–17)*.

BILATERAL LAPAROSCOPIC ADRENALECTOMY

Bilateral laparoscopic adrenalectomy is an excellent treatment option for patients with ACTH-dependent Cushing's syndrome after failed pituitary surgery or when the ACTH source cannot be resected or localized in patients with ectopic ACTH syndrome *(5, 18–20)*. When compared to the open approach, bilateral laparoscopic adrenal surgery is associated with much less tissue injury in patients who are immunocompromised and/or are predisposed to delayed wound healing. An additional advantage – because of the magnification – is better visibility of the surgical field, thus decreasing the risk for retained remnants and adrenal rest tissue.

Although transsphenoidal surgery for resection of an ACTH-secreting pituitary tumor is the treatment of choice in patients with pituitary-dependent disease, this surgery is not always successful *(21–24)* because the pituitary adenoma may invade areas that are not surgically accessible (e.g., cavernous sinuses) or it is so small that it escapes detection and resection at the time of pituitary surgery. Thus, transsphenoidal surgery for pituitary-dependent Cushing's syndrome is associated with a 20–40% failure rate *(23–27)*. Because reoperation in these patients carries an increased risk of causing panhypopituitarism, bilateral adrenalectomy has an important therapeutic role in this setting.

Radiation therapy to the sella is not an optimal therapy for Cushing's disease because its onset of action is slow and the failure rate is unacceptably high *(28)*. The main side effect is varying degrees of pituitary insufficiency *(29)*. Because bilateral laparoscopic adrenalectomy results in immediate cure of hypercortisolism, the role of pituitary irradiation should be limited to those that demonstrate pituitary tumor growth following bilateral adrenalectomy (Nelson's syndrome) – in this setting sellar radiation therapy or gamma knife radiosurgery are used to prevent a locally invasive pituitary tumor from further encroaching on surrounding structures. However, the clinician should recognize that a fear of Nelson's syndrome should never dissuade proceeding with a definitive cure for Cushing's syndrome.

Patients with the syndrome of ectopic ACTH secretion often have an unresectable, metastatic, or occult source of ACTH secretion *(30, 31)* (see also Chap. 14). In these patients, the metabolic manifestations of cortisol excess may appear suddenly and progress rapidly. However, most patients with clinically evident ectopic ACTH syndrome have more indolent tumors, such as bronchial or thymic carcinoid tumors, islet cell tumors, or medullary carcinoma of the thyroid. Carcinoid tumors that secrete ACTH may not be apparent even with careful radiological investigation and may take up to 20 years to localize *(31)*. When the source of ACTH is unresectable or occult, bilateral laparoscopic adrenalectomy is a life-saving treatment option because of the minimal morbidity associated with the procedure, especially when compared with conventional adrenalectomy *(5, 18, 19)*. Laparoscopic adrenalectomy is also superior to medical therapy in regard to tolerance, efficacy, and safety *(19)*. Bilateral laparoscopic adrenalectomy offers improved quality of life and palliation of hypercortisolism-related symptoms even in patients with disseminated, untreatable malignancy *(18)*.

Long-term medical management of Cushing's syndrome is not an optimal treatment option. The adrenal enzyme inhibitors, aminogluthetimide, metyrapone, mitotane, and ketoconazole, are the pharmaceuticals used most often to treat Cushing's syndrome medically. However, complete blockade of adrenal steroid synthesis is typically achieved only transiently; ACTH levels usually increase and override the blockade – leading to additional increases in the dosage of the enzyme inhibitor. The frequency of patient intolerance and side effects (e.g., liver enzyme abnormalities) of these medications is high and few patients are able to tolerate long-term pharmacologic therapy (see Chap. 13).

Since the description of laparoscopic adrenalectomy in 1992 *(1, 2)*, multiple centers have described their experience with bilateral laparoscopic adrenalectomy for the treatment of Cushing's syndrome *(3–5, 32–38)*. Increased experience with the technique has resulted in a decreased conversion rate to open adrenalectomy as well as decreased complications. At our center – between January of 1995 and October of 2006 – bilateral laparoscopic adrenalectomy was attempted in 68 patients with ACTH-dependent Cushing's syndrome (26, ectopic ACTH syndrome; 42, persistent pituitary-dependent Cushing's syndrome following pituitary surgery) and was successfully completed in 59 of 68 patients (87%); 9 (13%) required conversion to open adrenalectomy *(5)*. Intra-operative complications occurred in 3 patients (4.4%) and non-operative complications occurred in 11 (16%) patients. There were no perioperative deaths. In patients with follow-up data available, all achieved biochemical resolution and at least partial clinical resolution of signs and symptoms associated with hypercortisolism. Resolution of hypertension, diabetes, and obesity was achieved in 64, 29, and 35% of patients carrying those diagnoses prior to surgery, respectively *(5)*.

SURGICAL APPROACHES TO THE ADRENAL GLAND

In the past, the open posterior retroperitoneal approach was favored by many adrenal surgeons because, when compared to the open anterior approach, it resulted in less pain, a shortened period of ileus, fewer pulmonary complications, and less blood loss *(39)*. For laparoscopic adrenalectomy, the lateral transabdominal approach is preferred by most surgeons – the lateral decubitus position of the patient and the medial rotation of the viscera allow gravity to keep the liver, bowel, and spleen away from the surgical field. The posterior retroperitoneoscopic approach to the adrenal has not been found to be superior to the lateral transabdominal approach. However, this approach may be indicated in patients who have had prior upper abdominal surgery *(40)*. Some surgeons prefer the posterior retroperitoneoscopic approach because of shorter operating time, reduced blood loss, reduced risk of injury to the viscera, and lack of interference from previous abdominal surgery *(41, 42)*.

Regardless of the approach, the keys to successful adrenalectomy are knowledge of the anatomy, delicate tissue handling, and meticulous hemostasis. Since clinical outcomes are similar amongst the different approaches for endoscope-based adrenalectomy *(4)*, the choice of the approach is dependent upon surgeon preference and the clinical setting.

LAPAROSCOPIC TECHNIQUE

General endotracheal anesthesia is used. The patient is placed in the lateral decubitus position with the affected adrenal gland placed in the upper position. The operating table placed in the flexed position so that the patient's flank is maximally exposed. The initial skin incision – 1 cm in length – is 2 cm below and parallel to the costal margin and the pneumoperitoneum is established with carbon dioxide. Then the surgeon places three to four 10-mm trocar ports – the laparoscope is initially placed through the most anterior trocar and working instruments through the other ports (camera and instruments are interchangeable throughout the dissection). The right adrenal gland approach involves: mobilization of the lateral attachments of the liver for medial rotation and elevation; inferior retraction of the kidney; exposure of adrenal vein and vena cava. The left adrenal gland approach involves: mobilization of the splenic flexure of the colon along its attachments to the spleen; mobilization of the spleen and pancreas to allow for medial visceral rotation; exposure of left adrenal vein/inferior phrenic vein junction; and mobilization of the adrenal gland along Gerota's fascia. For both the right and left adrenal glands, the main adrenal is vein identified, clipped and transected; the adrenal gland and tumor are resected and placed in a retrieval pouch and delivered via a port site. The adrenal vein may be transected early or late in the dissection depending on the ease of exposure.

Most patients begin a clear liquid diet the evening of surgery and a regular diet the next day. Patients are encouraged to ambulate the evening of surgery. Most patients undergoing unilateral adrenalectomy may be dismissed from the hospital on postoperative day 1 or 2. Bilateral adrenalectomy patients and patients with severe Cushing's syndrome may require more than a 2-day hospitalization.

EFFICACY OF LAPAROSCOPIC ADRENALECTOMY

Prospective human randomized controlled trials comparing laparoscopic adrenalectomy to any of the open surgical approaches has not and will not be done *(3)*. In a prospective randomized study done at the Mayo Clinic, we examined the acute-phase response and wound healing in laparoscopic adrenalectomy vs. open adrenalectomy in a cushingoid porcine model *(17)*. Nitrogen balance, wound scores, and tensile strength at 24 h and 1 week were more favorable in the laparoscopic adrenalectomy group than the open adrenalectomy group. At least 20 case–control retrospective comparative studies in humans have evaluated the efficacy of laparoscopic adrenalectomy *(3)*. All of the studies reported less analgesia requirement, less blood loss, lower complication rate, and shorter hospital stay for laparoscopic than open adrenalectomy *(3)*. At Mayo Clinic, we performed a matched case–control study comparing 50 patients having laparoscopic adrenalectomy to 50 patients having adrenalectomy through the open posterior approach *(6)*. We found that laparoscopic adrenalectomy, compared to open adrenalectomy, was associated with shorter hospital stay, less postoperative narcotic use, more rapid return to normal activity, increased patient satisfaction, and less late morbidity. The late morbidity associated with posterior open adrenalectomy includes chronic pain, marked laxity involving the oblique muscles, and bothersome flank numbness *(6)*. The average conversion rate from laparoscopic to open adrenalectomy in a total of 2,550 patients from 28 reports was 3.6% *(3)*. The reasons for conversion included bleeding, adhesions, difficulty of dissection, unexpected malignancy, large size of tumor, vascular invasion, inadvertent pancreatic injury, damage to the pleura, failure to identify the adrenal tumor, and unsuspected Bochdalek hernia *(6, 43–46)*.

RISKS OF LAPAROSCOPIC ADRENALECTOMY

The surgeon sacrifices some tactile sensation, when compared to open surgery, and the small, flat, friable adrenal gland is manipulated with instruments in a two-dimensional plane. The overall complication rate associated with laparoscopic adrenalectomy from a summary of 2,550 procedures was 9.5% *(3)*. Some complications of laparoscopic adrenalectomy include bleeding, gland fragmentation, wound hematomas, organ injury, port site incisional hernia *(47)*, and port site pain *(48)*. Nerve root pain has been reported with the posterior retroperitoneoscopic adrenalectomy approach *(42)*. There is risk of violating the tumor capsule and organ parenchyma during manipulation with the laparoscopic instruments. In one series involving 88 patients *(43)* there was a 12% postoperative complication rate (e.g., deep venous thrombosis, hematomas, anemia), a 3% conversion rate to open adrenalectomy, and no mortality. In a series of 560 adrenalectomies by the posterior retroperitoneoscopic approach the mortality was zero; conversions to open or laparoscopic lateral surgery were necessary in nine patients (1.7%); major complications occurred in 1.3% of patients; minor complications in 14.4% *(40)*.

In patients with ACTH-dependent Cushing's syndrome, any viable cortical cells left behind in the patient will result in persistent/recurrent hypercortisolism *(4)*. The mortality rate for 2,550 laparoscopic adrenalectomies was 0.2% *(3)*; four of the seven deaths occurred in patients with Cushing's disease who underwent bilateral laparoscopic adrenalectomy *(3)*.

SUMMARY

Laparoscopic adrenalectomy is safe, effective, curative, and shortens hospitalization and convalescence. Laparoscopic adrenalectomy is the procedure of choice for the surgical management of Cushing's syndrome patients who have ACTH-dependent Cushing's syndrome and failed surgery for the removal of the source of ACTH. The keys to successful laparoscopic adrenalectomy are appropriate patient selection, knowledge of anatomy, delicate tissue handling, meticulous hemostasis, and experience with advanced laparoscopic surgery.

REFERENCES

1. Gagner M, Lacroix A, Bolte E. Laparoscopic adrenalectomy in Cushings syndrome and pheochromocytoma [Letter]. N Engl J Med 1992;327:1033.
2. Higashihara E, Tanaka Y, Horie S, Aruga S, Nutahara, K, Homma Y, et al. A case report of laparoscopic adrenalectomy. Nippon Hinyokika Gakkai Zassh 1992;83:1130–1133.
3. Assalia A, Gagner M. Laparoscopic adrenalectomy. Br J Surg 2004;91:1259–1274.
4. Chapuis Y, Chastanet S, Dousset B, Luton J-P. Bilateral laparoscopic adrenalectomy for disease. Br J Surg 1997;84:1009.
5. Chow JT, Thompson GB, Grant CS, Farley DR, Richards ML, Young WF Jr. Bilateral laparoscopic adrenalectomy for corticotrophin-dependent Cushing's syndrome: a review of the Mayo Clinic experience. Clin Endocrinol (Oxf) 2008;68:513–519.
6. Thompson GB, Grant CS, van Heerden JA, Schlinkert RT, Young WF Jr, Farley DR, et al. Laparoscopic versus open posterior adrenalectomy: a case-control study of 100 patients. Surgery 1997;122:1132–1136.
7. Korman JE, Ho T, Hiatt JR, Phillips EH Comparison of laparoscopic and open adrenalectomy. Am Surg. 1997;63:908–912.
8. Guazzoni G, Montorsi F, Bocciardi A, Da Pozzo L, Rigatti P, Lanzi R, et al. Transperitoneal laparoscopic versus open adrenalectomy for benign hyperfunctioning adrenal tumors: a comparative study. J Urol 1995;153:1597–1600.
9. Prinz RA,. A comparison of laparoscopic and open adrenalectomies. Arch Surg 1995;130:489–494.
10. MacGillivray DC, Shichman SJ, Ferrer FA, Malchoff CD. A comparison of open vs laparoscopic adrenalectomy. Surg Endoscopy 1996;10:987–990.
11. Hansen P, Bax T, Swanstrom L. Laparoscopic adrenalectomy: history, indications, and current techniques for a minimally invasive approach to adrenal pathology. Endoscopy 1997;29:309–314.
12. Horgan S, Sinanan M, Helton WS, Pellegrini CA. Use of laparoscopic techniques improves outcome from adrenalectomy. Am J Surg 1997;173:371–374.
13. Buell JF, Alexander HR, Norton JA, Yu KC, Fraker DL. Bilateral adrenalectomy for Cushings syndrome. Anterior versus posterior surgical approach. Ann Surg 1997;225:63–68.
14. van Heerden JA, Young, Jr. WF, Grant CS, Carpenter PC. Adrenal surgery for hypercortisolism: surgical aspects. Surgery 1995;117:466–472.
15. Watson RG, van Heerden JA, Northcutt RC, Grant CS, Ilstrup DM. Results of adrenal surgery for Cushings syndrome: 10 years experience. World J Surg 1986;10:531–538.
16. O'Riordain DS, Farley DR, Young WF Jr, Grant CS, van Heerden JA. Long-term outcome of bilateral adrenalectomy in patients with Cushings syndrome. Surgery 1994;116:1088–1093.
17. Kollmorgen CF, Thompson GB, Grant CS, van Heerden JA, Byrne J, Davies ET, et al. Laparoscopic versus open posterior adrenalectomy: comparison of acute-phase response and wound healing in the cushingoid porcine model. World J Surg 1998;22:613–620.
18. Thompson SK, Hayman AV, Ludlam WH, Deveney CW, Loriaux DL, Sheppard BC. Improved quality of life after bilateral laparoscopic adrenalectomy for Cushing's disease: a 10-year experience. Ann Surg 2007;245:790–794.
19. Mikhail AA, Tolhurst SR, Orvieto MA, Stockton BR, Zorn KC, Weiss RE, Kaplan EL, Shalhav AL. Open versus laparoscopic simultaneous bilateral adrenalectomy. Urology 2006;67:693–696.
20. Takata MC, Kebebew E, Clark OH, Duh QY. Laparoscopic bilateral adrenalectomy: results for 30 consecutive cases. Surg Endosc 2008;22:202–207.
21. Swearingen B, Biller BM, Barker FG, Katznelson L, Grinspoon S, Klibanski A, et al. Long-term mortality after transsphenoidal surgery for Cushing disease. Ann Intern Med 1999;130:821–824.
22. Mampalam TJ, Tyrrell JB, Wilson CB. Transsphenoidal microsurgery for Cushing disease: a report of 216 cases. Ann Intern Med 1988;109:487–493.
23. Patil CG, Prevedello DM, Lad SP, Vance ML, Thorner MO, Katznelson L, Laws ER Jr. Late recurrences of Cushing's disease after initial successful transsphenoidal surgery. J Clin Endocrinol Metab 2008;93:358–362.
24. Biller BM, Grossman AB, Stewart PM, Melmed S, Bertagna X, Bertherat J, Buchfelder M, Colao A, Hermus AR, Hofland LJ, Klibanski A, Lacroix A, Lindsay JR, Newell-Price J, Nieman LK, Petersenn S, Sonino N, Stalla GK,

Swearingen B, Vance ML, Wass JA, Boscaro M. Treatment of adrenocorticotropin-dependent Cushing's syndrome: a consensus statement. J Clin Endocrinol Metab 2008;93:2454–2462.
25 McCance DR, Russell CF, Kennedy TL, Hadden DR, Kennedy L, Atkinson AB. Bilateral adrenalectomy: low mortality and morbidity in Cushings disease. Clin Endocrinol (Oxf) 1993;39:315–321.
26 Tahir AH, Sheeler LR Recurrent Cushings disease after transsphenoidal surgery. Arch Intern Med 1992;152:977–981.
27. Toms GC, McCarthy MI, Niven MJ, Orteu CH, King TT, Monson JP. Predicting relapse after transsphenoidal surgery for Cushings disease. J Clin Endocrinol Metab 1993;76:291–294.
28. Orth DN, Liddle GW. Results of treatment in 108 patients with Cushings syndrome. N Engl J Med 1972;285:243–247.
29. Estrada J, Boronat M, Mielgo M, Magallon R, Millan I, Diez S, et al. The long-term outcome of pituitary irradiation after unsuccessful transsphenoidal surgery in Cushings disease. N Engl J Med 1997;336:172–177.
30. Ilias I, Torpy DJ, Pacak K, Mullen N, Wesley RA, Nieman LK. Cushing's syndrome due to ectopic corticotropin secretion: twenty years' experience at the National Institutes of Health. J Clin Endocrinol Metab 2005;90:4955–4962.
31. Aniszewski JP, Young WF Jr, Thompson GB, Grant CS, van Heerden JA. Cushing syndrome due to ectopic adrenocorticotropic hormone secretion. World J Surg 2001;25:934–940.
32. Chapuis Y. Laparoscopic versus Young–Mayor open posterior adrenalectomy: a case-control study of 100 patients. Chirurgie 1998;123:322–323.
33. Chapuis Y, Pitre J, Conti F, Abboud B, Pras-Jude N, Luton JP. Role and operative risk of bilateral adrenalectomy in hypercortisolism. World J Surg 1996;20:775–779.
34. Ferrer FA, MacGillivray DC, Malchoff CD, Albala DM, Shichman SJ. Bilateral laparoscopic adrenalectomy for adrenocorticotropic dependent Cushings syndrome. J Urol 1997;157:16–18.
35. Bax TW, Marcus DR, Galloway GO, Swanstrom LL, Sheppard BC. Laparoscopic bilateral adrenalectomy following failed hypophysectomy. Surg Endosc 1996;10:1150–1153.
36. Lanzi R, Montorsi F, Losa M, Centemero A, Manzoni MF, Rigatti P, et al. Laparoscopic bilateral adrenalectomy for persistent Cushing's disease after transsphenoidal surgery. Surgery 1998;123:144–150.
37. Acosta E, Pantoja JP, Famino R, Rull JA, Herrera MF. Laparoscopic versus open adrenalectomy in Cushing's syndrome and disease. Surgery 1999;126:1111–1116.
38. Hawn MT, Cook D, Deveney C, Sheppard BC. Quality of life after laparoscopic bilateral adrenalectomy for Cushing's disease. Surgery 2002;132:1064–1069.
39. Proye CA, Huart JY, Cuvillier XD, Assez NM, Gambardella B, Carnaille BM. Safety of the posterior approach in adrenal surgery: experience in 105 cases. Surgery 1993;114:1126–1131.
40. Walz MK, Alesina PF, Wenger FA, Deligiannis A, Szuczik E, Petersenn S, et al. Posterior retroperitoneoscopic adrenalectomy – results of 560 procedures in 520 patients. Surgery. 2006;140:943–950.
41. Miyake O, Yoshimura K, Yoshioka T, Honda M, Kokado Y, Miki T, et al. Laparoscopic adrenalectomy. Comparison of the transperitoneal and retroperitoneal approach. Eur Urol 1998;33:303–307.
42. Duh QY, Siperstein AE, Clark OH, Schecter WP, Horn JK, Harrison MR, et al. Laparoscopic adrenalectomy. Comparison of the lateral and posterior approaches. Arch Surg. 1996;131:870–876.
43. Gagner M, Pomp A, Haeniford BT, Pharand D, Lacroix A. Laparoscopic adrenalectomy: lessons learned from 100 consecutive procedures. Ann Surg 1997;226:238–247.
44. Higashihara E, Baba S, Nakagawa K, Murai M, Go H, Takeda M, et al. Learning curve and conversion to open surgery in cases of laparoscopic adrenalectomy and nephrectomy. J Urol. 1988;159:650–653.
45. Bonjer HJ, Lange JF, Kazemier G, de Herder WW, Steyerberg EW, Bruining HA. Comparison of three techniques for adrenalectomy. Br J Surg 1997;84:679–682.
46. Shen WT, Kebebew E, Clark OH, Duh Q-Y. Reasons for conversion from laparoscopic to open or hand-assisted adrenalectomy: review of 261 laparoscopic adrenalectomies from 1993 to 2003. World J Surg 2004;28:1176–1179.
47. Rutherford JC, Stowasser M, Tunny TJ, Klemm SA, Gordon RD. Laparoscopic adrenalectomy. World J Surg 1996;20: 758–761.
48. Vargas HI, Kavoussi LR, Bartlett DL, Wagner JR, Venzon DJ, Fraker DL, et al. Laparoscopic adrenalectomy: a new standard of care. Urology 1997;49:673–678.

12 Radiation Therapy and Stereotactic Radiosurgery for Cushing's Disease

Jay Jagannathan, Edward R. Laws, and Jason P. Sheehan

CONTENTS

SUMMARY

Although transsphenoidal resection is the mainstay of treatment, recurrent or residual ACTH-secreting adenomas are well suited for radiosurgery. Using a stereotactic device, radiation can be focused on a well-circumscribed region such as an adenoma and shielding of the nerves and eloquent structures in the suprasellar and parasellar regions. Radiosurgery is effective in inducing endocrine remission, even in cases where magnetic resonance (MR)-imaging is negative. This chapter reviews the indications and outcomes of stereotactic radiosurgery for Cushing's Disease.

Key Words: Cushing's disease, adenoma, pituitary, radiosurgery, stereotactic

INTRODUCTION AND EVOLUTION OF RADIATION TECHNIQUES

Pituitary adenomas represent 10–20% of all primary brain tumors *(1, 2)*. Lesions are broadly classified into two groups, depending on the presence or absence of secreted pituitary hormones. Tumors that secrete an excessive amount of a hormone are associated with various clinical syndromes. One of the most challenging pituitary adenomas from a treatment standpoint is ACTH-secreting adenomas. These tumors can be difficult to discern on magnetic resonance (MR) imaging *(3)*, and, even in the hands of an experienced surgical team, a significant number of patients may not achieve remission after transsphenoidal or transcranial resection of the adenoma *(4)*.

From: *Contemporary Endocrinology: Cushing's Syndrome: Pathophysiology, Diagnosis and Treatment*
Edited by: M.D. Bronstein (ed.), DOI 10.1007/978-1-60327-449-4_12,

Historically, external beam radiation therapy was the adjuvant treatment of choice for recurrent or residual pituitary adenomas. In their landmark series on the utility of conventional radiotherapy for pediatric Cushing's disease, Jennings et al. *(5)* reviewed the results of this radiotherapy in 15 Cushing's disease patients, successfully achieving remission in 12 (80%) within 18 months of radiation treatment, and 10 of the 15 were cured within 9 months of radiation. The remaining three patients however, required bilateral adrenalectomy for treatment failure. In another article by Estrada et al. *(6)*, external beam radiation therapy (mean 50 Gy) was used to treat 30 patients with persistent or recurrent Cushing's disease. Eighty-three percent of patients achieved remission within a 6–60-month period following radiation therapy; 57% developed growth hormone deficiency (Table 1).

Since this initial work, more contemporary data has demonstrated serious limitations of conventional radiotherapy in treating Cushing's disease – the time to hormonal normalization is slow and the rate of post-procedural hypopituitarism is high. Long-term sequelae such as cognitive deficits, visual dysfunction, radiation induced necrosis, radiation induced neoplasia, optic neuropathy, and stroke have been well described *(7)*. The incidence of cerebrovascular accidents and radiation induced neoplasia at 20 years for pituitary patients following radiation therapy are 21 and 2.4% *(8–10)*. Although Cushing's disease is a serious health problem if left untreated, many physicians became concerned that with radiation therapy that the "cure" was worse than the disease.

These aforementioned disadvantages with conventional radiation therapy led to the investigation of stereotactic radiosurgery as a treatment option for persistent Cushing's disease. The advantages of stereotactic radiosurgery over conventional radiation therapy include a higher biologic equivalent dose, steep fall off, image guidance, and small treatment volume. Moreover, the serious risks of hypopituitarism, stroke, and radiation-induced neoplasia appear to be substantially less with radiosurgery *(11)*.

Shortly after radiosurgery's development, Lars Leksell treated patients with pituitary tumors using the Gamma Knife (GK); original localization was achieved through use of plain radiographs of the sella *(12)*. With more recent advances in neuro-imaging including positron emission tomography (PET) scans and fat saturation MRI, the Gamma Knife and other radiosurgical

Table 1
Conventional Radiation in Pediatric Cushing's Disease

Series	*Patients (n)*	*Follow-up (months)*	*Remission rate (%)*	*Remission criteria*
Estrada et al. *(6)*	30	42	83	24-UFC
Pandey et al. *(76)*	11	34	100	24-UFC
Storr et al. *(77)*	7	83	86	Post-operative serum cortisol
Thoren et al. *(78)*	8	56	86	24-UFC
Minniti et al. *(79)*	40	113	73 (3 years) 84 (10 years)	Plasma Cortisol
Jennings et al. *(5)*	15	18	80	24-UFC

devices have been utilized to control adenoma growth and normalize hormone over-production for many Cushing's patients *(7, 13, 14)*. This chapter reviews the current status of radiosurgery for Cushing's disease.

ESTABLISHED RADIOSURGICAL MODALITIES FOR PITUITARY TUMORS

A variety of radiosurgical treatment options exist for the pituitary, each with potential advantages and limitations. Proton beam radiosurgery was one of the earliest modalities used for the treatment of pituitary tumors *(15, 16)*. This technique takes advantage of the superior dose distribution of protons vs. photons, due to the peak in the energy distribution of protons ("Bragg-peak") before they come to rest at the treatment depth *(17)*. This gives the theoretical advantage of producing very little lateral disruption and essentially no exit dose, and proton beam therapy can be used in the treatment of deep-seated lesions in the sella or near the cavernous sinus. Early studies on proton beam radiosurgery were complicated by high rates of hypopituitarism, a factor likely related to the nascent treatment planning of the time *(15)*. Reports on modern proton beam therapy have a lower rate of hypopituitarism, although even more contemporary reports demonstrate that more than half of all patients treated with the Proton Beam for Cushing's Disease developed endocrine deficits – a number that is significantly higher than those seen with other radiosurgical modalities *(18)*. However the major limitation of the technique is that proton beam (cyclotron) facilities are only available at a very limited number of centers worldwide *(19)*. Recent technological advances with more compact cyclotrons and dielectric wall accelerator technology may make proton technology more cost effective. However, in the absence of compelling clinical studies to demonstrate superiority for cranial radiosurgery, the reduction of the price of a unit from greater than $100 million to $20–30 million will likely do little to stimulate the widespread adoption of proton-based radiosurgery *(20)*.

In LINAC-based radiosurgery, multiple radiation arcs are used to crossfire photon beams at a target defined in stereotactic space *(21–23)*. LINAC-based radiosurgery devices include the Cyberknife (Accuray), Trilogy (Varian), Synergy (Elekta), Tomotherapy (Tomotherapy, Inc.), and X-Knife (Radionics). Most of the current systems use non-dynamic techniques in which the patient couch is set at an angle and the arc is moved around its radius to deliver radiation that enters the skull through many different points. Numerous techniques have been developed to enhance conformity of dose planning and delivery using LINAC-based systems. These include beam shaping and intensity modulation *(24–26)*. Newer developments include the introduction of jaws, noncircular, and mini- and micro-leaf collimators *(27)*. The conformal beam can be delivered with the micromultileaf collimator or conformal blocks.

Gamma Knife radiosurgery usually involves multiple isocenters of different beam diameter to achieve a dose plan that conforms to the irregular three-dimensional volumes of most mass lesions (Fig. 1). The total number of isocenters varies depending upon the size and shape of the adenoma and the proximity of surrounding at-risk structures (e.g., the optic nerves or chiasm). The most recent version of the Gamma Knife, the Perfexion, combines advances in dose planning, beam collimation, and robotic engineering, and it eliminates the need to set coordinates manually for each isocenter.

No published comparisons of GK multiple isocenter techniques, linear accelerator or proton beam has shown a clear advantage of one technique over another with regard to sparing normal tissue, achieving endocrine remission or reducing complications *(28, 29)*. As with other neurosurgical procedures, the outcome may depend less on the radiosurgical device utilized and more upon the approach taken by an experienced radiosurgical team.

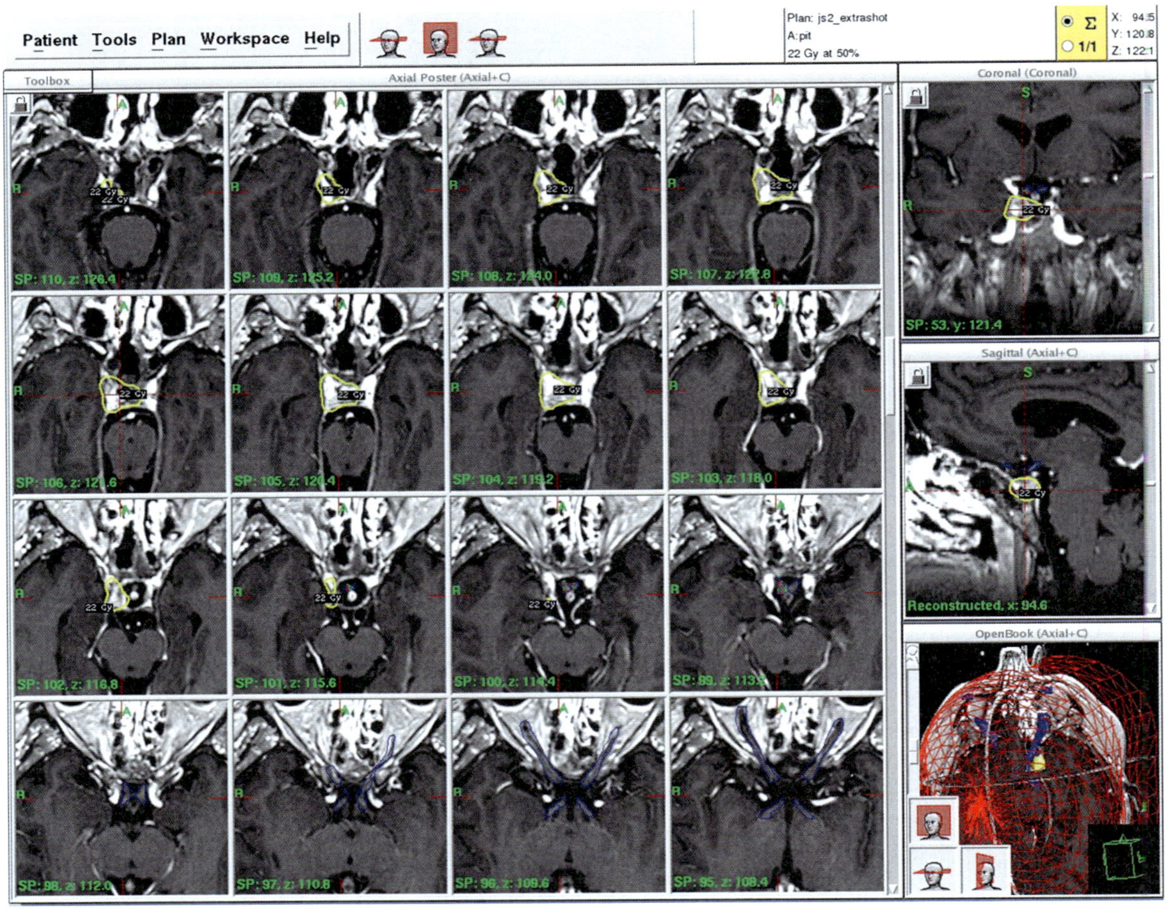

Fig. 1. A Gamma Knife dose plan for a patient with persistent Cushing's Disease. The patient had a prior trans-sphenoidal resection of her pituitary adenoma. Unfortunately, the adenoma was found to invade the right cavernous sinus. A Gamma Knife dose plan was developed to treat the residual adenoma and 22 Gy was delivered to the adenoma margin (*yellow*). The optic apparatus is outlined in *blue* and less than 8 Gy was delivered to it.

RADIOSURGICAL PLANNING AND TECHNIQUE

Treatment Planning

Most patients undergo immobilization either with a stereotactic frame or aquaplast mask. Once the target is immobilized, planning neuro-imaging studies are obtained. In the current era, stereotactic MR imaging using pre and post-contrast T1 sequences with fat suppression techniques are utilized for patients with pituitary adenomas. Axial and coronal slices are performed. Stereotactic CT imaging can be performed so as to co-register to MRI and may help in minimizing registration error; it can also be utilized for those that are unable to have an MRI (e.g., a patient with a cardiac pacemaker). PET imaging can also be employed and may have some utility in functional adenomas such as those in Cushing's patient *(30)*. Careful attention should also be paid to pre-resection imaging studies, intra-operative observations from the neurosurgeon, and petrosal sinus sampling *(31)*.

After the acquisition of stereotactic images, multiple isocenter dose planning is performed to enclose the borders of the tumor within the prescription isodose line *(32,33)*. The 50% isodose is the most common prescription isodose line for Gamma Knife radiosurgery because this line is generally where dose gradient is the steepest *(34)*. However, one should analyze the dose gradient and determine the optimal fall off isodose, which generally varies between 40 and 60% *(35)*.

There does not appear to be a direct correlation between the effect on adenoma volume and the endocrine remission rate following radiosurgery *(7, 36, 37)*. Fortunately, since most ACTH-secreting pituitary adenomas are small enough to be well-suited for stereotactic radiosurgery, radiosurgical dose–volume constraints are not usually a limiting factor. Since the systemic effects of Cushing's disease can be so devastating, it seems intuitive to deliver a reasonably high dose (equal to or greater than 20 Gy to the margin) to allow rapid hormonal normalization and control of adenoma growth. For improved rates of hormonal normalization in functioning adenomas, margin dose of 25 or 30 Gy may even be chosen.

In cases of Cushing's disease with radiologically identifiable targets in the cavernous sinus, radiosurgical plans can be devised with higher range treatment doses while shielding much of the normal stalk, gland, and optic apparatus, in other cases, particularly when MR-imaging is negative, the entire sellar contents and bilateral cavernous sinuses are targeted.

Neuro-Anatomical Considerations: Radiation Effects on the Optic Apparatus, Structures Within the Cavernous Sinus, and the Normal Pituitary Gland

Visual deterioration following radiosurgery is rare and can generally be avoided if the dose to the optic apparatus is restricted to less than 8 Gy, although reports of 10–12 Gy have been described by some groups *(38)*. Traditionally, a distance of 3 mm or more between the adenoma and the optic apparatus is desirable. The absolute distance between the optic apparatus is not the limiting factor, but rather defines how steeply the radiosurgical gradient must be constructed so that a tolerable dose is delivered to the optic apparatus while still delivering an effective dose to the adenoma. If an acceptable dose gradient cannot be constructed, then an alternative treatment (e.g. cytoreductive surgery or radiation therapy) should be considered. The Gamma Knife Perfexion permits treatment of some adenoma with as little clearance as 1–2 mm from the optic apparatus *(7, 39–42)*. Ultimately, the tolerable absolute dose permitted to the optic apparatus likely varies from patient to patient, and it may be affected by factors such as previous damage to the optic apparatus by pituitary adenoma compression, ischemic changes, type and timing of previous interventions (e.g., fractionated radiation therapy and surgery), the patient's age, and the presence or absence of other co-morbidities *(43, 44)*.

The majority of cranial nerves in the cavernous sinus appear to be more resistant to radiation effects than the optic nerve, but reports of cranial neuropathy, particularly after repeat radiosurgery are well-documented *(43)*. Although the tolerable limit to the cavernous sinus nerves is unknown, authors have described effective margin radiosurgical doses of between 15–25 Gy to this region without major side effects *(7, 45–49)*. Injury to the cavernous segment of the carotid artery is rare after radiosurgery, with a few isolated case reports *(50)*.

EFFECTIVENESS OF RADIOSURGERY FOR PITUITARY ADENOMAS

The goals of stereotactic radiosurgery in the treatment of Cushing's disease pituitary tumors are to inactivate adenoma cells, controlling tumor growth and to normalize hormone overproduction. Ideally, these goals are met without damaging the residual normal pituitary gland and surrounding vascular and neuronal structures. Moreover, radiosurgery should be carried out in such a way so as to avoid delayed radiation injury and secondary tumor formation.

Most centers define an endocrine remission for Cushing's disease as a 24 h urine-free cortisol (UFC) in the normal range associated with the resolution of clinical stigmata or a series of normal post-radiosurgical serum cortisol levels obtained throughout the day *(37, 51)*.

Reported endocrine remission rates following transsphenoidal vary from 10% to 100%, with higher remission rates when radiosurgery follows surgical debulking (Table 2) *(13, 14, 42, 43, 52–56)*. In series with at least ten patients and a median follow-up of 2 years, endocrine remission rates range from 17 to 83% *(54–57)*. Rähn and associates *(53, 54)* reported their experience at the Karolinska Institute involving 59 patients with Cushing's disease who were treated using the Gamma Knife and followed for 2–15 years. The efficacy rate of the initial treatment was 50%, with retreatment eventually providing normalization of cortisol production in 76% of patients *(58)*.

In our experience treating 107 patients with Cushing's disease, the remission rate was 53%, with the rate of remission statistically correlated with tumor volume, but not tumor invasion into the cavernous sinus or suprasellar region *(43)*. The mean prescription (margin) dose in Cushing's patients was 23 Gy, and we typically lowered the margin dose in patients who had prior radiation therapy. As reported by others, the rate of hormone normalization after radiosurgery for Cushing's disease appears to be difficult to predict, with remission occurring as early as 2 months and as late as 8 years *(59, 60)*. Our general experience is that most patients who ultimately have hormonal normalization do so within the first 2 years following radiosurgery, and patients with persistent disease should consider alternative treatments such as adrenalectomy, or repeat surgery (although this may be associated with a higher rate of cranial nerve damage) *(43)*. Recent work by the Marseille group suggests that ketaconazole and other cortisol-suppressive medications may adversely affect the endocrine outcome following radiosurgery *(61)*. As such, a temporary cessation of such cortisol-lowering agents at the time of radiosurgery seems prudent.

Table 2
Published Series on Radiosurgery for Cushing's Disease with 20 or More Patients

Authors	*Type of radiosurgery*	*Patients (n)*	*Remission criteria*	*Endocrine remission (%)*
Levy *(65)*	Proton beam	64	Normal basal cortisol and dexamethasone test	86
Witt *(42)*	Gamma Knife	25	Normal 24-UFC	28
Laws *(1)*	Gamma Knife	50	Normal 24-UFC	58
Sheehan *(37)*	Gamma Knife	43	Normal 24-UFC	63
Kobayashi *(54)*	Gamma Knife	20	ACTH <50 pg/ml; cortisol <10 microg/dl	35
Devin *(80)*	Linear accelerator	35	Normal cortisol	49
Castinetti *(61)*	Gamma Knife	40	Normal 24-UFC and dexamethasone suppression test	42.5
Jagannathan *(43)*	Gamma Knife	90	Normal 24-UFC	54
Petit *(18)*	Proton beam	33	Normal 24-UFC	52

Despite a conformal dose plan and appropriate dose delivery, some Cushing's patients do not achieve hormone normalization following microsurgery and radiosurgery, and require adrenalectomy as a "salvage" treatment for their disease. Although adrenalectomy is the definitive treatment for cortisol overproduction, a small subset of patients may develop Nelson's syndrome, characterized by rapid adenoma growth, hyperpigmentation, and tumor invasion into the parasellar structures *(62)*.

There are relatively few studies detailing the results of radiosurgery for Nelson's syndrome *(1, 54, 63–68)*. These studies report a mean tumor dose from between 12 and 28.7 Gy, and an endocrine remission rate ranging from 0 to 36%, although only a minority of these studies defined what was meant by endocrine remission. Even cases where endocrine remission was not achieved, tumor growth control rates were favorable, ranging from 82 to 100%.

Pollock and Young reported on 11 patients who underwent GKS for Nelson's syndrome. They reported control of tumor growth in 9 of 11 patients, with ACTH normalization in four patients (36%) *(67)*. Our experience involves 23 patients with at least 6 months follow-up, and a rate of tumor control of 90%. Decrease in ACTH levels occurred in 67% of patients, but normalization only occurred in four patients *(66)*.

COMPLICATIONS FOLLOWING RADIOSURGERY FOR CUSHING'S DISEASE

Side-effects following radiosurgery for pituitary adenomas are typically rare. However, the latency of such effects may be long (i.e., greater than 10 years) and warrants continued neurological, endocrine, and radiological follow-up. The most common problem after radiosurgery is new hypopituitarism. Well-respected groups have reported a low incidence (0–36%) of pituitary dysfunction following radiosurgery *(7, 43, 69, 70)*. This incidence is likely higher when patients are followed long-term, with the Karolinska Institute reporting a 72% incidence of hypopituitarism when patients were followed longer than 10 years *(60)*. We have observed an overall risk of 20–30% for development of hypopituitarism following radiosurgery.

Ultimately, total dose prescribed and the prescription (margin) dose are likely the major factors determining the risk and onset of radiation induced hypopituitarism. The GH axis is the most sensitive to the late effects of radiation, with the radiation induced defect believed to occur largely at the hypothalamic level *(71, 72)*. The gonadotropin and corticotrophin axes are the next most sensitive to radiation damage, and the TSH axis is least sensitive. Diabetes insipidus is extremely uncommon after radiosurgery with only sporadic case reports *(73)*.

Cranial neuropathies following Gamma Knife surgery for Cushing's disease are exceedingly rare following the first procedure, although the incidence may increase on re-treatment *(43)*. Visual injury in general can be avoided if the dose to the optic apparatus is restricted to less than 8 Gy (see discussion above).

Injury to the cavernous segment of the carotid artery or brain parenchymal is uncommon following radiosurgery. The exact incidence of radiosurgical induced neoplasms is unknown at present. To date, there are no reports of radiation-induced neoplasms following stereotactic radiosurgery to treat a pituitary adenoma.

PROGNOSIS AND FOLLOW-UP

Prognosis for a pituitary adenoma is dependent upon the pre-radiosurgical status, comorbid conditions, adenoma size and extension, and functional nature of the tumor. Patients being treated for Cushing's disease must be followed long-term with serial clinical, ophthalmological, endocrine, and radiological evaluations after radiosurgery. In particular, height, weight, and pubertal status must be carefully monitored in relevant age groups. Serial visual field examinations and screening should be performed. Questioning directed at assessing hormone function (screening for hypothyroidism, adrenal insufficiency, diabetes insipidus, etc.) should be directed to the patient and family. Serial testing of adrenal, thyroid function, and GH status (with IGF-1 levels and provocative testing when applicable) should be undertaken. Patients receiving hormone replacement should have their replacement therapy adjusted as necessary. Finally, serial MR imaging should be performed to assess for tumor recurrence. Generally, an initial post-radiosurgical neuro-imaging is performed 6 months following treatment and yearly thereafter (or more frequently as indicated). Endocrine and ophthalmologic follow-up should typically occur at these same time points.

Just as with extirpation, delayed recurrence following radiosurgical induced endocrine remission with normalization of 24 h UFC and resolution of Cushing's disease stigmata have been documented. Careful longitudinal follow-up of these patients will facilitate early detection and therapeutic intervention for patients with a recurrence of their Cushing's disease. Treatment options include repeat radiosurgery, adenoma resection, and adrenalectomy. A repeat MRI or other neuro-imaging study at the time of a recurrence is necessary to help select the appropriate treatment.

CONCLUSIONS

Stereotactic radiosurgery is a safe and effective modality in the treatment of Cushing's patients with either a recurrent or residual pituitary adenoma. In most patients, radiosurgery controls adenoma growth and normalizes ACTH and cortisol levels. Several challenges persist, including the optimal timing of radiosurgery, the identification of other factors that can improve the response of adenomas to radiosurgery, and the optimal target of the adenoma.

REFERENCES

1. Laws ER Jr, Vance ML. Radiosurgery for pituitary tumors and craniopharyngiomas. Neurosurg Clin N Am 1999;10:327–336.
2. Laws ER, Sheehan JP. Pituitary Surgery: A Modern Approach. New York: Basel;Karger, 2006.
3. Jagannathan J, Sheehan JP, Jane JA, Jr. Evaluation and management of Cushing syndrome in cases of negative sellar magnetic resonance imaging. Neurosurg Focus 2007;23:E3.
4. Mampalam TJ, Tyrrell JB, Wilson CB. Transsphenoidal microsurgery for Cushing disease. A report of 216 cases. Ann Intern Med 1988;109:487–493.
5. Jennings AS, Liddle GW, Orth DN. Results of treating childhood Cushing's disease with pituitary irradiation. N Engl J Med 1977;297:957–962.
6. Estrada J, Boronat M, Mielgo M, Magallon R, Millan I, Diez S, Lucas T, Barcelo B. The long-term outcome of pituitary irradiation after unsuccessful transsphenoidal surgery in Cushing's disease. N Engl J Med 1997;336:172–177.
7. Sheehan JP, Jagannathan J, Pouratian N, Steiner L. Stereotactic radiosurgery for pituitary adenomas: a review of the literature and our experience. Front Horm Res 2006;34:185–205.
8. Brada M, Burchell L, Ashley S, Traish D. The incidence of cerebrovascular accidents in patients with pituitary adenoma. Int J Radiat Oncol Biol Phys 1999;45:693–698.
9. Minniti G, Jaffrain-Rea ML, Osti M, Cantore G, Enrici RM. Radiotherapy for nonfunctioning pituitary adenomas: from conventional to modern stereotactic radiation techniques. Neurosurg Rev 2007;30:167–175; discussion 175–166.
10. Minniti G, Jaffrain-Rea ML, Osti M, Esposito V, Santoro A, Solda F, Gargiulo P, Tamburrano G, Enrici RM. The long-term efficacy of conventional radiotherapy in patients with GH-secreting pituitary adenomas. Clin Endocrinol (Oxf) 2005;62:210–216.
11. Sheehan JP, Niranjan A, Sheehan JM, Jane JA Jr, Laws ER, Kondziolka D, Flickinger J, Landolt AM, Loeffler JS, Lunsford LD. Stereotactic radiosurgery for pituitary adenomas: an intermediate review of its safety, efficacy, and role in the neurosurgical treatment armamentarium. J Neurosurg. 2005;102:678–691.
12. Leksell L. The stereotaxic method and radiosurgery of the brain. Acta Chir Scand. 1951;102:316–319.

13. Izawa M, Hayashi M, Nakaya K, Satoh H, Ochiai T, Hori T, Takakura K. Gamma knife radiosurgery for pituitary adenomas. J Neurosurg 93 Suppl 2000;3:19–22.
14. Jackson IM, Noren G. Gamma knife radiosurgery for pituitary tumours. Baillieres Best Pract Res Clin Endocrinol Metab 1999;13:461–469; 1999:Neurosurg Focus 2007;23:E3.
15. Braunstein GD, Loriaux DL. Proton-beam therapy. N Engl J Med 1971;284:332–333.
16. Dawson DM, Dingman JF. Hazards of proton-beam pituitary irradiation. N Engl J Med 1970;282:1434.
17. Lyman JT, Phillips MH, Frankel KA, Levy RP, Fabrikant JI. Radiation physics for particle beam radiosurgery. Neurosurg Clin N Am 1992;3:1–8.
18. Petit JH, Biller BM, Yock TI, Swearingen B, Coen JJ, Chapman P, Ancukiewicz M, Bussiere M, Klibanski A, Loeffler JS. Proton stereotactic radiotherapy for persistent adrenocorticotropin-producing adenomas. J Clin Endocrinol Metab 2008;93:393–399.
19. Ronson BB, Schulte RW, Han KP, Loredo LN, Slater JM, Slater JD. Fractionated proton beam irradiation of pituitary adenomas. Int J Radiat Oncol Biol Phys 2006;64:425–434.
20. Lundkvist J, Ekman M, Ericsson SR, Jonsson B, Glimelius B. Cost-effectiveness of proton radiation in the treatment of childhood medulloblastoma. Cancer 2005;103:793–801.
21. Podgorsak EB, Pike GB, Pla M, Olivier A, Souhami L. Radiosurgery with photon beams: physical aspects and adequacy of linear accelerators. Radiother Oncol 1990;17:349–358.
22. Popescu GF, Rodgers JE, von Hanwehr R. Optimization of dose distribution for LINAC based radiosurgery using elliptical collimators. Acta Neurochir Suppl 1995;63:35–39.
23. Schell MC, Smith V, Larson DA, Wu A, Flickinger JC. Evaluation of radiosurgery techniques with cumulative dose volume histograms in linac-based stereotactic external beam irradiation. Int J Radiat Oncol Biol Phys 1991;20: 1325–1330.
24. Andrews DW, Suarez O, Goldman HW, Downes MB, Bednarz G, Corn BW, Werner-Wasik M, Rosenstock J, Curran WJ Jr. Stereotactic radiosurgery and fractionated stereotactic radiotherapy for the treatment of acoustic schwannomas: comparative observations of 125 patients treated at one institution. Int J Radiat Oncol Biol Phys 2001;50:1265–1278.
25. Dong L, Shiu A, Tung S, Hogstrom K. A pencil-beam photon dose algorithm for stereotactic radiosurgery using a miniature multileaf collimator. Med Phys 1998;25:841–850.
26. Glasgow GP, Corrigan KW. Installation of 60Co 100 cm source-to-axis distance teletherapy units in vaults designed for 80-cm units. Health Phys. 1995;68:411–415.
27. Wang S, Wang R, Zhang X, Lin C, Wong Z, Li X. Dose distributions of linac-based radiosurgery for pineal region mass. Sheng Wu Yi Xue Gong Cheng Xue Za Zhi 1997;14:279–282.
28. Cheung JY, Yu KN, Ho RT, Yu CP. Monte Carlo calculations and GafChromic film measurements for plugged collimator helmets of Leksell Gamma Knife unit. Med Phys 1999;26:1252–1256.
29. Yu C, Luxton G, Jozsef G, Apuzzo ML, Petrovich Z. Dosimetric comparison of three photon radiosurgery techniques for an elongated ellipsoid target. Int J Radiat Oncol Biol Phys 1999;45:817–826.
30. Tang BN, Levivier M, Heureux M, Wikler D, Massager N, Devriendt D, David P, Dumarey N, Corvilain B, Goldman S. 11C-methionine PET for the diagnosis and management of recurrent pituitary adenomas. Eur J Nucl Med Mol Imaging 2006;33:169–178.
31. Oldfield EH, Doppman JL, Nieman LK, Chrousos GP, Miller DL, Katz DA, Cutler GB Jr, Loriaux DL. Petrosal sinus sampling with and without corticotropin-releasing hormone for the differential diagnosis of Cushing's syndrome. N Engl J Med 1991;325:897–905.
32. Alexander E III, Loeffler JS. Radiosurgery using a modified linear accelerator. Neurosurg Clin N Am 1992;3: 167–190.
33. Flickinger JC, Lunsford LD, Wu A, Maitz AH, Kalend AM. Treatment planning for gamma knife radiosurgery with multiple isocenters. Int J Radiat Oncol Biol Phys 1990;18:1495–1501.
34. Wu A, Lindner G, Maitz AH, Kalend AM, Lunsford LD, Flickinger JC, Bloomer WD. Physics of gamma knife approach on convergent beams in stereotactic radiosurgery. Int J Radiat Oncol Biol Phys 1990;18:941–949.
35. Paddick I. A simple scoring ratio to index the conformity of radiosurgical treatment plans. Technical note. J Neurosurg 2000;93(Suppl 3):219–222.
36. Sheehan JM, Lopes MB, Sheehan JP, Ellegala D, Webb KM, Laws ER Jr. Results of transsphenoidal surgery for Cushing's disease in patients with no histologically confirmed tumor. Neurosurgery 2000;47:33–36; discussion 37–39.
37. Sheehan JM, Vance ML, Sheehan JP, Ellegala DB, Laws ER Jr. Radiosurgery for Cushing's disease after failed transsphenoidal surgery. J Neurosurg 2000;93:738–742.
38. Leber KA, Bergloff J, Pendl G. Dose-response tolerance of the visual pathways and cranial nerves of the cavernous sinus to stereotactic radiosurgery. J Neurosurg 1998;88:43–50.

39. Chen JC, Giannotta SL, Yu C, Petrovich Z, Levy ML, Apuzzo ML. Radiosurgical management of benign cavernous sinus tumors: dose profiles and acute complications. Neurosurgery 2001;48:1022–30; discussion 1030–1032.
40. Lim YL, Leem W, Kim TS, Rhee BA, Kim GK. Four years' experiences in the treatment of pituitary adenomas with gamma knife radiosurgery. Stereotact Funct Neurosurg 1998;70(Suppl 1):95–109.
41. Witt TC. Stereotactic radiosurgery for pituitary tumors. Neurosurg Focus 2003;14:e10.
42. Witt TC, Kondziolka D, Flickinger JC, Lunsford LD. Gamma Knife radiosurgery for pituitary tumors. In: Lunsford LD, Kondziolka D, Flickinger J, eds. Gamma Knife Brain Surgery Progress in Neurological Surgery. Basel: Karger, 1998: 114–127.
43. Jagannathan J, Sheehan JP, Pouratian N, Laws ER, Steiner L, Vance ML. Gamma Knife surgery for Cushing's disease. J Neurosurg 2007;106:980–987.
44. Pouratian N, Sheehan J, Jagannathan J, Laws ER Jr, Steiner L, Vance ML. Gamma knife radiosurgery for medically and surgically refractory prolactinomas. Neurosurgery 2006;59:255–266; discussion 255–266.
45. Kuo JS, Chen JC, Yu C, Zelman V, Giannotta SL, Petrovich Z, MacPherson D, Apuzzo ML. Gamma knife radiosurgery for benign cavernous sinus tumors: quantitative analysis of treatment outcomes. Neurosurgery 2004;54:1385–1393; discussion 1393–1384.
46. Liu AL, Wang C, Sun S, Wang M, Liu P. Gamma knife radiosurgery for tumors involving the cavernous sinus. Stereotact Funct Neurosurg 2005;83:45–51.
47. Nakamura N, Shin M, Tago M, Terahara A, Kurita H, Nakagawa K, Ohtomo K. Gamma knife radiosurgery for cavernous hemangiomas in the cavernous sinus. Report of three cases. J Neurosurg 2002;97:477–480.
48. Peker S, Kilic T, Sengoz M, Pamir MN. Radiosurgical treatment of cavernous sinus cavernous haemangiomas. Acta Neurochir (Wien) 2004;146:337–341; discussion 340.
49. Sheehan JP, Kondziolka D, Flickinger J, Lunsford LD. Radiosurgery for residual or recurrent nonfunctioning pituitary adenoma. J Neurosurg 2002;97:408–414.
50. Lim YJ, Leem W, Park JT, Kim TS, Rhee BA, Kim GK. Cerebral infarction with ICA occlusion after Gamma Knife radiosurgery for pituitary adenoma: a case report. Stereotact Funct Neurosurg 72(Suppl) 1999;1:132–139.
51. Nieman LK. Medical therapy of Cushing's disease. Pituitary 2002;5:77–82.
52. Arnaldi G, Angeli A, Atkinson AB, Bertagna X, Cavagnini F, Chrousos GP, Fava GA, Findling JW, Gaillard RC, Grossman AB, Kola B, Lacroix A, Mancini T, Mantero F, Newell-Price J, Nieman LK, Sonino N, Vance ML, Giustina A, Boscaro M. Diagnosis and complications of Cushing's syndrome: a consensus statement. J Clin Endocrinol Metab 2003;88:5593–5602.
53. Chu JW, Matthias DF, Belanoff J, Schatzberg A, Hoffman AR, Feldman D. Successful long-term treatment of refractory Cushing's disease with high-dose mifepristone (RU 486). J Clin Endocrinol Metab 2001;86:3568–3573.
54. Kobayashi T, Kida Y, Mori Y. Gamma knife radiosurgery in the treatment of Cushing disease: long-term results. J Neurosurg 2002;97:422–428.
55. Morange-Ramos I, Regis J, Dufour H, Andrieu JM, Grisoli F, Jaquet P, Peragut JC. Gamma-knife surgery for secreting pituitary adenomas. Acta Neurochir (Wien) 1998;140:437–443.
56. Petrovich Z, Yu C, Giannotta SL, Zee CS, Apuzzo ML. Gamma knife radiosurgery for pituitary adenoma: early results. Neurosurgery 2003;53:51–59; discussion 59–61.
57. Mahmoud-Ahmed AS, Suh JH. Radiation therapy for Cushing's disease: a review. Pituitary 2002;5:175–180.
58. Rahn T, Thoren M, Hall K, Backlund EO. Stereotactic radiosurgery in Cushing's syndrome: acute radiation effects. Surg Neurol 1980;14:85–92.
59. Hayashi M, Taira T, Ochiai T, Chernov M, Takasu Y, Izawa M, Kouyama N, Tomida M, Tokumaru O, Katayama Y, Kawakami Y, Hori T, Takakura K. Gamma knife surgery of the pituitary: new treatment for thalamic pain syndrome. J Neurosurg 2005;102(Suppl):38–41.
60. Hoybye C, Grenback E, Rahn T, Degerblad M, Thoren M, Hulting AL. Adrenocorticotropic hormone-producing pituitary tumors: 12- to 22-year follow-up after treatment with stereotactic radiosurgery. Neurosurgery 2001;49:284–291; discussion 291–282.
61. Castinetti F, Nagai M, Dufour H, Kuhn JM, Morange I, Jaquet P, Conte-Devolx B, Regis J, Brue T. Gamma knife radiosurgery is a successful adjunctive treatment in Cushing's disease. Eur J Endocrinol 2007;156:91–98.
62. Nagesser SK, van Seters AP, Kievit J, Hermans J, Krans HM, van de Velde CJ. Long-term results of total adrenalectomy for Cushing's disease. World J Surg 2000;24:108–113.
63. Ganz JC. Gamma knife radiosurgery and its possible relationship to malignancy: a review. J Neurosurg 2002;97:644–652.
64. Ganz JC, Backlund EO, Thorsen FA. The effects of Gamma Knife surgery of pituitary adenomas on tumor growth and endocrinopathies. Stereotact Funct Neurosurg. 1993;61(Suppl 1):30–37.

65. Levy RP, Fabrikant JI, Frankel KA, Phillips MH, Lyman JT, Lawrence JH, Tobias CA. Heavy-charged-particle radiosurgery of the pituitary gland: clinical results of 840 patients. Stereotact Funct Neurosurg 1991;57:22–35.
66. Mauermann WJ, Sheehan JP, Chernavvsky DR, Laws ER, Steiner L, Vance ML. Gamma Knife surgery for adrenocorticotropic hormone-producing pituitary adenomas after bilateral adrenalectomy. J Neurosurg 2007;106:988–993.
67. Pollock BE, Young WF Jr. Stereotactic radiosurgery for patients with ACTH-producing pituitary adenomas after prior adrenalectomy. Int J Radiat Oncol Biol Phys 2002;54:839–841.
68. Wolffenbuttel BH, Kitz K, Beuls EM. Beneficial gamma-knife radiosurgery in a patient with Nelson's syndrome. Clin Neurol Neurosurg 1998;100:60–63.
69. Jane JA, Jr, Vance ML, Woodburn CJ, Laws ER Jr. Stereotactic radiosurgery for hypersecreting pituitary tumors: part of a multimodality approach. Neurosurg Focus 2003;14:e12.
70. Pollock BE, Kondziolka D, Lunsford LD, Flickinger JC. Stereotactic radiosurgery for pituitary adenomas: imaging, visual and endocrine results. Acta Neurochir Suppl 1994;62:33–38.
71. Blacklay A, Grossman A, Ross RJ, Savage MO, Davies PS, Plowman PN, Coy DH, Besser GM. Cranial irradiation for cerebral and nasopharyngeal tumours in children: evidence for the production of a hypothalamic defect in growth hormone release. J Endocrinol 1986;108:25–29.
72. Shalet SM. Radiation and pituitary dysfunction. N Engl J Med 1993;328:131–133.
73. Piedra MP, Brown PD, Carpenter PC, Link MJ. Resolution of diabetes insipidus following gamma knife surgery for a solitary metastasis to the pituitary stalk. Case report. J Neurosurg 2004;101:1053–1056.
76. Pandey P, Ojha BK, Mahapatra AK. Pediatric pituitary adenoma: a series of 42 patients. J Clin Neurosci 2005;12: 124–7.
77. Storr HL, Plowman PN, Carroll PV, et al. Clinical and endocrine responses to pituitary radiotherapy in pediatric Cushing's disease: an effective second-line treatment. J Clin Endocrinol Metab 2003;88:34–7.
78. Thoren M, Rahn T, Hallengren B, et al. Treatment of Cushing's disease in childhood and adolescence by stereotactic pituitary irradiation. Acta Paediatr Scand 1986;75:388–95.
79. Minniti G, Osti M, Jaffrain-Rea ML, Esposito V, Cantore G, Maurizi Enrici R. Long-term follow-up results of postoperative radiation therapy for Cushing's disease. J Neurooncol 2007;84:79–84.
80. Devin JK, Allen GS, Cmelak AJ, Duggan DM, Blevins LS. The efficacy of linear accelerator radiosurgery in the management of patients with Cushing's disease. Stereotact Funct Neurosurg 2004;82:254–62.

13 Medical Management of Cushing's Syndrome

Cuong Dang and Peter J. Trainer

CONTENTS

SUMMARY

The treatment of choice for Cushing's syndrome remains surgical. Medical therapy may be used to control hypercortisolaemia before surgery to optimize patient's preoperative state and where surgery has failed and radiotherapy has not taken effect. The most effective agents are those that inhibit steroidogenesis and include metyrapone, ketoconazole, and mitotane. Drugs targeting the hypothalamic-pituitary axis have been investigated but their roles in clinical practice remain limited although PPAR-γ agonists and somatostatin analogue SOM-230 (pasireotide) need further investigation. The only drug acting at the periphery targeting the glucocorticoid receptor remains mifepristone (RU486) but it is uncertain because of the challenge of monitoring disease activity. For the foreseeable future, the place of medical treatment will remain as an interim measure while waiting for definitive treatment.

Key Words: Cushing's syndrome, drug therapy, steroidogenesis inhibitor, hypothalamic-pituitary modulator

INTRODUCTION

The definitive management for Cushing's syndrome is surgical excision of the underlying cause of the hypercortisolaemia, with the exception of ACTH-independent bilateral macronodular hyperplasia where pharmacological treatment directed against the aberrant receptor can be effective *(1)* (see chap. 17).

From: *Contemporary Endocrinology: Cushing's Syndrome: Pathophysiology, Diagnosis and Treatment*
Edited by: M.D. Bronstein (ed.), DOI 10.1007/978-1-60327-449-4_13,

However, there is a role for medical therapy in the following circumstances:

1) To prepare patients with severe hypercortisolaemia for surgery by lowering circulating cortisol levels, thereby reversing the metabolic consequence of cortisol excess and by implication reduce the complications of surgery. This clearly depends on the interval to surgery and disease severity.
2) When it is not possible to make a definitive diagnosis at first investigation, then medical therapy can be used as a stop gap to control signs and symptoms before re-investigation.
3) After unsuccessful pituitary surgery while considering further definitive surgery, such as bilateral adrenalectomy.
4) To relieve signs and symptoms in patients with metastatic adrenocortical carcinoma.
5) While waiting for pituitary radiotherapy to be effective, which can be several years.
6) If at presentation psychiatric symptoms are so severe as to make systematic investigation or definitive treatment impossible.

MEDICAL THERAPY TARGETS

Medical therapy can be separated into agents that inhibit adrenal steroidogenesis, those that modulate pituitary ACTH release, or block glucocorticoid action. Currently in clinical practice, the most effective, reliable and widely used agents are those that inhibit steroidogenesis.

PITUITARY DIRECTED TREATMENT

Pituitary ACTH secretion is regulated by a number of neurotransmitters including catecholamines, serotonin, acetylcholine, GABA and peptides. In Cushing's disease, the pituitary tumour still remains partially responsive to hypothalamic stimuli, illustrated by responsiveness to exogenous CRH and dexamethasone. Reports exist advocating the virtues of various agents (vide infra) but to-date, none have gained widespread acceptance. However, recent data have renewed interest in the possibility of treating Cushing's disease with centrally acting drugs that modulate ACTH secretion through dopamine, somatostatin and PPAR-γ receptors.

Dopamine Agonists

Bromocriptine and cabergoline are dopamine agonists that have been widely used in the treatment of hyperprolactinaemia and acromegaly. It is unclear if the action in lowering ACTH secretion by bromocriptine is via CRH or directly on the pituitary *(2–4)*. A single dose of bromocriptine will cause a fall in ACTH in half of the patients with Cushing's disease, but unfortunately this effect is not maintained in the long term *(4, 5)*. There are reports that suggest with high-dose bromocriptine (40 mg/day) may result in clinical improvement in up to 50% of patients but others have found response rate of only 1–2% in the long term *(6, 7)*. Potential side effects of bromocriptine include nasal congestion, nausea, postural hypotension, headaches and hallucination.

The use of cabergoline in the management of Cushing's disease has been more encouraging. In an open labelled, uncontrolled study, Pivonello et al. found that in 20 patients with Cushing's disease that remained active after pituitary surgery, cabergoline at a dose of up to 7 mg per week for three months, normalised urinary free cortisol (UFC) in 7 (35%) patients, and a further 8 (40%) patients had partial response (defined as achieving >25% reduction in 24 h UFC from baseline) *(8)*. After 12 months, 6 out of the 8 partial responder achieve normalisation of the UFC. After 24 month, 8 of the 20 patients remained fully controlled on cabergoline treatment, with a median dose of cabergoline 3.5 mg/week. Two patients withdrew from the study because of hypotension. Although a number of uncertainties remain, it is still not known what determines responsiveness although initial response appear to be related to hyperprolactinaemia. There is concern regarding that cabergoline can cause valvular heart disease, but no side effects were detected with 7 mg/week of cabergoline *(9, 10)*. The result of the study is encouraging, but controlled studies using better measures of disease activity are required.

PPAR-γ Receptor Agonists

In 2002, the nuclear hormone receptor, peroxisome proliferator-activated receptor-γ (PPAR-γ), was identified in ACTH-secreting pituitary tumour *(11)*. In vivo experiments in mice inoculated with corticotroph AtT20 tumour cells demonstrated that treatment with an extremely high dose of the PPAR-γ agonist rosiglitazone (150 mg/kg/day) prevented the development of tumours. In mice with already established corticotroph tumours, rosiglitazone treatment decreased tumour volume in 75% and prevented signs of hypercortisolaemia in all cases, with a 75% reduction in ACTH level and 96% reduction in cortisol levels *(11)*. These observations caused great interest but are yet to impact on clinical practice.

A series of uncontrolled studies in humans have been performed with variable results. In a study of two patients with pituitary-dependent Cushing's syndrome treated with rosiglitazone 8 mg daily for 33 and 20 days (the second patient was also taking metyrapone 1 g/day), 24 h UFC fell in both patients[12]. In a second study of ten patients (four before surgery, four after relapse after surgery and two immediately after failed surgery) treated with 4–16 mg/day of rosiglitazone for a median 3 months, there was no consistent reduction in urinary-free cortisol, plasma ACTH or serum cortisol levels *(13)*. Side effects reported included oedema, weight increase, somnolence and increased hirsutism. In one of the larger studies, 14 patients with active Cushing's disease (7 untreated and 7 post-unsuccessful transsphenoidal surgery) were treated with 8—16 mg of rosiglitazone for 1–7 months *(14)*. In six patients, plasma ACTH, serum cortisol and 24 h UFC were lowered but only UFC reached significance. Two of the six patients also noted clinical improvement on follow-up at seven months. No clinical side effects were noted, but one patient developed hypercholesterolaemia. In a study of seven patients with Nelson's syndrome who took 8 mg of rosiglitazone for 12 weeks, no significant fall in ACTH was seen *(15)*. Similarly, in another study of six patients with Nelson's syndrome given rosiglitazone 12 mg/day for 14 weeks, there was no fall in ACTH levels *(16)*. In a study of five patients with Cushing's disease treated with pioglitazone 45 mg for 30 days, no alteration in 24 h UFC, or ACTH and cortisol responses to CRH administration was seen *(17)*.

In summary, the PPAR-γ agonists has been a disappointment in the treatment of Cushing's disease and have failed to reproduce the success seen in the in vitro and mouse models. The discrepancy between the in vitro and human experience may reflect the differences in the order of magnitude in the dose of PPAR- γ agonists used i.e. 150 mg/kg in mouse verses ≈0.1 mg/kg in human. It is a disappointment that no PPAR- γ agonists manufacturer has invested in the dose finding or controlled studies to provide definitive evidence of efficacy or the lack of it.

Somatostatin Analogues

Octreotide and lanreotide are analogues of somatostatin, which act mainly on somatostatin receptor subtype 2 (sst2), and are used extensively to treat neuroendocrine tumours and acromegaly and have been tried with limited success in ACTH-dependent Cushing's syndrome. The lack of efficacy may reflect that corticotrophs do not reliably express sst2 *(18)*.

Initial reports did show that somatostatin infusion decreases plasma ACTH level by between 40% and 70% in patients with Nelson's syndrome *(19)*. However, subsequent studies in Nelson's syndrome using somatostatin and octreotide have been less impressive and most patients with Cushing's disease have failed to respond *(20–24)*. The lack of clinical efficacy of octreotide may be due to the down regulation of somatostatin receptors by glucocorticoids. In the mouse, sst2 gene promoter sequence is the only somatostatin receptor shown to be directly transcriptionally regulated by glucocorticoids *(25, 26)*. There have been occasional reports that octreotide may have a role in treating ectopic ACTH producing tumours or in Cushing's disease in combination with ketoconazole, but the available evidence suggests that such patients are the exception rather than the rule *(27, 28)*.

There is renewed interest in somatostatin analogues in Cushing's disease because of encouraging data emerging from early studies with pasireotide (Novartis), a somatostatin analogue with affinity to the somatostatin receptor subtypes 1-, 2-, 3- and 40-fold higher affinity for sst5 than octreotide *(29–31)*. In vitro, compared to octreotide, pasireotide is more potent at suppressing ACTH release and at inhibiting CRH-induced ACTH release in corticotroph tumour cells *(32–34)*. Dexamethasone (10 nM) pre-treatment of mouse corticotroph cells fails to suppress pasireotide inhibition of CRH-induced ACTH release, whereas the suppressive effect of octreotide is blocked *(33)*.

A recent open-labelled, uncontrolled, single-arm phased II study 39 patients with ACTH-dependent Cushing's disease and 24 h UFC at least twice the upper limit of normal were treated with pasireotide 600 mcg twice daily subcutaneous injection for 15 days *(35)*. Analysed data are available in 29 patients, of which, 5 (17%) normalised 24 h UFC and 22 (76%) had a reduction in 24 h UFC. A reduction in serum cortisol and plasma ACTH were also seen. Side effects were common with 92% experiencing problems predominantly, affecting gastrointestinal tract. Hyperglycaemia was experienced by 14 (36%) patients, of which three were already known to suffer from diabetes mellitus (one patient withdrew from the study) and two from impaired fasting glycaemia. Although the result of this study is encouraging, larger and longer studies are still required to confirm safety and continued efficacy.

Retinoic Acid

Since the 1980s retinoic acid derivatives have been widely used by dermatologists in the treatment of acne and psoriasis, as well as in certain malignancy such as acute promyelocytic leukaemia *(36, 37)*. Retinoic acid is a ligand for Nur77/Nurr1 receptor, which is involved in the physiological stimulation of ACTH by CRH *(38)*. In vitro retinoic acid inhibits cell proliferation and induces cell death in ACTH-secreting tumours but not in normal pituitary cells. In the adrenal cortex it inhibits corticosterone secretion and cell proliferation, whereas in a mouse model, it blocks tumour growth and reduces circulating ACTH and cortisol. The dose was 10 mg/kg, which is within the dose range in human cancer therapy *(38)*. Studies in rodent and dog models of Cushing's disease are encouraging, but there are to date no published data in human *(38, 39)*.

Other Agents

A number of agents have also been investigated in the past with initially encouraging results, but all eventually have been dismissed. Cyproheptadine is a non-selective histamine and serotonin antagonist. In a series of three patients, at a dose of 24 mg/day, it was effective at reducing ACTH in Cushing's disease *(40)*. There is disagreement on whether cyproheptadine acts either directly on the pituitary or through the inhibition of CRH *(41–44)*. Subsequent studies failed to confirm its effectiveness, but it caused sedation and it no longer has a place in the current practice. Ritanserin is a specific 5-HT_2 antagonist which has been used in a few patients, but its effects do not appear to be sustained *(45, 46)*. There are conflicting results on the effectiveness of sodium valproate in treating Cushing's disease remain. There are reports suggesting that it is successful at suppressing ACTH at a daily dose of 600 mg, but subsequent data failed to demonstrate benefit either as primary therapy or after failed pituitary surgery *(47, 48)*.

DRUGS DIRECTED AT THE ADRENAL

Currently, these agents are the most consistently effective means of controlling cortisol secretion (Table 1).

Metyrapone

In the era before it was possible to measure plasma ACTH, the metyrapone test was used to investigate suspected Cushing's syndrome and hypoadrenalism, but its use now is exclusively therapeutic *(49, 50)*. It acts primarily on the final step in cortisol synthesis, namely, the conversion of 11-deoxycortisol to cortisol and therefore, results in a dramatic increase in circulating 11-deoxycortisol levels, which can cross-react in serum and urine cortisol immunoassays *(51)*. This cross-reactivity may result in spuriously elevated cortisol levels and a failure to appreciate that a patient is over-treated and hypoadrenal.

Metyrapone is a potent, short-acting inhibitor of cortisol synthesis with a rapid onset of action. Serum cortisol levels fall within four hours of an initial dose and care is required to avoid over-treatment. The routine starting dose is 250 mg three times per day with reassessment of cortisol levels 72 h later and dose titration as appropriate until a mean cortisol level of between 150 and 300 nmol/l (5.5—11 μg/dl) is achieved *(52)*. In patients with severe hypercortisolaemia up to 8 g/day in 3–4 divided doses may be necessary. Most patients tolerate the drug without difficulty as long as hypoadrenalism is avoided. Nausea, anorexia and abdominal pain can occur, but usually this is a sign of over-treatment. The major limitation of metyrapone is in women as the accumulation of cortisol precursors results in elevated androgens that frequently is manifested as hirsutism and acne. Although mineralcorticoid precursors levels are elevated, hypokalaemia, hypertension and oedema are not problems, presumably because of the benefits of lower circulating cortisol levels *(53, 54)*. In patients with pituitary-dependent Cushing's disease, ACTH levels rise but there is no evidence that this results in tachyphylaxis *(53, 55)*.

Ketoconazole

Ketoconazole is an imidazole derivative developed as an oral antifungal agent that inhibits cholesterol, sex steroid and cortisol synthesis by acting on the 11β-hydroxylase and C17-20 lyase enzymes *(56–59)*. It is the most frequently used agent in the treatment of Cushing's syndrome with starting

Table 1
Agents Inhibiting Steroidogenesis in Clinical Use

Agent	*Dose*	
Metyrappone	750–8,000 mg daily	Hypoadrenalism Side effects: nausea, abdominal pain, hirsutism, acne
Ketoconazole	400–1,200 mg daily	Slow onset of action Side effects: gastro-intestinal upset, rashes, abnormal LFT, gynaecomastia and reduced libido in men
Mitotane	500–4,000 mg daily	Gradual dose titration, taken with meal Side effects: gastro-intestinal upset, neurological disturbances, abnormal LFT, hypercholesterolaemia Avoid pregnancy up to five years after stopping the drug

dose being 200 mg twice daily increasing as necessary to 1,200 mg/day in four divided doses *(60, 61)*. In contrast to metyrapone it can take several weeks to see the full benefit of a dose adjustment and there is less risk of over-treatment and hypoadrenalism. With time it is effective at controlling the symptoms of Cushing's syndrome and in women its antiandrogenic properties are a virtue but in men, gynaecomastia and reduced libido have been reported. The most common side effects are gastrointestinal upset and skin rashes, but liver enzyme dysfunction can occur in up to 10% of cases, which rarely has proceeded to acute liver failure and fatality *(62–65)*. Ketoconazole has the added benefit of reducing the total cholesterol and LDL cholesterol *(66)*.

Metyrapone and ketoconazole can be very successfully co-administered as the former controls cortisol secretion while waiting for the slower onset of action of the latter agent, which in turn lowers androgens and thus negates one of the major limitations of the former.

Mitotane

Mitotane was introduced in 1960 as a cytotoxic agent for the treatment of adrenocortical carcinoma, which remains its main use today but it has also been used to control hypercortisolaemia for the treatment in benign causes of Cushing's syndrome. Mitotane reduces cortisol production by blocking cholesterol side-chain cleavage and 11 β-hydroxylase *(67–69)*. The onset of mitotane action is slow with sustained action maintained after discontinuation in up to a third of patient *(70)*. When used to control serum cortisol levels in benign disease, mitotane is initiated at a dose of 0.5—1 g/day, which is increased gradually by 0.5—1 g every few weeks to minimise side effects. Adverse effects such as nausea, anorexia and diarrhoea are common with doses of 2 g/day and almost universal at doses greater than 4 g/day *(71)*. Adrenal insufficiency and neurological side effects including abnormal gait, dizziness, vertigo, confusion and problem of language expression are often seen at higher dose *(70)*. Abnormal liver enzymes, hypercholesterolaemia, skin rash, hypouricaemia, gynaecomastia in male and prolonged bleeding time are also well recognized *(72, 73)*. Changes in hormone binding globulins may result in total hormone measurement being unreliable during treatment and thus caution is required when interpreting serum cortisol levels *(74, 75)*. Mitotane increases the metabolic clearance of exogenously administered steroid and the replacement dose of steroid is increased by about a third *(76)* To minimise side effects, mitotane dose should be gradually titrated up, taken with meals or at bedtime with food. Changing the schedule to once a day or alternate days may help with gastrointestinal problems. If side effects are severe, mitotane can be stopped for a week and restarted at a lower dose. Mitotane may induce spontaneous abortion and is a teratogen. Its effect may persist for a number of months after discontinuation and so a female patient should avoid pregnancy for up to five years after stopping the drug *(77)*. Ketoconazole and metyrapone are more effective and better tolerated agents and therefore the use of mitotane should be confined to the treatment of resistant patients.

Aminoglutethimide

Aminoglutethimide, which was introduced in 1959 as an anticonvulsant, was used in the treatment of breast cancer and noticed to induce adrenal insufficiency. It inhibits the side-chain cleavage of cholesterol to pregnenolone and therefore inhibits cortisol, oestrogen and aldosterone production *(78, 79)*. Even when effective the benefit may be transient either because of an increase in ACTH overcoming the enzymatic blockade or it may be induction of hepatic enzyme accelerating aminoglutethimide metabolism *(80, 81)*. Adverse effects such as lethargy, dizziness, ataxia and rashes are common on initiation and limit its use although they do resolve with time *(82, 83)*. There are better agents for controlling hypercortisolaemia and aminoglutethimide does not have a place in the modern treatment of Cushing's syndrome *(84)*.

Trilostane

Trilostane is a competitive inhibitor of 3β-hydroxysteroid dehydrogenase, which is an essential enzyme in the synthesis of cortisol, aldosterone and androstenedione *(51)*. It is an effective inhibitor of steroid synthesis in vitro but in man the results have been disappointing *(85)*. However, it is used in veterinary practice as it is very effective in controlling pituitary-dependent Cushing's in dogs *(86)*. The maximum daily dose is 1,440 mg and patients may experience side effects such as abdominal discomfort, diarrhoea and paraesthesia. Trilostane has largely fallen out of clinical use, but the very fact that it is so effective in dogs may mean it justifies reconsideration in man.

Etomidate

Etomidate is a parenteral anaesthetic agent which when first introduced was associated with excessive mortality in patients in intensive care, which was ultimately explained by the recognition that it induced hypoadrenalism by inhibiting 11β-hydroxylase, 17-hydroxylase, c17-20 lyase as well as cholesterol side chain cleavage *(87–89)*. A number of case reports have shown etomidate at 2.5 mg/h to be effective at correcting hypercortisolaemia in seriously ill patients with ectopic ACTH production *(90–92)*. Etomidate's use is limited by the need to be given intravenously but it has a place in acutely sick patients unable to be treated orally where rapid correction of hypercortisolaemia may be life saving.

AGENTS BLOCKING CORTISOL ACTION

Mifepristone (RU486) is a potent antagonist of the glucocorticoid and progesterone receptors *(93)*. In man, mifepristone blocks glucocorticoid action, resulting in negative feedback at the hypothalamic–pituitary level, leading to a rise in ACTH, arginine–vasopressin and therefore cortisol *(94)*. Recently, there has been renewed interest in using mifepristone for the management of ectopic ACTH syndrome. Mifepristone, at doses of up to 20 mg/kg, has been successfully used to treat a small number of patients with ectopic ACTH syndrome and there is every reason to believe that it could be successfully used in all patients if it were not for the problem of monitoring therapy *(95)*. As a receptor antagonist it does not lower circulating cortisol levels, which in fact rise, and therefore, it is very difficult to dose titrate and judge the effectiveness. The GH receptor antagonist pegvisomant has gained widespread acceptance as a treatment for acromegaly because its effectiveness can be judge by monitoring IGF-1. Unfortunately, the HPA axis lacks a marker analogous to IGF-1. Even with short-term use, a number of patients did develop symptoms of hypoadrenalism which is problematic as there is no effective method of monitoring over treatment *(96)*. There has also been report of a case of mifepristone causing severe hypokalaemia that is attributed to excess cortisol activation of mineralcorticoid receptor which responds to spironolactone therapy *(97)*. With caution, Mifepristone may have a role in the treatment of Cushing's syndrome and could be first line treatment if a biochemical measure of disease were identified *(98)*.

MONITORING OF TREATMENT

A major challenge of medical therapy is the monitoring of its effectiveness. UFC measurement is widely used, but has several major limitations and is intrinsically a poor solution to the problem. Only a small proportion of cortisol is excreted unaltered in urine and UFC immunoassays, to varying extents, detect biologically inactive cortisol metabolites, which may be raised in patients treated with agents such as metyrapone. UFC has the additional disadvantages of relying on complete collection and of being unable to detect over-treatment-induced hypoadrenalism. Although more labour-intensive, measurement of serum cortisol is a more appropriate means of assessing disease activity. The best validated technique is the calculation of a mean serum cortisol from multiple measurements taken during a single day. Studies comparing isotopically calculated cortisol production rates to serum levels indicate that a mean serum cortisol in the range 150–300 nmol/l (5.5—11 μg/dl) equates to a normal cortisol production rate, and this should be the target of medical therapy *(52)*.

Steroid analysis in saliva has been developed over 30 years now with salivary cortisol measurement popular in sports, stress and psychiatry research *(99–101)*. The advantages of salivary cortisol is that it offer a stress free and non-invasive method of collection that can be collected by patient themselves. Salivary cortisol correlate with plasma free cortisol and have been useful in the investigation of the HPA axis *(102–105)*. There are a few case reports using salivary cortisol to monitor Cushing's syndrome but major obstacles remain, the absence of a reference range and the lack of standardisation of assay methods *(106, 107)*. Salivary cortisol by mass spectrometry has the potential to monitor therapy without the problem of cross reactivity and contamination but there are no published data looking specifically at monitoring of Cushing's treatment *(108, 109)*. At the moment it is a research tool and is not yet use in routine clinical setting.

The cyclical nature of Cushing's syndrome in some patients means that even after disease control has been achieved regular treatment monitoring is required.

SUMMARY

A number of drugs have been used in the management of Cushing's syndrome. Regardless of the aetiology the most reliably effective treatments are metyrapone or ketoconazole as monotherapy, or in combination. However, the recent advances in understanding the role of the PPAR- γ and sst receptors in corticotrophs has raised the prospect of novel mode of treatment but enthusiasm must be tempered by the poor clinical results to date. Recent data suggests cabergoline may have greater role than previously appreciated, but it must be balanced against the increasing concern about valvulopathy.

REFERENCES

1. Christopoulos S, Bourdeau I, Lacroix A. Aberrant expression of hormone receptors in adrenal Cushing's syndrome. Pituitary 2004;7(4):225–235.
2. Lamberts SW, de Lange SA, Stefanko SZ. Adrenocorticotropin-secreting pituitary adenomas originate from the anterior or the intermediate lobe in Cushing's disease: differences in the regulation of hormone secretion. J Clin Endocrinol Metab 1982;54(2):286–291.
3. Croughs RJ, Koppeschaar HP, van't Verlaat JW, McNicol AM. Bromocriptine-responsive Cushing's disease associated with anterior pituitary corticotroph hyperplasia or normal pituitary gland. J Clin Endocrinol Metab 1989;68(2): 495–498.
4. Boscaro M, Benato M, Mantero F. Effect of bromocriptine in pituitary-dependent Cushing's syndrome. Clin Endocrinol (Oxf) 1983;19(4):485–491.
5. Lamberts SW, Klijn JG, de Quijada M, Timmermans HA, Uitterlinden P, de Jong FH et al. The mechanism of the suppressive action of bromocriptine on adrenocorticotropin secretion in patients with Cushing's disease and Nelson's syndrome. J Clin Endocrinol Metab 1980;51(2):307–311.
6. Mercado-Asis LB, Yasuda K, Murayama M, Mune T, Morita H, Miura K. Beneficial effects of high daily dose bromocriptine treatment in Cushing's disease. Endocrinol Jpn 1992;39(4):385–395.
7. Morris D, Grossman A. The medical management of Cushing's syndrome. Ann N Y Acad Sci 2002;970:119–133.
8. Pivonello R, De Martino MC, Cappabianca P, De Leo M, Faggiano A, Lombardi G et al. The Medical Treatment of Cushing's Disease: Effectiveness of Chronic Treatment with the Dopamine Agonist Cabergoline in Patients Unsuccessfully Treated by Surgery. J Clin Endocrinol Metab 2009;94(1):223–230.
9. Zanettini R, Antonini A, Gatto G, Gentile R, Tesei S, Pezzoli G. Valvular heart disease and the use of dopamine agonists for Parkinson's disease. N Engl J Med 2007;356(1):39–46.

10. Schade R, Andersohn F, Suissa S, Haverkamp W, Garbe E. Dopamine agonists and the risk of cardiac-valve regurgitation. N Engl J Med 2007;356(1):29–38.
11. Heaney AP, Fernando M, Yong WH, Melmed S. Functional PPAR-gamma receptor is a novel therapeutic target for ACTH-secreting pituitary adenomas. Nat Med 2002;8(11):1281–1287.
12. Hull SSA, Sheridan B, Atkinson AB. Pre-operative medical therapy with rosiglitazone in two patients with newly diagnosed pituitary-dependent Cushing's syndrome. Clin Endocrinol (Oxf) 62:259–261.
13. Giraldi FP, Scaroni C, Arvat E, Martin M, Giordano R, Albiger N et al. Effect of protracted treatment with rosiglitazone, a PPARgamma agonist, in patients with Cushing's disease. Clin Endocrinol (Oxf) 2006;64(2):219–224.
14. Ambrosi B, Dall'Asta C, Cannavo S, Libe R, Vigo T, Epaminonda P et al. Effects of chronic administration of PPAR-gamma ligand rosiglitazone in Cushing's disease. Eur J Endocrinol 2004;151(2):173–178.
15. Mullan KR, Leslie H, McCance DR, Sheridan B, Atkinson AB. The PPAR-gamma activator rosiglitazone fails to lower plasma ACTH levels in patients with Nelson's syndrome. Clin Endocrinol (Oxf) 2006;64(5):519–522.
16. Munir A, Song F, Ince P, Walters SJ, Ross R, Newell-Price J. Ineffectiveness of rosiglitazone therapy in Nelson's syndrome. J Clin Endocrinol Metab 2007;92(5):1758–1763.
17. Suri D, Weiss RE. Effect of pioglitazone on adrenocorticotropic hormone and cortisol secretion in Cushing's disease. J Clin Endocrinol Metab 2005;90(3):1340–1346.
18 Weckbecker G, Lewis I, Albert R, Schmid HA, Hoyer D, Bruns C. Opportunities in somatostatin research: biological, chemical and therapeutic aspects. Nat Rev Drug Discov 2003;2(12):999–1017.
19 Tyrrell JB, Lorenzi M, Gerich JE, Forsham PH. Inhibition by somatostatin of ACTH secretion in Nelson's syndrome. J Clin Endocrinol Metab 1975;40(6):1125–1127.
20 Lamberts SW, Uitterlinden P, Klijn JM. The effect of the long-acting somatostatin analogue SMS 201–995 on ACTH secretion in Nelson's syndrome and Cushing's disease. Acta Endocrinol (Copenh) 1989;120(6):760–766.
21. Julesz J, Laczi F, Janaky T, Laszlo F. Effects of somatostatin and bromocryptine on the plasma ACTH level in bilaterally adrenalectomized patients with Cushing's disease. Endokrinologie 1980;76(1):68–72.
22. Petrini L, Gasperi M, Pilosu R, Marcello A, Martino E. Long-term treatment of Nelson's syndrome by octreotide: a case report. J Endocrinol Invest 1994;17(2):135–139.
23. Ambrosi B, Bochicchio D, Fadin C, Colombo P, Faglia G. Failure of somatostatin and octreotide to acutely affect the hypothalamic-pituitary-adrenal function in patients with corticotropin hypersecretion. J Endocrinol Invest 1990;13(3):257–261.
24. Stalla GK, Brockmeier SJ, Renner U, Newton C, Buchfelder M, Stalla J et al. Octreotide exerts different effects in vivo and in vitro in Cushing's disease. Eur J Endocrinol 1994;130(2):125–131.
25. Kraus J, Woltje M, Hollt V. Regulation of mouse somatostatin receptor type 2 gene expression by glucocorticoids. FEBS Lett 1999;459(2):200–204.
26. Kraus J, Woltje M, Schonwetter N, Hollt V. Alternative promoter usage and tissue specific expression of the mouse somatostatin receptor 2 gene. FEBS Lett 1998;428(3):165–170.
27. Bertagna X, Favrod-Coune C, Escourolle H, Beuzeboc P, Christoforov B, Girard F et al. Suppression of ectopic adrenocorticotropin secretion by the long-acting somatostatin analog octreotide. J Clin Endocrinol Metab 1989;68(5):988–991.
28. Vignati F, Loli P. Additive effect of ketoconazole and octreotide in the treatment of severe adrenocorticotropin-dependent hypercortisolism. J Clin Endocrinol Metab 1996;81(8):2885–2890.
29. Boerlin V, van der HJ, Beglinger C, Poon KW, Hartmann S, Dutreix C et al. New insights on SOM230, a universal somatostatin receptor ligand. J Endocrinol Invest 2003;26(8 Suppl):14–16.
30. Lewis I, Bauer W, Albert R, Chandramouli N, Pless J, Weckbecker G et al. A novel somatostatin mimic with broad somatotropin release inhibitory factor receptor binding and superior therapeutic potential. J Med Chem 2003;46(12): 2334–2344.
31. Bruns C, Lewis I, Briner U, Meno-Tetang G, Weckbecker G. SOM230: a novel somatostatin peptidomimetic with broad somatotropin release inhibiting factor (SRIF) receptor binding and a unique antisecretory profile. Eur J Endocrinol 2002;146(5):707–716.
32. Hofland LJ, van der HJ, Feelders R, van Aken MO, van Koetsveld PM, Waaijers M et al. The multi-ligand somatostatin analogue SOM230 inhibits ACTH secretion by cultured human corticotroph adenomas via somatostatin receptor type 5. Eur J Endocrinol 2005;152(4):645–654.
33. van der HJ, Waaijers M, van Koetsveld PM, Sprij-Mooij D, Feelders RA, Schmid HA et al. Distinct functional properties of native somatostatin receptor subtype 5 compared with subtype 2 in the regulation of ACTH release by corticotroph tumor cells. Am J Physiol Endocrinol Metab 2005;289(2):E278-E287.
34. Strowski MZ, Dashkevicz MP, Parmar RM, Wilkinson H, Kohler M, Schaeffer JM et al. Somatostatin receptor subtypes 2 and 5 inhibit corticotropin-releasing hormone-stimulated adrenocorticotropin secretion from AtT-20 cells. Neuroendocrinology 2002;75(6):339–346.

35. Boscaro M, Ludlam WH, Atkinson B, Glusman JE, Petersenn S, Reincke M et al. Treatment of Pituitary-Dependent Cushing's Disease with the Multireceptor Ligand Somatostatin Analog Pasireotide (SOM230): A Multicenter, Phase II Trial. J Clin Endocrinol Metab 2009;94(1):115–122.
36. New hope in acne. Lancet 1979;1(8128):1222–1223.
37. Tallman MS, Nabhan C, Feusner JH, Rowe JM. Acute promyelocytic leukemia: evolving therapeutic strategies. Blood 2002;99(3):759–767.
38. Paez-Pereda M, Kovalovsky D, Hopfner U, Theodoropoulou M, Pagotto U, Uhl E et al. Retinoic acid prevents experimental Cushing syndrome. J Clin Invest 2001;108(8):1123–1131.
39. Castillo V, Giacomini D, Paez-Pereda M, Stalla J, Labeur M, Theodoropoulou M et al. Retinoic acid as a novel medical therapy for Cushing's disease in dogs. Endocrinology 2006;147(9):4438–4444.
40. Krieger DT, Amorosa L, Linick F. Cyproheptadine-induced remission of Cushing's disease. N Engl J Med 1975;293(18):893–896.
41. Suda T, Tozawa F, Mouri T, Sasaki A, Shibasaki T, Demura H et al. Effects of cyproheptadine, reserpine, and synthetic corticotropin-releasing factor on pituitary glands from patients with Cushing's disease. J Clin Endocrinol Metab 1983;56(6):1094–1099.
42. Waveren Hogervorst CO, Koppeschaar HP, Zelissen PM, Lips CJ, Garcia BM. Cortisol secretory patterns in Cushing's disease and response to cyproheptadine treatment. J Clin Endocrinol Metab 1996;81(2):652–655.
43. Tanakol R, Alagol F, Azizlerli H, Sandalci O, Terzioglu T, Berker F. Cyproheptadine treatment in Cushing's disease. J Endocrinol Invest 1996;19(4):242–247.
44. Whitehead HM, Beacom R, Sheridan B, Atkinson AB. The effect of cyproheptadine and/or bromocriptine on plasma ACTH levels in patients cured of Cushing's disease by bilateral adrenalectomy. Clin Endocrinol (Oxf) 1990;32(2):193–201.
45. Sonino N, Boscaro M, Fallo F, Fava GA. Potential therapeutic effects of ritanserin in Cushing's disease. JAMA 1992;267(8):1073.
46. Sonino N, Fava GA, Fallo F, Franceschetto A, Belluardo P, Boscaro M. Effect of the serotonin antagonists ritanserin and ketanserin in Cushing's disease. Pituitary 2000;3(2):55–59.
47. Koppeschaar HP, Croughs RJ, Thijssen JH, Schwarz F. Sodium valproate and cyproheptadine may independently induce a remission in the same patient with Cushing's disease. Acta Endocrinol (Copenh) 1983;104(2):160–163.
48. Colao A, Pivonello R, Tripodi FS, Orio F, Jr., Ferone D, Cerbone G et al. Failure of long-term therapy with sodium valproate in Cushing's disease. J Endocrinol Invest 1997;20(7):387–392.
49. Newell-Price J, Grossman AB. The differential diagnosis of Cushing's syndrome. Ann Endocrinol (Paris) 2001;62(2):173–179.
50. Liddle GW, Estepe HL, Kendall JWJ, Williams WCJ, Townes A. Clinical application of a new test of pituitary reserve. J Clin Endocrinol Metab 1959;19:875–894.
51. ABPI. Medicines Compendium. Datapharm Communications Ltd, 2008.
52. Trainer PJ, Eastment C, Grossman AB, Wheeler MJ, Perry L, Besser GM. The relationship between cortisol production rate and serial serum cortisol estimation in patients on medical therapy for Cushing's syndrome. Clin Endocrinol (Oxf) 1993;39(4):441–443.
53. Verhelst JA, Trainer PJ, Howlett TA, Perry L, Rees LH, Grossman AB et al. Short and long-term responses to metyrapone in the medical management of 91 patients with Cushing's syndrome. Clin Endocrinol (Oxf) 1991;35(2):169–178.
54. Connell JM, Cordiner J, Davies DL, Fraser R, Frier BM, McPherson SG. Pregnancy complicated by Cushing's syndrome: potential hazard of metyrapone therapy. Case report. Br J Obstet Gynaecol 1985;92(11):1192–1195.
55. Orth DN. Metyrapone is useful only as adjunctive therapy in Cushing's disease. Ann Intern Med 1978;89(1):128–130.
56. Engelhardt D, Dorr G, Jaspers C, Knorr D. Ketoconazole blocks cortisol secretion in man by inhibition of adrenal 11 beta-hydroxylase. Klin Wochenschr 1985;63(13):607–612.
57. Oelkers W, Bahr V, Hensen J, Pickartz H. Primary adrenocortical micronodular adenomatosis causing Cushing's syndrome. Effects of ketoconazole on steroid production and in vitro performance of adrenal cells. Acta Endocrinol (Copenh) 1986;113(3):370–377.
58. Sonino N. The endocrine effects of ketoconazole. J Endocrinol Invest 1986;9(4):341–347.
59. Weber MM, Luppa P, Engelhardt D. Inhibition of human adrenal androgen secretion by ketoconazole. Klin Wochenschr 1989;67(14):707–712.
60. Angeli A, Frairia R. Ketoconazole therapy in Cushing's disease. Lancet 1985;1(8432):821.
61. Sonino N, Boscaro M, Paoletta A, Mantero F, Ziliotto D. Ketoconazole treatment in Cushing's syndrome: experience in 34 patients. Clin Endocrinol (Oxf). 1991;35(4):347–352.

62. Zollner E, Delport S, Bonnici F. Fatal liver failure due to ketoconazole treatment of a girl with Cushing's syndrome. J Pediatr Endocrinol Metab 2001;14(3):335–338.
63. Lewis JH, Zimmerman HJ, Benson GD, Ishak KG. Hepatic injury associated with ketoconazole therapy. Analysis of 33 cases. Gastroenterology 1984;86(3):503–513.
64. Stricker BH, Blok AP, Bronkhorst FB, Van Parys GE, Desmet VJ. Ketoconazole-associated hepatic injury. A clinicopathological study of 55 cases. J Hepatol 1986;3(3):399–406.
65. Knight TE, Shikuma CY, Knight J. Ketoconazole-induced fulminant hepatitis necessitating liver transplantation. J Am Acad Dermatol 1991;25(2 Pt 2):398–400.
66. Miettinen TA. Cholesterol metabolism during ketoconazole treatment in man. J Lipid Res 1988;29(1):43–51.
67. Hart MM, Straw JA. Effect of 1-)0-chlorophenyl)-1-(p-chlorophenyl)-2,2-dichloroethane on adrenocorticotropic hormone-induced steroidogenesis in various preparations in vitro of dog adrenal cortex. Biochem Pharmacol 1971;20(7): 1679–1688.
68. Young RB, Bryson MJ, Sweat ML, Street JC. Complexing of DDT and o,p'DDD with adrenal cytochrome P-450 hydroxylating systems. J Steroid Biochem 1973;4(6):585–591.
69. Caticha O, Odell WD, Wilson DE, Dowdell LA, Noth RH, Swislocki AL et al. Estradiol stimulates cortisol production by adrenal cells in estrogen-dependent primary adrenocortical nodular dysplasia. J Clin Endocrinol Metab 1993;77(2):494–497.
70. Luton JP, Cerdas S, Billaud L, Thomas G, Guilhaume B, Bertagna X et al. Clinical features of adrenocortical carcinoma, prognostic factors, and the effect of mitotane therapy. N Engl J Med 1990;322(17):1195–1201.
71. Hutter AM, Jr., Kayhoe DE. Adrenal cortical carcinoma. Results of treatment with o,p'DDD in 138 patients. Am J Med 1966;41(4):581–592.
72. Maher VM, Trainer PJ, Scoppola A, Anderson JV, Thompson GR, Besser GM. Possible mechanism and treatment of o,p'DDD-induced hypercholesterolaemia. Q J Med 1992;84(305):671–679.
73. Haak HR, Caekebeke-Peerlinck KM, van Seters AP, Briet E. Prolonged bleeding time due to mitotane therapy. Eur J Cancer 1991;27(5):638–641.
74. Bledsoe T, Island DP, Ney RL, Liddle GW. An effect of o,p'-DDD on the extra-adrenal metabolism of cortisol in man. J Clin Endocrinol Metab 1964;24:1303–1311.
75. van Seters AP, Moolenaar AJ. Mitotane increases the blood levels of hormone-binding proteins. Acta Endocrinol (Copenh) 1991;124(5):526–533.
76. Hague RV, May W, Cullen DR. Hepatic microsomal enzyme induction and adrenal crisis due to o,p'DDD therapy for metastatic adrenocortical carcinoma. Clin Endocrinol (Oxf) 1989;31(1):51–57.
77. Leiba S, Weinstein R, Shindel B, Lapidot M, Stern E, Levavi H et al. The protracted effect of o,p'-DDD in Cushing's disease and its impact on adrenal morphogenesis of young human embryo. Ann Endocrinol (Paris) 1989;50(1):49–53.
78. Dexter RN, Fishman LM, Ney RL, Liddle GW. Inhibition of adrenal corticosteroid synthesis by aminoglutethimide: studies of the mechanism of action. J Clin Endocrinol Metab 1967;27(4):473–480.
79. Shaw MA, Nicholls PJ, Smith HJ. Aminoglutethimide and ketoconazole: historical perspectives and future prospects. J Steroid Biochem 1988;31(1):137–146.
80. Zachmann M, Gitzelmann RP, Zagalak M, Prader A. Effect of aminoglutethimide on urinary cortisol and cortisol metabolites in adolescents with Cushing's syndrome. Clin Endocrinol (Oxf) 1977;7(1):63–71.
81. Sonino N, Boscaro M. Medical therapy for Cushing's disease. Endocrinol Metab Clin North Am 1999;28(1): 211–222.
82. Miller JW, Crapo L. The medical treatment of Cushing's syndrome. Endocr Rev 1993;14(4):443–458.
83. Misbin RI, Canary J, Willard D. Aminoglutethimide in the treatment of Cushing's syndrome. J Clin Pharmacol 1976;16(11–12):645–651.
84. Child DF, Burke CW, Burley DM, Rees LH, Fraser TR. Drug controlled of Cushing's syndrome. Combined aminoglutethimide and metyrapone therapy. Acta Endocrinol (Copenh) 1976;82(2):330–341.
85. Dewis P, Anderson DC, Bu'lock DE, Earnshaw R, Kelly WF. Experience with trilostane in the treatment of Cushing's syndrome. Clin Endocrinol (Oxf) 1983;18(6):533–540.
86. Sieber-Ruckstuhl NS, Boretti FS, Wenger M, Maser-Gluth C, Reusch CE. Cortisol, aldosterone, cortisol precursor, androgen and endogenous ACTH concentrations in dogs with pituitary-dependant hyperadrenocorticism treated with trilostane. Domest Anim Endocrinol 2006;31(1) 63–75.
87. Ledingham IM, Watt I. Influence of sedation on mortality in critically ill multiple trauma patients. Lancet 1983;1(8336):1270.
88. Weber MM, Lang J, Abedinpour F, Zeilberger K, Adelmann B, Engelhardt D. Different inhibitory effect of etomidate and ketoconazole on the human adrenal steroid biosynthesis. Clin Investig 1993;71(11):933–938.

89. Allolio B, Stuttmann R, Fischer H, Leonhard W, Winkelmann W. Long-term etomidate and adrenocortical suppression. Lancet 1983;2(8350):626.
90. Allolio B, Schulte HM, Kaulen D, Reincke M, Jaursch-Hancke C, Winkelmann W. Nonhypnotic low-dose etomidate for rapid correction of hypercortisolaemia in Cushing's syndrome. Klin Wochenschr 1988;66(8):361–364.
91. Drake WM, Perry LA, Hinds CJ, Lowe DG, Reznek RH, Besser GM. Emergency and prolonged use of intravenous etomidate to control hypercortisolemia in a patient with Cushing's syndrome and peritonitis. J Clin Endocrinol Metab 1998;83(10):3542–3544.
92. Krakoff J, Koch CA, Calis KA, Alexander RH, Nieman LK. Use of a parenteral propylene glycol-containing etomidate preparation for the long-term management of ectopic Cushing's syndrome. J Clin Endocrinol Metab 2001;86(9): 4104–4108.
93. Baulieu EE. The steroid hormone antagonist RU486. Mechanism at the cellular level and clinical applications. Endocrinol Metab Clin North Am 1991;20(4):873–891.
94. Healy DL, Chrousos GP, Schulte HM, Gold PW, Hodgen GD. Increased adrenocorticotropin, cortisol, and arginine vasopressin secretion in primates after the antiglucocorticoid steroid RU 486: dose response relationships. J Clin Endocrinol Metab 1985;60(1):1–4.
95. Nieman LK, Chrousos GP, Kellner C, Spitz IM, Nisula BC, Cutler GB et al. Successful treatment of Cushing's syndrome with the glucocorticoid antagonist RU 486. J Clin Endocrinol Metab 1985;61(3):536–540.
96. Bertagna X, Bertagna C, Laudat MH, Husson JM, Girard F, Luton JP. Pituitary-adrenal response to the antiglucocorticoid action of RU 486 in Cushing's syndrome. J Clin Endocrinol Metab 1986;63(3):639–643.
97. Chu JW, Matthias DF, Belanoff J, Schatzberg A, Hoffman AR, Feldman D. Successful long-term treatment of refractory Cushing's disease with high-dose mifepristone (RU 486). J Clin Endocrinol Metab 2001;86(8):3568–3573.
98. Sartor O, Cutler GB, Jr. Mifepristone: treatment of Cushing's syndrome. Clin Obstet Gynecol 1996;39(2):506–510
99. de Weerth C, Graat G, Buitelaar JK, Thijssen JH. Measurement of cortisol in small quantities of saliva. Clin Chem 2003;49(4):658–660.
100. Paccotti P, Minetto M, Terzolo M, Ventura M, Ganzit GP, Borrione P et al. Effects of high-intensity isokinetic exercise on salivary cortisol in athletes with different training schedules: relationships to serum cortisol and lactate. Int J Sports Med 2005;26(9):747–755.
101. Abercrombie HC, Speck NS, Monticelli RM. Endogenous cortisol elevations are related to memory facilitation only in individuals who are emotionally aroused. Psychoneuroendocrinology 2006;31(2):187–196.
102. Umeda T, Hiramatsu R, Iwaoka T, Shimada T, Miura F, Sato T. Use of saliva for monitoring unbound free cortisol levels in serum. Clin Chim Acta 1981;110(2–3):245–253.
103. Vining RF, McGinley RA, Maksvytis JJ, Ho KY. Salivary cortisol: a better measure of adrenal cortical function than serum cortisol. Ann Clin Biochem 1983;20 (Pt 6):329–335.
104. Gozansky WS, Lynn JS, Laudenslager ML, Kohrt WM. Salivary cortisol determined by enzyme immunoassay is preferable to serum total cortisol for assessment of dynamic hypothalamic–pituitary–adrenal axis activity. Clin Endocrinol (Oxf) 2005;63(3):336–341.
105. Patel RS, Shaw SR, McIntyre HE, McGarry GW, Wallace AM. Morning salivary cortisol versus short Synacthen test as a test of adrenal suppression. Ann Clin Biochem 2004;41(Pt 5):408–410.
106. Wong V, Yan T, Donald A, McLean M. Saliva and bloodspot cortisol: novel sampling methods to assess hydrocortisone replacement therapy in hypoadrenal patients. Clin Endocrinol (Oxf) 2004;61(1):131–137.
107. Myhill PC, Sillars BA, Starkstein S, Annus T, Yeap BB. Reduction in salivary cortisol concentration correlates with resolution of psychosis in Cushing's syndrome. J Neuropsychiatry Clin Neurosci 2008;20(1):113–115.
108. Gotelli GR, Wall JH, Kabra PM, Marton LJ. Fluorometric liquid-chromatographic determination of serum cortisol. Clin Chem 1981;27(3):441–443.
109. Guo T, Taylor RL, Singh RJ, Soldin SJ. Simultaneous determination of 12 steroids by isotope dilution liquid chromatography-photospray ionization tandem mass spectrometry. Clin Chim Acta 2006;372(1–2):76–82.

14 ACTH-Dependent Cushing Syndrome: Clinical and Diagnostic Aspects, and Treatment Approaches for Ectopic Cushing's Syndrome

Krystallenia I. Alexandraki, Andrea M. Isidori, and Ashley B. Grossman

Contents

Summary

Ectopic Cushing's syndrome (ECS) is represented mainly by the ectopic ACTH syndrome (EAS) and comprises ~20% of ACTH-dependent CS and ~10% of all types of CS. Nearly any neuroendocrine or non-endocrine tumour may be associated with EAS but the more prevalent tumours are bronchial carcinoids, small cell lung carcinomas (SCLC), islet cell tumours of the pancreas or pancreatic carcinoids, thymic carcinoids, medullary carcinomas of the thyroid, phaeochromocytomas and gastrinomas. Occult tumours are highly represented in all the series (12–37.5%) and constitute the more challenging cases of EAS, requiring long-term follow-up. Clinical features are often similar in ACTH-dependent CS, but the rapid onset and progress may suggest an ectopic source. A combination of biochemical tests and imaging studies seem the most appropriate approach for the prompt identification of EAS, even if there are several pitfalls to be avoided along the way. The most appropriate management for cure of EAS, when its source is identified, is surgical excision after control of hypercortisolaemia. Inhibitors of cortisol secretion and other newer modalities can be used alone or in

From: *Contemporary Endocrinology: Cushing's Syndrome: Pathophysiology, Diagnosis and Treatment*
Edited by: M.D. Bronstein (ed.), DOI 10.1007/978-1-60327-449-4_14,

combination, and bilateral adrenalectomy remains an alternative option. Tumour histology, the presence of metastases and effective control of hypercortisolaemia affect mortality and morbidity. The identification of a primary source for the EAS represents a considerable challenge for endocrinologists, requiring a careful and logical step-by-step approach of investigational protocols to avoid the calamity of misdiagnosis.

Key Words: Ectopic Cushing's syndrome, ACTH ectopic syndrome, Cushing's syndrome, neuroendocrine tumours, SCLC, hypercortisolaemia

INTRODUCTION

Ectopic Cushing's syndrome (ECS) is represented mainly by the ACTH ectopic syndrome (EAS) and comprises around 20% of ACTH-dependent CS and some 10% of all types of CS *(1)*. It can be associated with high malignant tumours or more indolent neuroendocrine tumours (NETs), and every effort should be made to localise its source by a meticulous diagnostic work-up followed by an attempt at complete resection, which represents the most appropriate treatment. However, a source cannot be always identified promptly, often requiring lifelong follow-up. Recently, we suggested a reclassification of EAS according to the clarity and timing of the identification of the source *(2)*. *Overt EAS* is associated with an obvious tumoural source at the time of the initial investigation, *covert EAS* with tumours that are identified during a subsequent evaluation or prolonged follow-up, and *occult EAS* with tumours that cannot be identified even after a meticulous diagnostic work-up, which is repeated during an extended follow-up period.

Another point of conflict in the definition is the presence of EAS before the diagnosis of the causative tumour or its emergence during follow-up *(3)*. The latter occurs in patients with high malignant tumours usually seen in oncological departments, and EAS represents a paraneoplastic syndrome appearing in the end-stage. Patients presenting with the EAS are usually seen in endocrine departments and is the most challenging, since it requires a structured diagnostic protocol for the identification of the tumoural source. We suggest that the type presenting with the syndrome ab initio should be defined as *classic EAS*, whereas the more oncologically presenting disorder should be considered as *paraneoplastic EAS* since its identification is used as a marker of disease progression and severity (Table 1). In addition, pathologic examination has shown that some tumours with positive immunostaining for ACTH may never present with clinical or biochemical evidence of excess hormone secretion *(4)*.

Table 1
Suggested Definitions of the Different ACTH Ectopic Syndrome (EAS) Types

Overt EAS when associated with an obvious tumoural source at the time of the initial investigation
Covert EAS when associated with tumours which are identified during a subsequent evaluation or prolonged follow-up
Occult EAS when associated with tumours that cannot be identified even after a meticulous diagnostic work-up which is repeated during an extended follow-up period
Classic EAS when presenting *ab initio* with the tumoural source
Paraneoplastic EAS when presenting during the natural history of an already known tumour

This review will focus on summarising our more recent knowledge regarding classic EAS as defined above. Furthermore, a brief description of the rare tumours that are the cause of EAS by secreting isolated CRH or the combination of CRH and ACTH will also be discussed *(1)*.

SOURCES OF EAS

The most frequently reported type of EAS is represented by Small cell lung carcinoma (SCLC) followed by neuroendocrine tumours (NETs), phaeochromocytomas and medullary carcinoma of the thyroid (MTC). The different percentages reported depend on the criteria used to characterise EAS in each study as well as by the referral pattern of the patients in oncological or endocrine departments; thus, the previous literature emphasises the high prevalence of SCLCs while nowadays NETs, and particularly bronchial carcinoids, seem to be more prevalent *(5, 6)*. Published series report as more frequent tumours associated with EAS bronchial carcinoids, SCLCs, islet cell tumours of the pancreas or pancreatic carcinoids, thymic carcinoids, MTC, phaeochromocytomas and gastrinomas, as well as cases in which the tumour was not identified *(2, 3, 6–17)*. However, the fact that, in some series SCLCs, MTC and phaechromocytomas were not included *(10, 11)* affected the reported percentages (Table 2). Other type of NETs and other miscellaneous tumours have also been rarely described *(2, 4, 6, 17–19)* (Table 2). Overall, the thorax and the neck remain the main sites of EAS, whereas the abdomen is the site of one-third of primary tumours *(6)*. It is of note that covert tumours are mainly represented by bronchial and appendiceal carcinoid tumours, NETs and SCLCs *(11, 12, 17)*, whereas the major occult source where tumours are eventually demonstrated remains the lung *(10)*.

Table 2
The Various Tumours that are Associated with Ectopic ACTH Syndrome

Tumour type (2–4, 6–19)	*Percentage reported (%)*
Bronchial carcinoids	5–40
SCLC	3.3–50
Islet cell tumours of the pancreas/pancreatic carcinoids	7.5–25
Thymic carcinoids	5–25
MTC	2–8
Phaeochromocytoma	2.5–25
Gastrinoma	5
Tumour not identified	12–37.5
Other neuroendocrine tumours (primary hepatic carcinoid tumours, spindle cell pancreatic endocrine tumours, olfactory esthesioneuroblastoma, paraganglioma, ectopic pituitary adenoma or disseminated with unknown primary)	<5
Other miscellaneous tumours (squamous cell cancer of the lung, mesothelioma, small cell colon carcinomas, tumours of the esophagus, stomach, pancreas, larynx, trachea, salivary gland, prostate, leydig cell, breast, ovary, uterine cervix, kidney, gallbladder and anorectal cancer, hepatocellular carcinoma, melanoma, leukaemia, lymphoma, and osteomyeloma)	

Regarding pathology, in a recent study, immunohistochemistry showed positive staining for chromogranin in 73% (10 carcinoids, 3 pancreatic tumours, 2 phaeochromocytomas, 1 glomus tumour), ACTH in 64% (10 carcinoids, 2 phaeochromocytomas, 1 pancreatic tumour, 1 glomus tumour), neuron-specific enolase (NSE) in 32% (4 carcinoids, 2 phaeochromocytomas, 1 glomus tumour), synaptophysin in 27% (5 carcinoids and 1 phaeochromocytoma), CK 8/18 in 23% (4 carcinoids, 1 phaeochromocytoma), calcitonin in 9% (phaeochromocytomas) and gastrin (pancreatic tumour), glucagon (pancreatic tumour), CD56 and TTF-1 (carcinoid) each on one occasion *(20)*. It has been suggested that the negative immunostaining for ACTH results from a high secretory capacity; however, negative in situ hybridization suggests that either a tumour identified is unrelated to the EAS or that it represents dedifferentiation of the original tumour *(21)*. Regarding bronchial carcinoids, approximately an equal number of typical and atypical carcinoids have been described *(17)*. In terms of tumour size, these have ranged from 0.3–4 cm in pulmonary carcinoids, 1–5 cm in thymic carcinoids, 1–4 cm in NETs, 3–7 cm in phaeochromocytomas and 1.5–5 cm in gastrinomas *(17)*.

DIAGNOSIS OF EAS

The diagnosis of ACTH-dependent CS requires stringent criteria for both EAS and CD *(1)*. The diagnosis of EAS requires reversal of the clinical picture after resection of the tumour and/or demonstration of ACTH immunohistochemical staining in the tumour tissue or in metastatic deposits, and/or complete/partial resolution of the hypercortisolaemia after tumour removal/debulking. However, these strict criteria are not applicable to many of the reported cases of EAS *(1, 6)*. There have been described cases that immunohistochemistry did not show ACTH in the tumoural cells, but a substantial post-operative fall in ACTH and cortisol was observed, suggesting that only a subpopulation of cells may actually secrete ACTH *(20)*. On the other hand, tumour resection might not be curative with disseminated tumours *(1)*.

Clinical Features, Signs and Symptoms

The age range of patients with EAS is at least one decade older than in CD, and the female-to-male ratio differs also, being from 1:1 to 2:1 in most studies *(2, 8–10, 17, 20)*. In addition, signs and symptoms seen in EAS cannot be characterised with accuracy since most data are provided from retrospective studies, and different departmental protocols have been used. However, there is general agreement that these depend on the tissue of origin and the type of tumour secreting ACTH. Generally, it has been shown that SCLCs have a more rapid onset of clinical signs than NETs, which generally have a gradual onset which is often indistinguishable from CD. However, it has been suggested that patients with SCLC, when evaluated at an early stage in their progression, may present in a similar manner to patients with other less malignant causes of EAS *(5)*. The time between the first clinical symptom of hypercortisolism and diagnosis of EAS was shorter in patients with SCLC and pancreatic islet cell tumours compared to bronchial carcinoids *(2, 6)*.

Concerning specific clinical features, weakness due to proximal myopathy, thinning of the skin and bruising were frequently present in all the studies, as well as hypertension, abnormalities in carbohydrate metabolism, hyperpigmentation and psychiatric features such as psychosis or major depression *(2, 16, 20)*. The rapidity of onset and the severity of the syndrome have been implicated for the more frequent presence of skin pigmentation and ankle oedema in SCLCs compared to other causes of EAS *(2)*. On the other hand, psychiatric disorders are prominent in NETs but less so in SCLCs, representing approximately 50% of patients with EAS *(2, 17)*. Furthermore systemic, local and even multiple infections, osteoporosis, osteopenia and/or fractures were features that correlated with the degree of hypercortisolaemia *(2, 9, 16, 17, 22)*. Groups of patients with overt or covert EAS did not differ in their clinical features, supporting the fact that the degree of hypercortisolaemia is the major determinant of the clinical features of the syndrome rather than its duration *(2)*.

Biochemical Work-up

Biochemical tests are considering crucial in the diagnostic work-up of EAS. Following confirmation of pathological hypercortisolaemia by the overnight dexamethasone test, low-dose dexamethasone test (LDDST), urinary free cortisol assessment and midnight serum or salivary cortisol assessments, testing focuses on differentiating between pituitary and ectopic ACTH production. This is dependent also on the demonstration of the detection of plasma ACTH to exclude primary adrenal disease. The subsequent selection of tests is based on the rationale that usually the corticotroph tumour cells in CD retain some responsiveness to the negative feedback effects of glucocorticoids or other regulatory mechanisms, whereas tumours ectopically secreting ACTH generally do not *(1, 23–25)*. The high-dose dexamethasone test (HDDST) and corticotropin-releasing hormone (CRH) (either alone or in combination with desmopressin) tests have been assessed. In the HDDST, cortisol suppression greater than 50% is indicative of CD with sensitivity of 60–100% and specificity of 65–100% *(23, 26–29)*; the sensitivity reaches 91% when the cut-off value for suppression is 50% of the baseline value and 97% when the cut-off value for suppression is 60%. Six to 40% of EAS patients have shown serum cortisol or urinary cortisol or 17-OHCS suppression on the HDDST *(9, 15, 17, 20, 24)*, but serum assessment is considered the more sensitive marker *(1, 24)*. Interestingly, when a cut-off for serum cortisol suppression was greater than 60% it occurred in 3% of patients with EAS, and when it was >80% it did not occur in any patients with EAS *(24, 26, 29)*. Patients with bronchial carcinoids have shown a higher incidence of cortisol suppression, approximately 60% following the HDDST *(15, 24)*. With the classic CRH stimulation test, an ACTH increase >35% and cortisol >20% above baseline levels is considered to be a specific response for CD when ovine CRH is used *(30)*, and an increase >105% and >14% respectively when human CRH is used *(31)*. The CRH test had a sensitivity of 94% for cortisol and ACTH responses, and overall approximately 5–17% of patients with EAS respond to CRH administration using a variety of cut-offs for cortisol and ACTH criteria *(23, 24, 26, 30, 31)*. In general, for a plasma ACTH increase >35% and cortisol >20% above baseline levels, the sensitivity is 70–93% and 85–92%, and specificity 100% and 88–100%, respectively; for an ACTH increase >50% and cortisol >20% the sensitivity is 93% and and 91% and the specificity 100% and 88%, respectively *(26, 31)*. Using desmopressin instead of CRH, 40% false-positive responses were observed in patients with EAS *(32)*, with a reported sensitivity of 77–84% and specificity 73–83% *(23, 26)*. Thus, looking at all the published data it appears that while each test on its own may be of relatively limited diagnostic accuracy, the combination of the results from HDDST and CRH tests is of clinical value, since the lack of response to *both* tests had a sensitivity of 100% and a diagnostic accuracy of 98% *(2, 5, 24, 33)*. The combination of these tests resulted in a 100% correct diagnosis for CD or 79% for EAS, while a 1% false-positive response was shown in patients with EAS *(17, 20, 26)*. Interestingly, a patient with EAS has been described associated with a lung carcinoid tumour with an absent response to desmopressin and CRH tests but with a significant increment in plasma ACTH and serum cortisol levels after the administration of GHRP-6 *(20)*, which is a potent ACTH secretagogue in normal individuals and patients with CD *(34)*.

The next step in the diagnostic work-up depends on the availability of bilateral inferior petrosal sinus sampling (BIPSS) with CRH stimulation, which represents the best diagnostic tool for differentiation of ACTH-dependent CS *(1, 23)*. Regarding BIPSS, the criteria used to identify CD is an inferior petrosal sinus-to-peripheral (IPS:P) ACTH ratio at baseline more than 2.0 and a gradient greater than 3.0 following CRH or desmopressin stimulation *(1)*. In patients with EAS, an IPS:P of less than 2.0 before and after CRH or desmopressin administration has been reported *(35, 36)*. However, there have been rare reports of false negative *(5, 36, 37)* as well as false-positive responses, even following CRH *(2, 17, 37–39)*, particularly when an adequate hypercortisolaemic state is not present *(10)*. Furthermore, this test demands experience and is performed only in specialised centres since its complications include stroke, perforation of the atrial wall, hematomas and transitory arrhythmias *(20)*.

The responses to these tests did not differ among patients with overt, covert and occult EAS *(2)*. In addition, no difference was seen among patients with NETs or other tumours or patients with occult tumours *(17)*. The importance of the combination of these tests has been proved by reported cases that showed disconcordance between HDDST/CRH and BIPSS in the presence of EAS *(5)*.

Whole-body venous catheterisation and sampling when an ectopic source is suspected has not been shown to be useful, and is no longer recommended, besides being clinically demanding, as modern imaging modalities have proved to be more useful *(10, 17, 40)*. However, selective venous sampling from suspected sources of EAS on the basis of an abnormal CT may still occasionally be useful to confirm the source of EAS *(2, 10)*.

Other discriminatory factors traditionally used to differentiate between EAS and CD are the absolute levels of plasma ACTH and the degree of hypokalaemia. With regard to ACTH levels, no cut-off limit has been defined to distinguish patients with EAS and CD even if some discriminatory values of baseline ACTH have been described previously *(2, 11, 17, 41)*. In 50–64% of patients with EAS ACTH levels were greater than 200 ng/L, but with considerable overlap between patients with CD and EAS *(9, 15, 26)*; 24–32% of patients with EAS had levels within the normal range *(17, 20)*. On the other hand, ACTH levels did not differ in patients with occult and overt EAS, suggesting that the dimension of a tumour is not correlated with the level of ACTH *(2, 17)*; however, higher levels were observed in patients where the source was identified within 6 months *(17)*. Biologically-inactive fragments or precursors not detected in conventional ACTH assays have been associated with EAS, such as pro-opiomelanocortin (POMC) *(42)*, and a high POMC/ACTH ratio has been considered a marker of tumour aggressiveness *(43)*. However, macroadenomas in CD also tend to produce a larger proportion of inactive ACTH-related molecules. Hypokalaemia is present in around 64–70% of patients with EAS *(9, 15, 17, 20)*, but is also seen in a minority of patients with CD. Severe systemic infection and/or sepsis were present in 35% of EAS patients *(22)*, but any grade of infection from mild to severe was reported in some 50% of patients *(17)*.

Additional biochemical markers may be associated with NETs and these have been assessed in several studies. Calcitonin and urinary catecholamines have been measured to exclude MTC and phaeochromocytoma as a source *(6)*. Calcitonin and gastrin have been both found to be the most commonly elevated tumour markers, regardless of tumour type, in all the recent series *(2, 20)*; calcitonin has been suggested to be particularly useful in differentiation between EAS and CD since in the latter it shows low levels *(17)*. Specifically, increased levels were seen in 75% and 38% patients with overt and occult tumours, respectively, and overall in 44–66% of EAS *(9, 11, 17)*. It has been also suggested that when tumour markers indicative of endocrine islet cell tumours were positive, such tumours were relatively large and radiologically evident. On the other hand, urinary 5-hydroxyindoleacetic acid levels were normal in the majority of patients since NETs arising from the embryonic foregut (such as the lung) are usually deficient in the enzyme aromatic L-amino acid decarboxylase *(44)*; however, they have been found to be increased in 26% of EAS patients *(18)*. Other tumour markers occasionally documented as elevated are the gut peptides such as glucagon, somatostatin, pancreatic polypeptide, vasoactive intestinal peptide, the placental marker β-human chorionic gonadotropin, and the oncofetal proteins α-fetoprotein, carcinoembryonic antigen, and other neuroendocrine or hormonal markers such as NSE, α-subunit and GHRH *(12, 21)*. In general, one or other of such tumour markers is increased in 72% of patients with EAS *(20)*.

Imaging

In searching for an ectopic source, axial imaging with thin-cut multislice imaging with chest, abdominal, and pelvic CT scanning, plus possibly MRI of the thorax and pelvis, are complementary and have the highest detection rate for EAS source identification *(2, 11, 17, 21)*. MRI of the abdomen is not used routinely, in part because of the problem of bowel movement artefact and because of the fact that calcification associated with the primary tumour is easier to identify on a CT scan; CT and MRI fail to localise the source of EAS in 8–50% of patients *(2, 10, 17, 20)*, but this rate reduces to 12.5% when an appropriate and meticulous technique is used and patients are followed-up long-term along with the additional newer imaging modalities *(2, 5)*.

Scintigraphy has been reported to be variably helpful, and in the absence of conventional imaging is often difficult to interpret *(21)*. Standard ^{111}In-octreotide scintigraphy (Octreoscan™) has been claimed by some groups as offering novel information, but while it may occasionally be useful on its own it generally has not shown a source undetectable on CT and MRI, although it does add supportive functional data *(16, 17, 45)*. However, even if the data do not support the superiority of the octreotide scintiscan over CT scanning, as shown in a direct comparison *(9, 12, 45)*, it has been proved useful to enhance their resolution for findings not seen on first assessment *(12, 20)*, and there are isolated cases that report its superiority *(46, 47)*. It has been recently suggested that its performance is useful as complementary modality to CT and MRI in specific cases *(20, 48, 49)* and should be considered when other imaging modalities fail to localise the ACTH-secreting tumour *(5, 49, 50)*. In one report, the octreotide scintiscan (using high doses - 180 mCi) identified a tumour in one patient with otherwise negative imaging *(51)*. It may be that PET scanning with the new isotope Ga-68 will be more sensitive.

The standard [^{18}F]Flurodeoxyglucose positron emission tomography (FDG-PET) scan usually does not add more information since such occult tumours have a low metabolic rate and FDG-PET did not detect tumours that were occult on CT/MRI *(51, 52)*. However, there are isolated cases where FDG-PET identified tumours not revealed by the other imaging studies, or were useful to confirm suspicious findings and recurrence *(53, 54)*. Furthermore, a bronchial carcinoid overlooked by planar indium-111 pentetreotide scintigraphy was accurately localised by SPECT/CT acquisition *(55)*. On the other hand, whole-body PET with ^{11}C-5-hydroxytryptophan has been used in few cases and it seems promising when the source of EAS cannot be identified and may thus identify an otherwise occult NET *(56, 57)*. ^{131}I- and ^{123}I meta-iodobenzylguanidine scans have also been used in occasional patients with or without success in primary tumour or metastasis identification *(2, 10)*. Other imaging studies such as selective abdominal angiography and endoscopic ultrasonography can be used in specific cases when there is a suspicion of a pancreatic NET *(12)*, and thyroid ultrasound to exclude an MTC *(21)*.

Finally, one additional imaging tool is the appearance of the adrenals on CT scanning, as these have been reported to be normal in size in only 7% of patients with EAS, while a moderate or marked hyperplasia is present in 56% and 37% respectively. By contrast, in CD 50% show either normal or mildly enlarged adrenals *(10)*. However, no difference was observed between EAS and CD regarding macronodular hyperplasia (11% vs. 10%, respectively). Of note, the search for a secretory phaeochromocytoma has to be included in the investigation of EAS, as well as the fact that the presence of adrenal hyperplasia might complicate the search for a source prior to control of the hypercortisolaemia *(10)*.

TREATMENT OF EAS

Surgical Approaches

When an ectopic source is identified the ideal treatment is radical excision of the tumour. In patients with a single primary lesion, curative resection with complete remission was found in 83% *(2)*. In most studies curative surgery was successful in 30–47% *(2, 17)*. Conversely, the surgical approach might be non-curative in disseminated tumours but may still supply useful diagnostic biopsies. On the other hand, multiple recurrences may be controlled by multiple surgical excisions *(58)*.

Another surgical approach in EAS is unilateral or complete bilateral adrenalectomy, performed in 30–56% of patients when hypercortisolaemia cannot be treated by other means, or when a source of EAS remains occult after a long-term follow-up. It has also been used when medical treatment was ineffective, not well tolerated, or rejected by the patient, as in young women desiring pregnancy *(2, 8, 17, 20)*. The recent advances in the technique of bilateral laparoscopic adrenalectomy make this alternative attractive, particularly in occult EAS *(59)*.

Medical Therapy

The medical management of a tumour associated with EAS should target the tumour or its consequences, namely the hypercortisolaemia. Consequently, inhibitors of cortisol secretion have to be used for the rapid control of the short-term sequelae of hypercortisolaemia, the metabolic consequences and poor healing *(60)*. The time to use these drugs is during the diagnostic work-up after the biochemical tests and before the surgical approach, or during the "waiting period" for the identification of a covert or occult tumour *(17, 61)*. This fact has to be considered in case of SCLCs, since the correction of hypercortisolism has to be achieved promptly to normalise serum cortisol rapidly since myelosuppressive cytotoxic chemotherapy creates a highly lethal combination with cortisol excess. It has been recently reported that in medical oncology departments, myelosuppressive regimens are often postponed for several weeks until cortisol has been normalised *(62)*. Additionally, etomidate infusions have been successfully used when a rapid control of hypercortisolaemia in severely ill patients with EAS is required *(63)*, or when severely ill patients are unable to take oral medications long-term *(64)*.

In some cases, somatostatin receptors (SSTRs) as well as dopamine receptors have been identified in tumour specimens or by imaging studies, and thus somatostatin analogues (SSAs) and dopamine agonists, alone or in combination, have been used in cases of recurrence, incomplete resection or occult tumours *(65, 66)*. The presence of SSTRs in EAS has been investigated and confirmed by octreotide scintiscanning *(67)*, and SSAs have been successfully used to reduce cortisol levels alone or in combination with inhibitors of cortisol secretion *(68–70)*. Interestingly, it has been demonstrated that aberrant functioning of the glucocorticoid receptor may be responsible for the sensitivity to SSAs in EAS opposed to CD *(65, 71, 72)*. In addition, D_2 and D_4 receptors were identified in NETs, and cabergoline treatment effectively reduced cortisol levels in some patients with persistent EAS after surgery *(73)*. However, each treatment alone was associated with an escape phenomenon *(73, 74)* although this was abrogated by the combination with SSA and the dopamine agonist treatment, as shown in a patient with EAS and an atypical carcinoid tumour *(75)*.

Complementary Therapy

Additional types of treatment have been used whenever surgery is not curative, and a multidisciplinary approach should be adopted to control tumour growth and associated symptoms *(6)*. External radiotherapy directed to the mediastinum has been used for carcinoids directed to the tumour bed or to metastatic deposits *(2, 17)*. Radiofrequency ablation was used to treat hepatic metastases of NETs, and intraoperative "octreoscanning" with a hand-held gamma detector probe has been proposed to increase the intraoperative detection rate *(76, 77)*. Interferon has also been used in metastatic NETs and SCLCs, as well as chemotherapy with 5-fluorouracil, streptozotocin, cisplatin, etoposide, and/or adriamycin *(17)*. Hormone analogues and/or radionuclide treatment, chemoembolisation and ^{131}I-MIBG treatment have also been used *(2)*.

Prognosis

The prognosis of patients with EAS is influenced by tumour histology and by hypercortisolaemia, since they both affect mortality and morbidity. Patients with SCLCs and thymic carcinoids seem to have the worst prognosis, while patients with tumours with endocrine differentiation have a better prognosis. Furthermore, patients with MTC, phaeochromocytoma and other carcinoid tumours have a worse prognosis compared to bronchial carcinoid tumours. Islet cell tumours and MTC are aggressive and frequently metastatic at the time of diagnosis *(2)*. Metastatic deposits imply a negative effect on overall survival in patients with NETs, while extrathoracic NETs, thymic carcinoids, SCLCs, MTC, and gastrinomas which usually were detected as overt tumours with metastatic disease caused death within 2 years *(17)*. On the other hand, pulmonary, appendiceal and pancreatic carcinoids, and pulmonary or mediastinal NETs, tended to be initially occult and were less likely to metastasise *(3, 17)*. Patients harbouring phaeochromocytomas or bronchial carcinoids, and those without local or lymph node metastases, seemed to have a better prognosis when compared with those with local or distant metastases *(20)*. Generally, patients with pulmonary EAS (besides SCLCs) survived longest *(17)*. Survival analysis revealed that tumour histology and, in the subgroup of NETs, the presence of non-lymph node metastases, are the most important prognostic factors predicting overall survival *(2)*. The mortality rate described was 18–63% depending on the duration of follow-up: 81% of patients died because of metastases *(2, 17)*. Interestingly, the observed mortality rate was 100% for SCLSs, 100% for MTC, 67% for gastrinoma, 67% for islet-cell tumours, 40% for thymic carcinoid, 20% for phaeochromocytomas, 15% for NETs, 9% for pulmonary carcinoids, and 12–40% for occult tumours *(2, 17)*. Thus, patients with occult tumours survived longer *(2, 17, 20)*, and in the longest follow-up study only patients with NETs were still alive *(2)*. Interestingly, the survival of patients with occult EAS was affected by the prompt and effective control of hypercortisolaemia *(5, 17)*. Hypercortisolaemia was associated with infections, pancreatitis, peritonitis with perforation, meningitis, cardiac failure and pulmonary embolism, these also being causes of death *(2, 17, 20)*. This fact implies the necessity for the rapid control of hypercortisolaemia and the prophylaxis of its complications.

OTHER TYPES OF ECS

Isolated CRH CS is a very rare cause of ECS and has been described with SCLCs, bronchial carcinoid, ectopic pituitary adenoma, intrasellar gangliocytomas, phaeochromocytomas, prostatic carcinomas and MTC or its metastases *(12, 78)*. Most patients had pituitary surgery with the demonstration of pituitary hyperplasia, and their diagnosis followed surgery or was post-mortem *(12)*. It has been suggested that some of those cases are tumours co-secreting CRH and ACTH, with negative immunostaining for ACTH because of the high ACTH secretion levels *(12, 79)*. Such combined CRH and ACTH secretion causing CS has been described with SCLCs, bronchial and thymic carcinoids, pancreatic carcinoma and MTC, phaeochromocytoma, paraganglioma and nephroblastoma *(12, 79)*.

PITFALLS IN DIFFERENTIAL DIAGNOSIS

As previously stated the diagnosis of EAS has to be carefully based on clinical, biochemical and imaging features of a patient with CS. A conclusive diagnosis may need to be deferred until there is clear-cut evidence of an ectopic source or the identification of a pituitary adenoma; the major pitfall is the interruption of follow-up of occult EAS, which has to be prolonged for more than 20 years *(21)*. The outcome of this management is a rate of 12–50% of patients with EAS undergoing transsphenoidal surgery, this rate being higher in occult EAS *(8, 10, 16, 17, 80)*.

However, improvements in imaging may demonstrate "lesions" which are unrelated to the source of ACTH, as they do in the pituitary *(81)*. On the other hand, the fact that bronchial carcinoids might be equal or less than 1cm *(23)*, and may be confused with vascular shadows, is a further pitfall for the unwary *(25)*. Octreotide scintiscanning should always be performed only in conjunction with conventional imaging studies since false-positive results have been reported in certain conditions, such as inflammation, granulomatous and autoimmune lesions, follicular thyroid adenomas, radiation fibrosis, lymphomas, and accessory spleens *(25)*.

With regard to biochemical testing, again all results must be judged in combination. Recently, it was reported that the clinical and biochemical features, and very high ACTH levels, seen in a cohort of patients with pituitary macroadenomas to some extent mimicked those of the EAS: the rate of cortisol suppression is lower in patients with CD caused by pituitary macroadenomas compared to microadenomas *(82, 83)*. Furthermore, technical problems during catheterisation, petrosal sinus hypoplasia, and anomalous venous drainage may result in false-negative results of BIPSS *(25)*, while ectopic CRH secretion or treatment with inhibitors of cortisol secretion result in false-positive results of BIPSS because of desuppression of the normal corticotrophs with consequent responsivity to CRH or desmopressin *(21, 25)*.

Finally, the cyclical secretion of ACTH in EAS has to be considered since the intercycle suppression of normal corticotroph production could lead to a false-negative BIPSS if sampled during an "off" phase *(37)*. Cyclic hypercortisolaemia has been described in association with typical bronchial and malignant carcinoid tumour of the lung, gastric carcinoid, oncocytic carcinoid of the kidney, bronchial adenoma, phaeochromocytoma, ectopic pituitary adenoma and in occult tumours *(47, 66, 84–86)*. A recent review reported a prevalence of 26% of EAS in patients with cyclic CS between published series and case reports *(85)*. However, in the most recent series of patients with EAS, 4–10% had "cyclic" CS as opposed to a prevalence of 15% recently described in CD *(2, 20, 87)*.

CONCLUSIONS

We would emphasise that nearly any neuroendocrine or non-endocrine tumour, including atypical tumours, may be associated with EAS. This is the reason why a multidisciplinary approach is required for both diagnostic work-up and therapeutic management. The lack of consistent endocrine evaluation and imaging to clearly reveal the source of EAS suggests the adoption of a step-by-step approach, particularly in the case of occult disease. It is important to consider a probabilistic approach to diagnostic testing in place of a linear algorithm. New technologies in imaging and nuclear medicine as well as new drugs that target the sources of EAS are continuously under exploration for better management of EAS. Survival of patients with EAS depends on the source of the primary tumour; those with SCLCs fare badly but the more indolent tumours, especially the bronchial carcinoids, show prolonged survival followed by pancreatic and appendiceal carcinoids. Furthermore, if a source repeatedly fails to be found, the prognosis is often favourable and the appearance of a malignant tumour, albeit of low grade, must be sought during follow-up, which should be lifelong.

REFERENCES

1. Newell-Price J, Bertagna X, Grossman AB, Nieman LK. Cushing's syndrome. Lancet 2006;367:1605–1617.
2. Isidori AM, Kaltsas GA, Pozza C, et al. The ectopic adrenocorticotrophin syndrome: clinical features, diagnosis, management and long-term follow-up. J Clin Endocrinol Metab 2006;91:371–377.
3. Aniszewski JP, Young WF Jr, Thompson GB, Grant CS, van Heerden JA. Cushing syndrome due to ectopic adrenocorticotropic hormone secretion.World J Surg 2001;25:934–940.
4. Imura H, Matsukura S, Yamamoto H, Hirata Y, Nakai Y. Studies on ectopic ACTH-producing tumors. II. Clinical and biochemical features of 30 cases. Cancer 1975;35:1430–1437.
5. Isidori AM, Kaltsas GA, Grossman AB. Ectopic ACTH syndrome. Front Horm Res 2006;35:143–156.
6. Isidori AM, Lenzi A. Ectopic ACTH syndrome. Arq Bras Endocrinol Metabol 2007;51:1217–1225.
7. Liddle GW, Nicholson WE, Island DP, Orth DN, Abe K, Lowder SC. Clinical and laboratory studies of ectopic humoral syndromes. Recent Prog Horm Res 1969;25:283–314.
8. Jex RK, van Heerden JA, Carpenter PC, Grant CS. Ectopic ACTH syndrome. Diagnostic and therapeutic aspects. Am J Surg 1985;149:276–282.
9. Howlett TA, Drury PL, Perry L, Doniach I, Rees LH, Besser GM. Diagnosis and management of ACTH-dependent Cushing's syndrome: comparison of the features in ectopic and pituitary ACTH production. Clin Endocrinol (Oxf). 1986;24:699–713.
10. Doppman JL, Nieman L, Miller DL, et al. Ectopic adrenocorticotropic hormone syndrome: localization studies in 28 patients. Radiology 1989;172:115–124.
11. Wajchenberg BL, Mendonca BB, Liberman B, et al. Ectopic adrenocorticotropic hormone syndrome. Endocr Rev 1994;15:752–787.
12. Wajchenberg BL, Mendonça B, Liberman B, Adelaide M, Pereira A, Kirschner MA. Ectopic ACTH syndrome. J Steroid Biochem Mol Biol 1995;53:139–151.
13. Tabarin A, Valli N, Chanson P, et al. Usefulness of somatostatin receptor scintigraphy in patients with occult ectopic adrenocorticotropin syndrome. J Clin Endocrinol Metab 1999;84:1193–1202.
14. Torpy DJ, Mullen N, Ilias I, Nieman LK. Association of hypertension and hypokalemia with Cushing's syndrome caused by ectopic ACTH secretion: a series of 58 cases. Ann NY Acad Sci 2002;970:134–144.
15 Beuschlein F, Hammer GD. Ectopic pro-opiomelanocortin syndrome. Endocrinol Metab Clin North Am 2002;31:191–234.
16 Hernández I, Espinosa-de-los-Monteros AL, Mendoza V, et al.Ectopic ACTH-secreting syndrome: a single center experience report with a high prevalence of occult tumor. Arch Med Res 2006;37:976–980.
17 Ilias I, Torpy DJ, Pacak K, Mullen N, Wesley RA, Nieman LK. Cushing's syndrome due to ectopic corticotropin secretion: twenty years' experience at the National Institutes of Health. J Clin Endocrinol Metab 2005; 90:4955–4962.
18 Chetty R, Serra S. Spindle cell pancreatic endocrine tumor associated with Cushing's syndrome. Endocr Pathol 2005;16:145–151.
19. Shah NA, Urusova IA, D'Agnolo A, et al. Primary hepatic carcinoid tumor presenting as Cushing's syndrome. J Endocrinol Invest 2007;30:327–333.
20. Salgado LR, Fragoso MC, Knoepfelmacher M, et al. Ectopic ACTH syndrome: our experience with 25 cases. Eur J Endocrinol 2006;155:725–733.
21. Grossman AB, Kelly P, Rockall A, Bhattacharya S, McNicol A, Barwick T. Cushing's syndrome caused by an occult source: difficulties in diagnosis and management. Nat Clin Pract Endocrinol Metab 2006;2:642–647.
22. Sarlis NJ, Chanock SJ, Nieman LK. Cortisolemic indices predict severe infections in Cushing syndrome due to ectopic production of adrenocorticotropin. J Clin Endocrinol Metab 2000;85:42–47.
23. Newell-Price J, Trainer P, Besser GM, Grossman A. The diagnosis and differential diagnosis of Cushing's syndrome and pseudo-Cushing's states. Endocr Rev 1998;19:647–672.
24. Isidori AM, Kaltsas GA, Mohammed S, et al. Discriminatory value of the low-dose dexamethasone suppression test in establishing the diagnosis and differential diagnosis of Cushing's syndrome. J Clin Endocrinol Metab 2003;88:5299–5306.
25. Vilar L, Freitas Mda C, Faria M, et al. Pitfalls in the diagnosis of Cushing's syndrome. Arq Bras Endocrinol Metabol 2007;51:1207–1216.
26. Vilar L, Naves LA, Freitas MC, et al. Endogenous Cushing's syndrome: Clinical and laboratorial features in 73 cases. Arq Bras Endocrinol Metab 2007;51:566–574.
27. Kaye TB, Crapo L. The Cushing syndrome: an update on diagnostic tests. Ann Intern Med 1990;112:434–444.
28. Meier CA, Biller BMK. Clinical and biochemical evaluation of Cushing's syndrome. Endocrinol Metab Clin North Am 1997;26:741–762.

29. Invitti C, Giraldi FP, de Martin M, Cavagnini F. Diagnosis and management of Cushing's syndrome: results of an Italian multicentre study. Study group of the Italian Society of Endocrinology on the pathophysiology of the hypothalamic-pituitaryadrenal axis. J Clin Endocrinol Metab 1999;84:440–448.
30. Nieman LK, Oldfield EH, Wesley R, Chrousos GP, Loriaux DL, Cutler GB Jr. A simplified morning ovine corticotropin-releasing hormone stimulation test for the differential diagnosis of adrenocorticotropin-dependent Cushing's syndrome. J Clin Endocrinol Metab 1993;77:1308–1312.
31. Newell-Price J, Morris DG, Drake WM, et al. Optimal response criteria for the human CRH test in the differential diagnosis of ACTH-dependent Cushing's syndrome. J Clin Endocrinol Metab 2002;87:1640–1645.
32. Terzolo M, Reimondo G, Ali A, et al. The limited value of the desmopressin test in the diagnostic approach to Cushing's syndrome. Clin Endocrinol (Oxf). 2001;54:609–616.
33. Nieman LK, Chrousos GP, Oldfield EH, Avgerinos PC, Cutler GB Jr, Loriaux DL. The ovine corticotropin-releasing hormone stimulation test and the dexamethasone suppression test in the differential diagnosis of Cushing's syndrome. Ann Intern Med 1986;105:862–867.
34. Ghigo E, Arvat E, Ramunni J, et al. Adrenocorticotropin- and cortisolreleasing effect of hexarelin, a synthetic growth hormonereleasing peptide, in normal subjects and patients with Cushing's syndrome. J Clin Endocrinol Metab 1997;82:2439–2444.
35. Castinetti F, Morange I, Dufour H, et al. Desmopressin test during petrosal sinus sampling: a valuable tool to discriminate pituitary or ectopic ACTH-dependent Cushing's syndrome. Eur J Endocrinol 2007;157:271–277.
36. Kaltsas GA, Giannulis MG, Newell-Price J, et al. A critical analysis of the value of simultaneous inferior petrosal sinus sampling in Cushing's disease and the occult ectopic adrenocorticotropin syndrome. J Clin Endocrinol Metab 1999;84:487–492.
37. Swearingen B, Katznelson L, Miller K, et al: Diagnostic errors after inferior petrosal sinus sampling. J Clin Endocrinol Metab 2004;89:3752–3763.
38. Oldfield EH, Doppman JL, Nieman LK, et al: Petrosal sinus sampling with and without corticotropin-releasing hormone for the differential diagnosis of Cushing's syndrome. N Engl J Med 1991;325:897–905.
39. Yamamoto Y, Davis DH, Nippoldt TB, Young WF Jr, Huston J III, Parisi JE: False-positive inferior petrosal sinus sampling in the diagnosis of Cushing's disease. Report of two cases. J Neurosurg 1995;83:1087–1091.
40. Doppman JL, Pass HI, Nieman LK, et al. Corticotropin-secreting carcinoid tumors of the thymus: diagnostic unreliability of thymic venous sampling. Radiology 1992;184:71–74.
41. Kuhn JM, Proeschel MF, Seurin DJ, Bertagna XY, Luton JP, Girard FL. Comparative assessment of ACTH and lipotropin plasma levels in the diagnosis and follow-up of patients with Cushing's syndrome: a study of 210 cases. Am J Med 1989;86:678–684.
42. Tabarin A, Corcuff JB, Rashedi M, Navarranne A, Ducassou D, Roger P. Comparative value of plasma ACTH and beta-endorphin measurement with three different commercial kits for the etiological diagnosis of ACTH-dependent Cushing's syndrome. Acta Endocrinol (Copenh). 1992;126:308–314.
43. Raffin-Sanson ML, Massias JF, Dumont C, et al. High plasma proopiomelanocortin in aggressive adrenocorticotropin-secreting tumors. J Clin Endocrinol Metab 1996;81:4272–4277.
44. Van Sickle DG. Carcinoid tumors. Analysis of 61 cases, including 11 cases of carcinoid syndrome. Cleve Clin Q. 1972;39:79–86.
45. Torpy DJ, Chen CC, Mullen N, et al. Lack of utility of (111)In-pentetreotide scintigraphy in localizing ectopic ACTH producing tumors: follow-up of 18 patients. J Clin Endocrinol Metab 1999;84:1186–1192.
46. Reincke M, Allolio B, Arlt W, Körber C. Comment on primary localization of an ectopic ACTH-producing bronchial carcinoid tumor by indium111 pentetreotide scintigraphy. J Clin Endocrinol Metab 1999;84:3399–3400.
47. Silva F, Vázquez-Sellés J, Aguilö F, Vázquez G, Flores C. Recurrent ectopic adrenocorticotropic hormone producing thymic carcinoid detected with octreotide imaging. Clin Nucl Med 1999;24:109–110.
48. De Herder WW, Lamberts SW. Octapeptide somatostatin-analogue therapy of Cushing's syndrome. Postgrad Med J 1999;75:65–66.
49. Fanti S, Farsad M, Battista G, et al. Somatostatin receptor scintigraphy for bronchial carcinoid follow-up. Clin Nucl Med 2003;28:548–552.
50. Tsagarakis S, Christoforaki M, Giannopoulou H, et al. A reappraisal of the utility of somatostatin receptor scintigraphy in patients with ectopic adrenocorticotropin Cushing's syndrome. J Clin Endocrinol Metab 2003;88:4754–4758.
51. Pacak K, Ilias I, Chen CC, Carrasquillo JA, Whatley M, Nieman LK. The role of [(18)F]fluorodeoxyglucose positron emission tomography and [(111)In]-diethylenetriaminepentaacetate-D-Phe-pentetreotide scintigraphy in the localization of ectopic adrenocorticotropin-secreting tumors causing Cushing's syndrome. J Clin Endocrinol Metab 2004;89:2214–2221.

52. Adams S, Baum RP, Stuckensen T, Bitter K, Hor G. Prospective comparison of 18F-FDG PET with conventional imaging modalities (CT, MRI, US) in lymph node staging of head and neck cancer. European Journal of Nuclear Medicine 1998;25:1255–1260.
53. Kumar J, Spring M, Carroll PV, Barrington SF, Powrie JK. 18Flurodeoxyglucose positron emission tomography in the localization of ectopic ACTH-secreting neuroendocrine tumours. Clin Endocrinol (Oxf). 2006;64:371–374.
54. Markou A, Manning P, Kaya B, Datta SN, Bomanji JB, Conway GS. [18F]fluoro-2-deoxy-D-glucose ([18F]FDG) positron emission tomography imaging of thymic carcinoid tumor presenting with recurrent Cushing's syndrome. Eur J Endocrinol 2005;152:521–525.
55. Aide N, Reznik Y, Icard P, Franson T, Bardet S. Paraneoplastic ACTH secretion: bronchial carcinoid overlooked by planar indium-111 pentetreotide scintigraphy and accurately localized by SPECT/CT acquisition. Clin Nucl Med 2007;32:398–400.
56. Nikolaou A, Thomas D, Kampanellou C, et al. The value of 11C-5-hydroxy-tryptophan (5HTP) positron emission tomography (PET) in neuroendocrine tumour diagnosis and management: experience from one center. J Endocrinol Invest 2010; Mar 22.
57. Orlefors H, Sundin A, Garske U, et al. Whole-body (11)C-5-hydroxytryptophan positron emission tomography as a universal imaging technique for neuroendocrine tumors: comparison with somatostatin receptor scintigraphy and computed tomography. J Clin Endocrinol Metab 2005;90:3392–3400.
58. Connor TB, Wood C, Lance BK, Orth DN, Williams JB. Multiple recurrent carcinoid tumors that secreted adrenocorticotropin (ACTH) over a period of 26 years. The Endocrinologist 1994;4:177–183.
59. Zografos GN, Markou A, Ageli C, et al. Laparoscopic surgery for adrenal tumors. A retrospective analysis. Hormones (Athens). 2006;5:52–56.
60. Morris D, Grossman A. The medical management of Cushing's syndrome. Ann N Y Acad Sci 2002;970:119–133.
61. Biller BM, Grossman AB, Stewart PM, et al. Treatment of adrenocorticotropin-dependent Cushing's syndrome: a consensus statement. J Clin Endocrinol Metab 2008;93:2454–2462.
62. Vassilopoulou-Sellin R. Paraneoplastic hypercortisolism as a risk factor for severe infections in patients with malignant diseases. J Clin Endocrinol Metab 2001;86:947–948.
63. Drake WM, Perry LA, Hinds CJ, Lowe DG, Reznek RH, Besser GM: Emergency and prolonged use of intravenous etomidate to control hypercortisolemia in a patient with Cushing's syndrome and peritonitis. J Clin Endocrinol Metab 1998;83:3542–3544.
64. Krakoff J, Koch CA, Calis KA, Alexander RH, Nieman LK. Use of a parenteral propylene glycol-containing etomidate preparation for the long-term management of ectopic Cushing's syndrome. J Clin Endocrinol Metab 2001;86:4104–4108.
65. de Bruin C, Feelders RA, Lamberts SW, Hofland LJ. Somatostatin and dopamine receptors as targets for medical treatment of Cushing's Syndrome. Rev Endocr Metab Disord 2009;10:91–102.
66. Peri A, Bemporad D, Parenti G, Luciani P, Serio M, Mannelli M. Cushing's syndrome due to intermittent ectopic ACTH production showing a temporary remission during a pulmonary infection. Eur J Endocrinol 2001;145:605–611.
67. de Herder WW, Krenning EP, Malchoff CD, et al. Somatostatin receptor scintigraphy: its value in tumor localization in patients with Cushing's syndrome caused by ectopic corticotropin or corticotropin-releasing hormone secretion. Am J Med 1994;96:305–312.
68. Phlipponneau M, Nocaudie M, Epelbaum J, et al. Somatostatin analogs for the localization and preoperative treatment of an adrenocorticotropin-secreting bronchial carcinoid tumor. J Clin Endocrinol Metab 1994;78:20–24.
69. Bertagna X, Favrod-Coune C, Escourolle H, et al. Suppression of ectopic adrenocorticotropin secretion by the long-acting somatostatin analog octreotide. J Clin Endocrinol Metab 1989;68:988–991.
70. Vignati F, Loli P. Additive effect of ketoconazole and octreotide in the treatment of severe adrenocorticotropin-depen. dent hypercortisolism. J Clin Endocrinol Metab 1996;81:2885–2890.
71. Lamberts SW, Tilanus HW, Klooswijk AI, Bruining HA, van der Lely AJ, de Jong FH. Successful treatment with SMS 201–995 of Cushing's syndrome caused by ectopic adrenocorticotropin secretion from a metastatic gastrin-secreting pancreatic islet cell carcinoma. J Clin Endocrinol Metab 1988;67:1080–1083.
72. Alexandraki KI, Grossman AB. Pituitary-targeted medical therapy of Cushing's disease. Expert Opin Investig Drugs 2008;17:669–677.
73. Pivonello R, Ferone D, de Herder WW, Faggiano A, et al. Dopamine receptor expression and function in corticotroph ectopic tumors. J Clin Endocrinol Metab 2007;92:65–69.
74. Hofland LJ, Lamberts SW. The pathophysiological consequences of somatostatin receptor internalization and resistance. Endocr Rev 2003;24:28–47.

75. Pivonello R, Ferone D, Lamberts SW, Colao A. Cabergoline plus lanreotide for ectopic Cushing's syndrome. N Engl J Med 2005;352:2457–2458.
76. Mansi L, Rambaldi PF, Panza N, Esposito D, Esposito V, Pastore V. Diagnosis and radioguided surgery with 111In-pentetreotide in a patient with paraneoplastic Cushing's syndrome due to a bronchial carcinoid. Eur J Endocrinol 1997;137:688–690.
77. Grossrubatscher E, Vignati F, Dalino P, et al. Use of radioguided surgery with [111In]-pentetreotide in the management of an ACTH-secreting bronchial carcinoid causing ectopic Cushing's syndrome. J Endocrinol Invest 2005;28:72–78.
78. Chrisoulidou A, Pazaitou-Panayiotou K, Georgiou E, et al. Ectopic Cushing's syndrome due to CRH secreting liver metastasis in a patient with medullary thyroid carcinoma. Hormones (Athens). 2008;7:259–262.
79. Orth DN. Cushing's syndrome. N Engl J Med 1995;332:791–803.
80. Findling JW, Tyrrell JB. Occult ectopic secretion of corticotropin. Arch Intern Med 1986;146:929–933.
81. Krikorian A, Aron D. Evaluation and management of pituitary incidentalomas—revisiting an acquaintance. Nat Clin Pract Endocrinol Metab 2006;2:138–145.
82. Vilar L, Freitas MC, Moura E, et al. Cushing's disease caused by macroadenomas – Report of 7 cases. Arq Bras Endocrinol Metab 1996;40:S221.
83. Woo YS, Isidori AM, Wat WZ, et al. Clinical and biochemical characteristics of adrenocorticotropin-secreting macroadenomas. J Clin Endocrinol Metab 2005;90:4963–4969.
84. Zerikly RK, Eray E, Faiman C, et al. Cyclic Cushing syndrome due to an ectopic pituitary adenoma. Nat Clin Pract Endocrinol Metab 2009;5:174–179.
85. Meinardi JR, Wolffenbuttel BH, Dullaart RP. Cyclic Cushing's syndrome: a clinical challenge. Eur J Endocrinol 2007;157(3):245–254.
86. Albiger NM, Scaroni CM, Mantero F. Cyclic Cushing's syndrome: an overview. Arq Bras Endocrinol Metabol 2007;51:1253–1260.
87. Alexandraki KI, Kaltsas GA, Isidori AM, et al. The prevalence and characteristic features of cyclicity and variability in Cushing's disease. Eur J Endocrinol 2009;160:1011–1018.

15 Revisiting the Nelson's Syndrome: Corticotroph Tumor Progression After Bilateral Adrenalectomy in Cushing's Disease

Guillaume Assie, Laurence Guignat, Jérôme Bertherat, and Xavier Bertagna

CONTENTS

SUMMARY

Since Don Nelson's first description in 1958 of a pituitary macroadenoma occurring after adrenalectomy in a patient with Cushing's disease, the "Nelson's syndrome" has long been feared. However, major medical advances, such as pituitary imaging with MRI, surgery by the transsphenoidal route, and safe radiotherapy, have changed the way corticotroph tumor progression (CTP) can be monitored and treated. Rather than "wait" for the late occurrence of Nelson's syndrome, as defined originally with the complications of macroadenomas, we can now detect, early and precisely, the possible occurrence of CTP long before the classical features of Nelson's syndrome have developed.

From: *Contemporary Endocrinology: Cushing's Syndrome: Pathophysiology, Diagnosis and Treatment*
Edited by: M.D. Bronstein (ed.), DOI 10.1007/978-1-60327-449-4_15,

In a recent study of 53 patients followed by MRI after bilateral adrenalectomy, we showed that 3 years after adrenalectomy, the proportion of patients showing evidence of CTP reached 39%; this number tended to plateau at 47% after 7 years. Thus, ca. 50% of the patients showed no evidence of CTP under this time period. Factors that were found to be significantly associated with a higher risk to develop CTP were duration of Cushing's disease, baseline ACTH plasma level in the year following adrenalectomy, and the rate of increase in ACTH plasma levels after adrenalectomy.

If necessary, pituitary surgery and/or radiotherapy can control the CTP in a majority of situations. The CTP does not seem accelerated during the pregnancy.

There is no question that pituitary surgery remains the first-line treatment in most patients with Cushing's disease. Yet, when complete removal of a corticotroph tumor is not achievable, total bilateral adrenalectomy can be considered among the various therapeutic options in Cushing's disease. The CTP is not constant and is manageable in most cases. There is a definite need for new pharmacologic agent directed against corticotroph tumors.

Key Words: Nelson's syndrome, Cushing's syndrome, Cushing's disease, bilateral adrenalectomy

A WORD OF HISTORY

In 1958, Don Nelson et al. *(1)* (Fig. 1) first reported on the occurrence of a pituitary macroadenoma secreting high amounts of ACTH after total bilateral adrenalectomy for Cushing's syndrome: a 33-year-old woman who developed marked skin hyperpigmentation, and evidence of pituitary tumor (enlarged sella on skull X-ray and visual field defects), 3 years after she had been subjected to

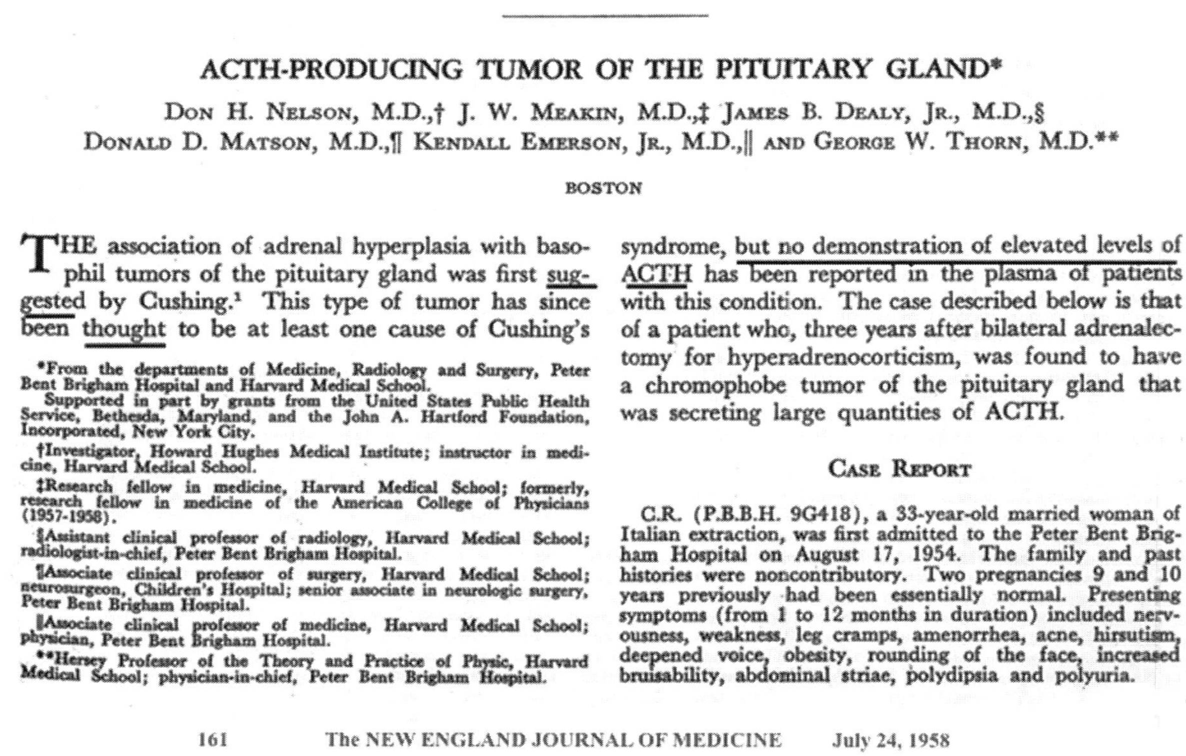

ACTH-PRODUCING TUMOR OF THE PITUITARY GLAND*

DON H. NELSON, M.D.,† J. W. MEAKIN, M.D.,‡ JAMES B. DEALY, JR., M.D.,§ DONALD D. MATSON, M.D.,¶ KENDALL EMERSON, JR., M.D.,‖ AND GEORGE W. THORN, M.D.**

BOSTON

THE association of adrenal hyperplasia with basophil tumors of the pituitary gland was first suggested by Cushing.[1] This type of tumor has since been thought to be at least one cause of Cushing's syndrome, but no demonstration of elevated levels of ACTH has been reported in the plasma of patients with this condition. The case described below is that of a patient who, three years after bilateral adrenalectomy for hyperadrenocorticism, was found to have a chromophobe tumor of the pituitary gland that was secreting large quantities of ACTH.

*From the departments of Medicine, Radiology and Surgery, Peter Bent Brigham Hospital and Harvard Medical School.

Supported in part by grants from the United States Public Health Service, Bethesda, Maryland, and the John A. Hartford Foundation, Incorporated, New York City.

†Investigator, Howard Hughes Medical Institute; instructor in medicine, Harvard Medical School.

‡Research fellow in medicine, Harvard Medical School; formerly, research fellow in medicine of the American College of Physicians (1957-1958).

§Assistant clinical professor of radiology, Harvard Medical School; radiologist-in-chief, Peter Bent Brigham Hospital.

¶Associate clinical professor of surgery, Harvard Medical School; neurosurgeon, Children's Hospital; senior associate in neurologic surgery, Peter Bent Brigham Hospital.

‖Associate clinical professor of medicine, Harvard Medical School; physician, Peter Bent Brigham Hospital.

**Hersey Professor of the Theory and Practice of Physic, Harvard Medical School; physician-in-chief, Peter Bent Brigham Hospital.

CASE REPORT

C.R. (P.B.B.H. 9G418), a 33-year-old married woman of Italian extraction, was first admitted to the Peter Bent Brigham Hospital on August 17, 1954. The family and past histories were noncontributory. Two pregnancies 9 and 10 years previously had been essentially normal. Presenting symptoms (from 1 to 12 months in duration) included nervousness, weakness, leg cramps, amenorrhea, acne, hirsutism, deepened voice, obesity, rounding of the face, increased bruisability, abdominal striae, polydipsia and polyuria.

161 The NEW ENGLAND JOURNAL OF MEDICINE July 24, 1958

Fig. 1. Publication of the first patient with "Nelson's syndrome" in the *New England Journal of Medicine* in 1958.

bilateral adrenalectomy for Cushing's syndrome. ACTH plasma levels were high enough to be measured by a bioassay in the hypophysectomized dog. Other authors independently reported similar cases *(2–5)*, demonstrating the existence of ACTH-secreting pituitary adenomas, as had been previously surmised by Harvey Cushing *(6)*. These observations came as an illuminating clue for the pathogenesis of Cushing's disease. They also raised the fear that adrenalectomy in Cushing's disease could induce the occurrence or trigger the growth of a pituitary adenoma, with the risk of subsequent complications related to the tumor burden. In 1960, Nelson et al. published the first series of patients *(7)*: "Nelson's syndrome" (NS) was born, which, 50 years later, still remains an "ill-defined" condition.

NELSON'S SYNDROME: IS THERE A DEFINITION?

About 50 series *(8, 9)* have reported on NS, grossly defined by the association of an "expanding" pituitary tumor and "high" ACTH secretion after adrenalectomy in Cushing's disease. Variable criteria have been used: (1) the presence of a pituitary macroadenoma either diagnosed on X-ray or sellar tomography, or on the occurrence of visual defects, is even not considered; (2) the diagnosis of "high ACTH plasma levels" based either on qualitative assessment of cutaneous pigmentation, or on various baseline plasma ACTH cutoffs; (3) the cohorts of patients received heterogeneous treatments, some directly interfering with the potential tumor growth such as pituitary irradiation. Moreover, major advances such as transsphenoidal surgery or pituitary MRI have often occurred during the inclusion period.

With these various and heterogeneous "definitions," the prevalence of NS ranged from 8 to 29% in the largest series, with a time interval between adrenalectomy and the diagnosis of NS ranging 0.5–24 years.

WE SHOULD RATHER LOOK AT "CORTICOTROPH TUMOR PROGRESSION"

Today we know that the corticotroph adenoma is indeed the cause of Cushing's disease, and we can use highly sensitive imaging and biological means to visualize it and assess its function through pituitary MRI and ACTH measurements with immunoassays. In these cases where bilateral adrenalectomy is eventually performed, these modern approaches are now routinely used for the diagnosis and/or the follow-up of patients with Cushing's disease (Fig. 2).

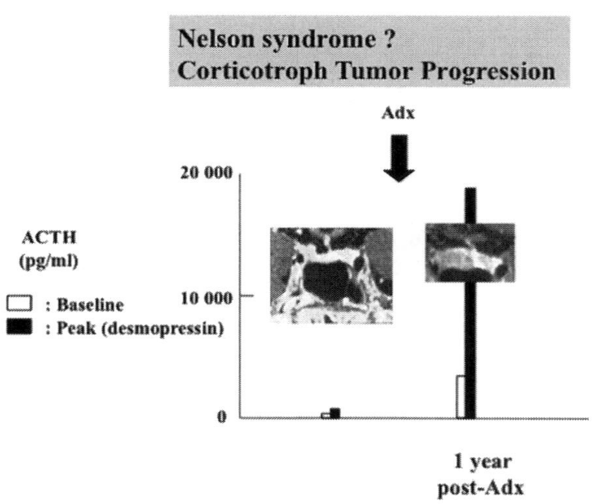

Fig. 2. Corticotroph tumor progresssion (CTP) as assessed by repeat pituitary MRI, 1 year after total bilateral adrenalectomy in a patient with Cushing's disease and a negative imaging initially. Parallel increases in ACTH plasma levels are shown, basally, and after stimulation (desmopressin).

Rather than "wait" for the late occurrence of NS, as "defined" originally (Fig. 3, upper), we can now "detect," early and precisely, the possible occurrence of CTP long before the "classical" features of NS have developed (Fig. 3, lower).

IS CORTICOTROPH TUMOR PROGRESSION INEVITABLE?

We recently studied *(9)* the rate of occurrence of CTP in a cohort of 53 patients with Cushing's disease who were carefully followed in a single center after bilateral adrenalectomy, using repeat MRI, for a median duration of follow-up after adrenalectomy of 4.6 years (range 0.5–13.5). None had received pituitary radiotherapy. The CTP was defined either by the occurrence of an adenoma at MRI or the growth of a pre-existing adenoma on pituitary MRI.

Three years after adrenalectomy, the proportion of patients showing evidence of CTP reached 39%; this number tended to plateau at 47% after 7 years (Fig. 4). Thus, ca. 50% of the patients showed no evidence of CTP under this time period.

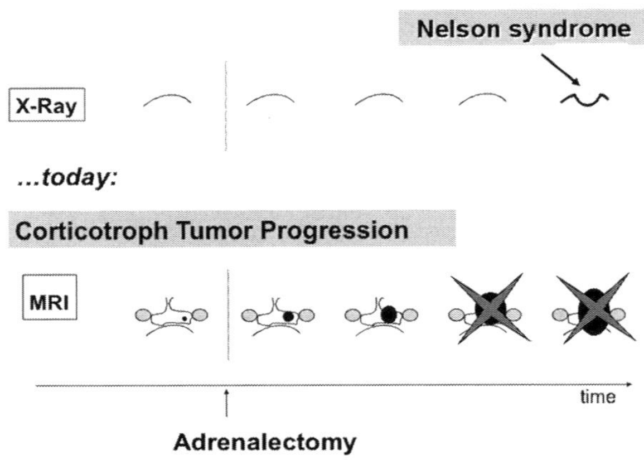

Fig. 3. Nelson's syndrome or Corticotroph Tumor Progression (CTP)? Late diagnosis of the Nelson's syndrome, originally, when the diagnosis means lacked sensitivity (*upper part*). Close follow-up of possible CTP, with modern tools such as pituitary MRI (*lower part*).

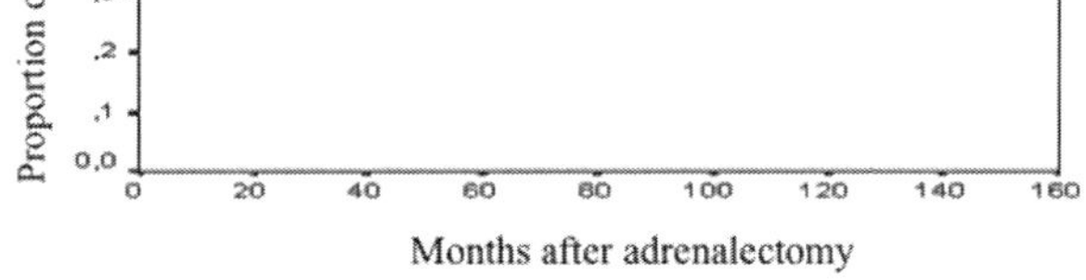

Fig. 4. Survival without evidence of CTP at MRI after total bilateral adrenalectomy in a cohort of 53 patients with Cushing's disease not subjected to pituitary irradiation.

CAN WE PREDICT CORTICOTROPH TUMOR PROGRESSION?

In the past, many studies *(9)* have attempted to identify predictive factors of the classical NS with contrasted results, such as young age at adrenalectomy in some studies but not all, lack of pituitary irradiation prior to adrenalectomy in some studies but not all, the surgical or morphological documentation of a pituitary adenoma before adrenalectomy, the existence of an adrenal remnant after adrenalectomy in some studies but not all, the duration of the Cushing's disease in some studies but not all, and free urinary cortisol before adrenalectomy in some studies but not all. Finally, some factors have never been demonstrated as predictive, such as the patient's sex, basal ACTH in the morning before adrenalectomy, the level of glucocorticoid substitution after adrenalectomy, and pregnancy.

Eventually many studies agreed that a high baseline ACTH plasma value in the year following adrenalectomy was the best validated predictive factor *(9)*.

In our recent study *(9)*, factors that were found to be significantly associated with a higher risk to develop CTP were duration of Cushing's disease, baseline ACTH plasma level in the year following adrenalectomy, and the rate of increase in ACTH plasma levels after adrenalectomy. Some of our patients had been treated by *o,p*'DDD at some time in the course of their disease; we showed that increases in plasma ACTH concentration during *o,p*'DDD-induced cortisol deprivation tended to predict CTP after adrenalectomy, but this relationship did not reach full significance ($p = 0.08$).

In those patients that have been subjected to pituitary surgery before adrenalectomy, pathological studies of the tissue until now have not unraveled predictors of CTP: in our recent study *(9)*, neither the presence of mitoses nor a high percentage of Ki67-immunopositive nuclei in the adenoma was predictive of CTP.

CAN WE DETECT CORTICOTROPH TUMOR PROGRESSION EARLY?

There is a definite need to improve the accuracy of our means to assess pituitary tumor growth by imaging. Pituitary MRI has brought a real revolution in the field *(10–12)*, yet little data are available that provide us with clear tools to evaluate subtle morphological changes. They will be useful not only to follow CTP after adrenalectomy in Cushing's disease, but also in other circumstances, when other types of adenomas are subjected to direct – medical or irradiation – treatments, or, when patients with acromegaly are treated with GH-receptor antagonists. We have thoroughly evaluated the performance of pituitary MRI to assess specifically pituitary ACTH secreting adenomas *(13)*.

The CTP can indeed be easily detected by repeat pituitary MRI. It is recommended that it be performed before and 6 months after adrenalectomy, then every year, at least for the next 5–6 years. In the absence of CTP, it seems reasonable to increase the time intervals of MRI surveillance thereafter.

Repeat determinations of ACTH plasma levels also add valuable information *(9)*. Yet there is no threshold, no accepted condition (baseline, before or after the morning glucocorticoid administration), stimulated, suppressed that has proven to be a valid and more sensitive detector of early CTP.

CAN WE PREVENT OR TREAT CORTICOTROPH TUMOR PROGRESSION?

The historical cases of Nelson's syndrome were characterized by large invasive pituitary macroadenomas presenting a major therapeutic challenge. Today with pituitary MRI the tumor could have been detected much earlier at a smaller size, and the surgical procedures have improved as well as the radiotherapy protocol.

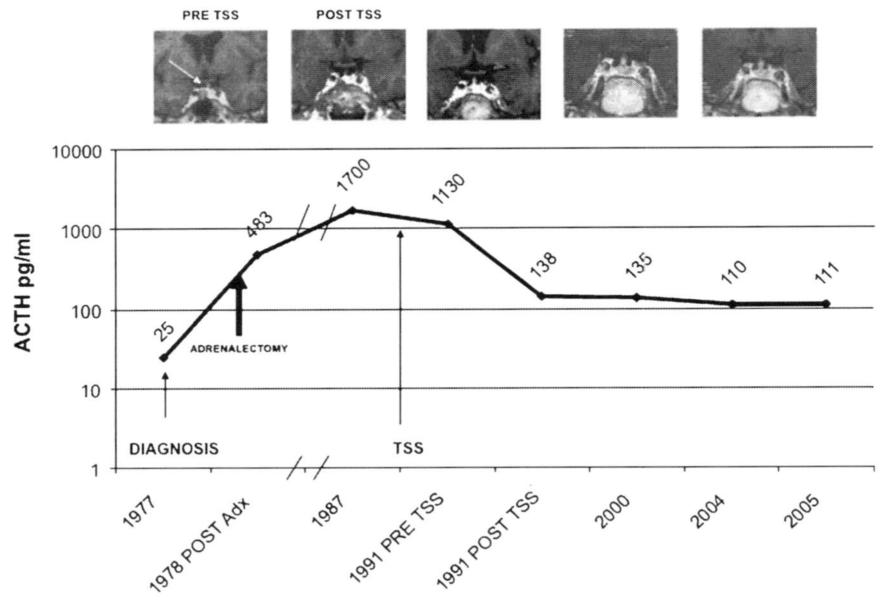

Fig. 5. Successful removal of a pituitary corticotroph adenoma that had appeared at MRI years after total bilateral adrenalectomy.

After adrenalectomy, the goal is not to cure the pituitary adenoma, but rather to manage CTP so that no complication related to the tumor burden occurs. Indeed, a microadenoma that appears on MRI after adrenalectomy may not be removed as far as it does not grow, especially in patients with high risk for pituitary surgery. Alternatively, it may be successfully removed in case of progression (Fig. 5). A close pituitary MRI follow-up is necessary for an early CTP diagnosis.

Some studies, but not all have shown some protective effect of radiotherapy performed immediately following bilateral adrenalectomy *(9)*.

The identification of clinical and molecular factors predicting aggressive CTP is needed. With such factors, we could adapt the pituitary MRI follow-up schedule, we could propose pituitary irradiation in high-risk patients, and we could better choose the right time for pituitary surgery in face of a growing pituitary adenoma. It is clear that further prospective studies would be ideally necessary to answer all these questions, a goal that is difficult to reach when we deal with a rare disease.

IS THERE A ROLE FOR BILATERAL ADRENALECTOMY IN CUSHING'S DISEASE?

Bilateral adrenalectomy is by no means the ideal treatment for Cushing's disease.

Pituitary surgery, usually by the transsphenoidal route, is indeed the first-line treatment. In case of failure or recurrence, the choice is generally between pituitary irradiation (inconstant and delayed success with the risk of pituitary insufficiency) and adrenal directed therapy, either pharmacological (usually ketoconazol *o,p'*DDD with their inconstant efficacy and frequent side effects, and precluding pregnancy) or surgical (constant and immediate success, but adrenal failure and the risk of NS).

In any case, we know that CTP is not constant, and modern follow-up with repeat MRI allows managing it before the classical NS develops. Under these conditions adrenalectomy is an efficient therapeutic means in difficult cases, particularly in young women who wish to get pregnant.

DOES PREGNANCY ACCELERATE CORTICOTROPH TUMOR PROGRESSION?

Because Cushing's disease often occurs in young female patients, the wish of pregnancy is frequently an issue that must be taken into account when one has to choose amongst a variety of therapeutical options when pituitary surgery has failed. We have thoroughly examined the hypothesis that pregnancy could unfavorably act on CTP:

A retrospective cohort study was performed on patients who underwent pregnancy after bilateral adrenalectomy, followed in a single center (Cochin Hospital, Paris): 20 pregnancies from 11 patients. None had pituitary irradiation: CTP was assessed by pituitary MRI. Plasma ACTH and corticotroph tumor volume variations before, around and after pregnancy, were monitored and compared using paired Wilcoxon rank test. Data on maternal and neonatal outcomes were recorded by phone and obstetrical correspondence. The CTP occurred in 8 out of 17 pregnancies, and ACTH increased in 8 out of 10 pregnancies. However, compared to before pregnancy, neither the corticotroph tumor variation nor the ACTH variation increased during pregnancy or after pregnancy. We concluded that pregnancy does not accelerate CTP after bilateral adrenalectomy. Pregnancy in these conditions is manageable provided the patients can be followed closely *(14)*.

WHAT WE ALL LOOK FOR IN CUSHING'S DISEASE

The corticotroph adenoma is an "orphan pituitary tumor."

In contrast with other secreting adenomas like PRL-, GH-, or TSH adenomas, there is, at this time, no pharmacological means that has unequivocally shown a therapeutic action at ACTH-secreting pituitary tumors.

Thorough studies are ongoing that may bear some promises: new dopaminergic and/or somatostatinergic drugs such as cabergoline and the preferential SST5 ligand SOM-230 are actively being studied, including in clinical trials in patients with Cushing's disease *(15, 16)*. The PPAR gamma agonists have not proved as active in human as in experimental studies *(17)*, and animal studies with retinoic acid may also shed some light *(18)*. Yet, one should remain very cautious.

PATHOPHYSIOLOGICAL HYPOTHESES

There are many questions that still have not found an answer.

Can we distinguish the adenomas of Nelson's syndrome from the micro adenomas of Cushing's disease?

Most approaches have shown that pituitary tissues obtained in patients with NS essentially show molecular features identical to that observed in corticotroph adenomas of Cushing's disease *(19–27)*: POMC gene transcription is qualitatively unaltered, generating the normal 1,200 nucleotide (nt) POMC mRNA; POMC is normally processed, generating intact ACTH, with no unanticipated POMC product; most tumors are loaded with CRH-R1 and vasopressin V3 receptors, and remain highly responsive to their ligands; they express a variety of nuclear factors that are associated with the corticotroph phenotype: Ptx1, Tpit, Neuro D, Nurr 77, Nur 1, the glucorticoid receptor type II; and they are monoclonal tumors. Yet these tumors, like corticotroph adenomas in general, show a set-point defect or partial resistance to glucocorticoids. This is best shown by in vivo studies showing that ACTH plasma levels are not normally suppressed by glucocorticoid administration in patients with Nelson's syndrome. Confirmation of this feature in vitro is difficult because the direct comparison with normal corticotroph cells is absent in most studies.

Does bilateral adrenalectomy actually trigger an accelerated growth of the pituitary corticotroph adenoma? And, if yes, by what mechanism?

That some adenomas do indeed grow after adrenalectomy is by no way a proof. We do not know if the adenoma – whose natural destiny is indeed to grow – would have grown slower if we had taken the time to observe it without treatment. There is no room here for a controlled trial, with a placebo group patients placed on anticortisolic drugs, particularly when they are under *o,p*'DDD, a drug that can really induce a "chemical adrenalectomy," often show evidence of CTP, both by imaging and increased ACTH plasma levels. Yet in both situations a common feature is the efficient cortisol deprivation that is chronically induced.

Corticotroph adenoma cells express the ubiquitous glucocorticoid receptor (GR), with no evidence for imbalance between its two isoforms *(28, 29)*. Cortisol lowers the proliferation rate of human corticotroph adenoma cells in primary culture *(30)*. In rats, dexamethasone induces apoptosis of a subpopulation of anterior pituitary cells that is expanded by adrenalectomy *(28)*. Whether these cells are corticotroph cells remains to be established. One case of somatic mutation of the GR in an aggressive corticotroph tumor in a patient with NS has been reported, but seems to be uncommon *(31)*. Furthermore, LOH at the GR locus was found in 6 of 22 corticotroph adenomas *(32)*, but haplo insufficiency was not established. Whether these abnormalities are more frequent in aggressive tumors of the Nelson's syndrome is not known. These data would plead for a direct glucocorticoid inhibition of the corticotroph tumor growth, but such an evidence in Cushing's disease is not demonstrable, as glucocorticoids have undissociable pleitrophic effects such as CRH downregulation. Thus, we cannot definitely conclude that abrogation of chronic glucocorticoid excess after adrenalectomy would boost the corticotroph tumor growth.

In both situations, "chemical" or surgical adrenalectomy, the cortisol deprivation is relative: patients are indeed substituted. And the endocrinologist has all the possibilities to monitor his treatment. Yet there are two fundamental differences compared with the untreated situation: (a) much less cortisol in blood and (b) because patients are usually on hydrocortisone replacement in the morning and noon, most likely no circulating cortisol overnight. It is conceivable therefore that in the latter situation, hypothalamic CRH activity can resume, possibly in an exaggerated manner, whereas it is thought to be totally suppressed in active Cushing's disease. It could be hypothesized that the recovered CRH production acting on a cortisol-deprived ACTH-producing pituitary adenoma may exert a growth promotion effect. Some animal models provide evidence for such a role of CRH: CRH excess induces an increase of corticotroph cells number, as seen in tumors with ectopic CRH secretion *(33)*, in rats with chronic CRH infusion *(34)* and in transgenic mouse overexpressing the CRH receptor *(35)*. CRH receptor 1 (CRH-R1) is abundantly expressed in corticotroph adenomas *(36, 37)*. However, no mutation of CRH-R1 was found in corticotroph adenomas *(36)*. Adrenalectomy in rats increases hypothalamic CRH transcription, and is followed by a moderate increase of corticotroph cell number *(38)*, and by a downregulation of CRH-R1 expression *(39, 40)*. To our knowledge no data are available on the kinetics of CRH-R1 expression in human corticotroph adenomas after adrenalectomy. Moreover, evaluating the CRH tone in humans after adrenalectomy is challenging, so that the role for CRH in stimulating the proliferation of corticotroph adenoma after adrenalectomy, although attractive, remains speculative. Compounds with anti-CRH activity might prove useful to test such a hypothesis.

BACK TO HISTORY

After our initial paper of 2004 *(9)* suggesting that NS should be "revisited," a more recent one appeared in the September 2007 issue of *Neurosurgical Focus (41)* which retrospectively analyzed the "historical perspectives and current concepts" in Nelson syndrome. Somehow acknowledging the need to reassess this condition, these authors eventually wrote "the authors believe this disease must be reevaluated in the contemporary era and a modern paradigm adapted."

Among the authors of this paper, Don Nelson himself (Fig. 6).

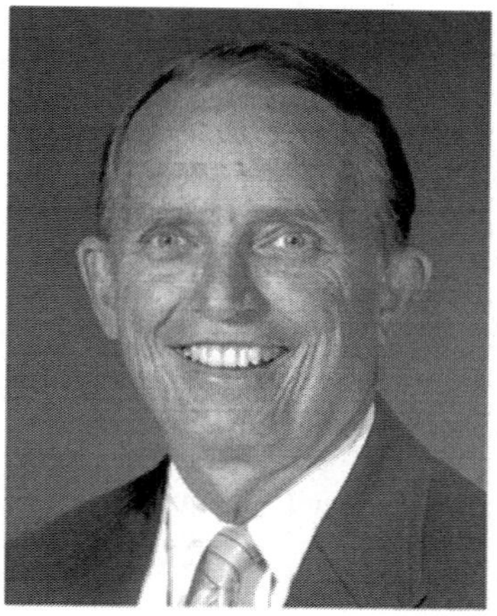

« Recent photograph of Dr. Don H. Nelson »

Nelson syndrome : historical perspectives and current concepts

Hornyak M, Weiss MH, Nelson DH, Couldwell WT

Neurosurg Focus 23:E12, September 2007

« …the authors believe this disease must be reevaluated in the contemporary era and a modern paradigm adopted. »

Fig. 6. Reassessment of Nelson's syndrome by Don H. Nelson.

ACKNOWLEDGMENTS

The authors are indebted to Stéphane Gaillard (Neurosurgery Department, Hôpital Foch), Hélène Bahurel, Marie Bienvenue, Paul Legmann (Radiology Department, Hôpital Cochin), Bertrand Dousset (Endocrine Surgery, Hôpital Cochin), and Michèle Kujas (Pathology Department, Hôpital La Pitié).

REFERENCES

1. Nelson DH, Meakin JW, Dealy JB, Jr, Matson DD, Emerson K, Jr, Thorn GW. ACTH-producing tumor of the pituitary gland. N Engl J Med 1958;259(4):161–164.
2. Salassa RM, Kearns TP, Kernohan JW, Sprague RG, Maccarty CS. Pituitary tumors in patients with Cushing's syndrome. J Clin Endocrinol Metab 1959;19:1523–1539.
3. Montgomery DA, Welbourn RB, McCaughey WT, Gleadhill CA. Pituitary tumours manifested after adrenalectomy for Cushing's syndrome. Lancet 1959;2:707–710.
4. Glenn F, Karl RC, Horwith M. The surgical treatment of Cushing's syndrome. Ann Surg 1958;148(3):365–374.
5. Rees JR, Zilva JF. Diabetes insipidus complicating total adrenalectomy. J Clin Pathol 1959;12:530–534.
6. Cushing H. The basophil adenomas of the pituitary body and their clinical manifestations (pituitary basophilism). Bull Johns Hopkins Hosp 1932;50:137–195.
7. Nelson DH, Meakin JW, Thorn GW. ACTH-producing pituitary tumors following adrenalectomy for Cushing's syndrome. Ann Intern Med 1960;52:560–569.
8. Assié G, Bahurel H, Bertherat J, Kujas M, Legmann P, Bertagna X. The Nelson's syndrome… revisited. Pituitary 2004;7(4):209–215; review.
9. Assié G, Bahurel H, Coste J, Silvera S, Kujas M, Dugué MA, Karray F, Dousset B, Bertherat J, Legmann P, Bertagna X. Corticotroph tumor progression after adrenalectomy in Cushing's disease: a reappraisal of Nelson's syndrome. J Clin Endocrinol Metab 2007;92(1):172–179.
10. Juliani G, Avataneo T, Potenzoni F, Sorrentino T. [CT and MR compared in the study of hypophysis]. Radiol Med (Torino) 1989;77(1–2):51–64.
11. Johnson MR, Hoare RD, Cox T, et al. The evaluation of patients with a suspected pituitary microadenoma: computer tomography compared to magnetic resonance imaging. Clin Endocrinol (Oxf) 1992;36(4):335–338.
12. Vest-Courtalon C, Ravel A, Perez N, et al. [Pituitary gland MRI and Cushing disease: report of 14 operated patients]. J Radiol 2000;81(7):781–786.

13. Bahurel-Barrera H, Assie G, Silvera S, Bertagna X, Coste J, Legmann P. Inter- and intra-observer variability in detection and progression assessment with MRI of microadenoma in Cushing's disease patients followed up after bilateral adrenalectomy. Pituitary 2008;11(3):263–269.
14. Jornayvaz FR, Assié G, Bienvenu M, Coste J, Legmann P, Bertherat J, Bertagna X. Pregnancy does not accelerate corticotroph tumor progression in Nelson's syndrome. Endocrine Society Annual Meeting 2009, P1–P610.
15. Pivonello R, De Martino MC, Cappabianca P, De Leo M, Faggiano A, Lombardi G, Hofland LJ, Lamberts SW, Colao A. The medical treatment of Cushing's disease: effectiveness of chronic treatment with the dopamine agonist cabergoline in patients unsuccessfully treated by surgery. J Clin Endocrinol Metab 2009;94(1):223–230.
16. Boscaro M, Ludlam WH, Atkinson B, Glusman JE, Petersenn S, Reincke M, Snyder P, Tabarin A, Biller BM, Findling J, Melmed S, Darby CH, Hu K, Wang Y, Freda PU, Grossman AB, Frohman LA, Bertherat J. Treatment of pituitary-dependent Cushing's disease with the multireceptor ligand somatostatin analog pasireotide (SOM230): a multicenter, phase II trial. J Clin Endocrinol Metab 2009;94(1):115–122.
17. Heaney AP, Fernando M, Yong WH, Melmed S. Functional PPAR-gamma receptor is a novel therapeutic target for ACTH-secreting pituitary adenomas. Nat Med 2002;8(11):1281–1287.
18. Paez-Pereda M, Kovalovsky D, Hopfner U, Theodoropoulou M, Pagotto U, Uhl E, Losa M, Stalla J, Grubler Y, Missale C, Arzt E, Stalla GK. Retinoic acid prevents experimental Cushing syndrome. J Clin Invest 2001;108(8):1123–1131.
19. Bertagna X, Raux-Demay MC, Guilhaume B, et al. Cushing's disease. In: Melmed S, (ed) The Pituitary. 2nd edition. Malden: Blackwell, 2002:496–560.
20. de Keyzer Y, Bertagna X, Lenne F, et al. Proopiomelanocortin gene expression in ACTH secreting non-pituitary tumors. J Clin Invest 1985;76:1892–1898.
21. Raffin-Sanson ML, de Keyzer Y, Bertagna X. Proopiomelanocortin, a polypeptide precursor with multiple functions: from physiology to pathological conditions. Eur J Endocrinol 2003;149(2):79–90; review
22. Dahia PL, Grossman AB. The molecular pathogenesis of corticotroph tumors. Endocr Rev 1999;20(2):136–155.
23. de Keyzer Y, Rene P, Lenne F, Auzan C, Clauser E, Bertagna X. V3 vasopressin receptor and corticotropic phenotype in pituitary and nonpituitary tumors. Horm Res 1997;47(4–6):259–262; review.
24. Herman V, Fagin J, Gonsky R, Kovacs K, Melmed S. Clonal origin of pituitary adenomas. J Clin Endocrinol Metab 1990;71(6):1427–1433.
25. Gicquel C, Le Bouc Y, Luton JP, Girard F, Bertagna X. Monoclonality of corticotroph macroadenomas in Cushing's disease. J Clin Endocrinol Metab 1992;75(2):472–475.
26. Wolfsen AR, Odell WD. The dose-response relationship of ACTH and cortisol in Cushing's disease. Clin Endocrinol (Oxf) 1980;12(6):557–568.
27. Suda T, Tozawa F, Dobashi I, Horiba N, Ohmori N, Yamakado M, Yamada M, Demura H. Corticotropin-releasing hormone, proopiomelanocortin, and glucocorticoid receptor gene expression in adrenocorticotropin-producing tumors in vitro. J Clin Invest 1993;92(6):2790–2795.
28. Resetic J, Reiner Z, Ludecke D, Riznar-Resetic V, Sekso M. The effects of cortisol, 11-epicortisol, and lysine vasopressin on DNA and RNA synthesis in isolated human adrenocorticotropic hormone-secreting pituitary tumor cells. Steroids 1990;55(3):98–100.
29. Dahia PL, Honegger J, Reincke M, et al. Expression of glucocorticoid receptor gene isoforms in corticotropin-secreting tumors. J Clin Endocrinol Metab 1997;82(4):1088–1093.
30. Nolan LA, Levy A. Temporally sensitive trophic responsiveness of the adrenalectomized rat anterior pituitary to dexamethasone challenge: relationship between mitotic activity and apoptotic sensitivity. Endocrinology 2003;144(1):212–219.
31. Karl M, Von Wichert G, Kempter E, et al. Nelson's syndrome associated with a somatic frame shift mutation in the glucocorticoid receptor gene. J Clin Endocrinol Metab 1996;81(1):124–129.
32. Huizenga NA, de Lange P, Koper JW, et al. Human adrenocorticotropin-secreting pituitary adenomas show frequent loss of heterozygosity at the glucocorticoid receptor gene locus. J Clin Endocrinol Metab 1998;83(3):917–921.
33. Carey RM, Varma SK, Drake CR, Jr, et al. Ectopic secretion of corticotropin-releasing factor as a cause of Cushing's syndrome. A clinical, morphologic, and biochemical study. N Engl J Med 1984;311(1):13–20.
34. Gertz BJ, Contreras LN, McComb DJ, Kovacs K, Tyrrell JB, Dallman MF. Chronic administration of corticotropin-releasing factor increases pituitary corticotroph number. Endocrinology 1987;120(1):381–388.
35. Stenzel-Poore MP, Cameron VA, Vaughan J, Sawchenko PE, Vale W. Development of Cushing's syndrome in corticotropin-releasing factor transgenic mice. Endocrinology 1992;130(6):3378–3386.
36. de Keyzer Y, Rene P, Beldjord C, Lenne F, Bertagna X. Overexpression of vasopressin (V3) and corticotrophin-releasing hormone receptor genes in corticotroph tumours. Clin Endocrinol (Oxf) 1998;49(4):475–482.

37. Dieterich KD, Gundelfinger ED, Ludecke DK, Lehnert H. Mutation and expression analysis of corticotropin-releasing factor 1 receptor in adrenocorticotropin-secreting pituitary adenomas. J Clin Endocrinol Metab 1998;83(9):3327–3331.
38. McNicol AM, Carbajo-Perez E. Aspects of anterior pituitary growth, with special reference to corticotrophs. Pituitary 1999;1(3–4):257–268.
39. Wynn PC, Harwood JP, Catt KJ, Aguilera G. Regulation of corticotropin-releasing factor (CRF) receptors in the rat pituitary gland: effects of adrenalectomy on CRF receptors and corticotroph responses. Endocrinology 1985;116(4):1653–1659.
40. Sakai K, Horiba N, Sakai Y, Tozawa F, Demura H, Suda T. Regulation of corticotropin-releasing factor receptor messenger ribonucleic acid in rat anterior pituitary. Endocrinology 1996;137(5):1758–1763.
41. Hornyak M, Weiss MH, Nelson DH, Couldwell WT. Nelson syndrome: historical perspectives and current concepts. Neurosurg Focus 2007;23(3):E12.

16 ACTH-Independent Cushing's Syndrome: Adrenocortical Tumors

Maria Candida Barisson Villares Fragoso, Sorahia Domenice, Ana Claudia Latronico, and Berenice Bilharinho Mendonca

Contents

Summary

Approximately 15–20% of endogenous Cushing's syndrome (CS) is secondary to adrenal gland disorders. Unilateral adrenocortical tumors (adenoma or carcinomas) are responsible for the majority of the cases of primary adrenal CS. Adrenocortical tumors are more common in the population above 50 years of age. Steroid-secreting adrenal tumors causing endocrine disease are rare, however, they correspond to 80% of all causes of ACTH-independent Cushing's syndrome. The most common clinical presentation in adults is CS, contrasting with pediatric patients in whom virilization syndrome is more frequent.

The incidence of adrenocortical carcinoma in the United States is estimated to be 0.2–0.4 per million population per year. Nevertheless, there is a high incidence of adrenocortical tumors in Southern and Southwestern region of Brazil, estimated to be approximately 10–15 times greater than the worldwide incidence.

From: *Contemporary Endocrinology: Cushing's Syndrome: Pathophysiology, Diagnosis and Treatment*
Edited by: M.D. Bronstein (ed.), DOI 10.1007/978-1-60327-449-4_16,

In this chapter, we review the clinical features, hormonal and imaging diagnosis, and treatment of ACTH-independent Cushing's syndrome due to adrenocortical tumors.

Key Words: Cushing's syndrome, adrenocortical tumors, adrenal adenoma, adrenal carcinoma

INTRODUCTION

Cushing's syndrome (CS) was described by Harvey Cushing in 1932 and since then a variety of disorders underlying CS has been identified. Endogenous CS is traditionally classified as either ACTH dependent, corresponding to around 80% of all cases, or ACTH independent, which accounts for 15–20% of cases *(1)*.

Unilateral functional tumors, adenomas, and less frequently adrenal cortical carcinomas (ACC) are responsible for the majority of adrenal CS (80–95%). Other causes, accounting for the remaining 10–15% of cases include primary pigmented nodular adrenocortical disease (PPNAD), primary non-pigmented micronodular hyperplasia, and ACTH-independent macronodular adrenal hyperplasia (AIMAH) *(2)*.

Here we will review the phenotype, the diagnosis, and treatment of ACTH-independent Cushing's syndrome due to adrenocortical tumors.

EPIDEMIOLOGY

Adrenocortical tumors are classified as functional (hormone secreting) or silent and either benign or malignant. Benign adrenocortical tumors are more frequent with a prevalence of at least 3% in individuals above 50 years of age, whereas ACC are rare, with estimations of prevalence ranging from 4 to 12 cases per million and incidence 1–2 per million population/year in adults of North America and Europe *(3)*. Nowadays, the majority of these tumors are discovered incidentally due to the increased number of radiological procedures performed in clinical practice. In children, the incidence is considered to be approximately ten times lower, with the notable exception of the Southern and Southwestern regions of Brazil, where an exceptionally high annual incidence of ACC has been reported (3.4–4.2 per million children under 15 years). The specific germline mutation (R337H) at TP53 tumor suppressor gene has been frequently identified in this population *(4)*.

Adrenocortical carcinomas can occur at all ages, from early infancy to the seventh and eight decades of life. A bimodal age distribution has been reported to ACC, with the first peak occurring before the age of 5 years, and a second and higher peak in the fourth and fifth decade *(5, 6)*. Women are commonly often affected than men accounting for 65–90% of reported cases *(7, 8)*. Some investigators have reported an increased left-sided prevalence, nevertheless others describe a right-sided preponderance in 2–10% of cases *(8)*. Epidemiologic studies have associated an increased risk of ACC to the use of oral contraceptives and smoking *(9, 10)*. The ACC has a heterogeneous presentation and a poor prognosis with high recurrence and mortality rates.

CLINICAL PRESENTATION

Patients with ACC present with signs and symptoms of excessive adrenal steroid output in approximately 60% of cases. Rapidly progressing CS with or without signs of virilization is the most common clinical presentation in adults.

Hypercortisolism induces centripetal obesity, protein wasting with skin thinning and striae, muscular atrophy (myopathy), and osteoporosis. Cortisol excess can also result in impaired defense against opportunist infection, glucose intolerance or diabetes mellitus, systemic hypertension, psychiatric disturbances, and gonadal dysfunction in both men and women (Table 1) *(1)*. The clinical presentation of adult and pediatric patients with adrenocortical tumors (adenoma or carcinoma) is considerably diverse (Figs. 1 and 2).

Out of 231 patients with adrenocortical tumors followed from 1976 to 2009 at Hospital das Clinicas University of Sao Paulo, Brazil, 48 adults (40 female; ranging from 16 to 71 years of age) and ten children (seven female; ranging from 3 months to 15 years of age) bore ACC. Autonomous cortisol secretion, either alone or in combination with other steroids, was detected in 81% of the adult patients. Hypercortisolism was identified in 48% of pediatric patients, although only 10% of them presented classical clinical CS (unpublished data).

Depending on duration and intensity of steroid production its manifestation can range widely from subclinical to overt Cushing's syndrome. In patients with adrenal incidentaloma, mild cortisol secretion can be misdiagnosed because symptoms such as obesity, systemic hypertension, and glucose intolerance are not exclusive manifestation of CS. An important clinical clue to the presence of glucocorticoid excess is the concurrent onset and increase of these symptoms simultaneously *(11, 12)*.

Table 1
Signs and Symptoms of Cushing's Syndrome

Signs or symptoms	*Reported incidence (%)*
Centripetal obesity	79–97
Facial plethora	50–94
Glucose intolerance	39–90
Weakness, proximal myopathy	29–90
Psychological changes	31–86
Easy bruisability	23–84
Hirsutism	64–81
Oligomenorrhea or amenorrhea	55–80
Impotence	55–80
Acne, oily skin	26–80
Abdominal striae	51–71
Ankle edema	28–60
Backache, vertebral collapse, fracture	40–50
Polydipsia, polyuria	25–44
Renal calculi	15–19
Hyperpigmentation	4–16
Headache	0–47
Exophthalmos	0–33
Tinea versicolor infection	0–30
Abdominal pain	0–21

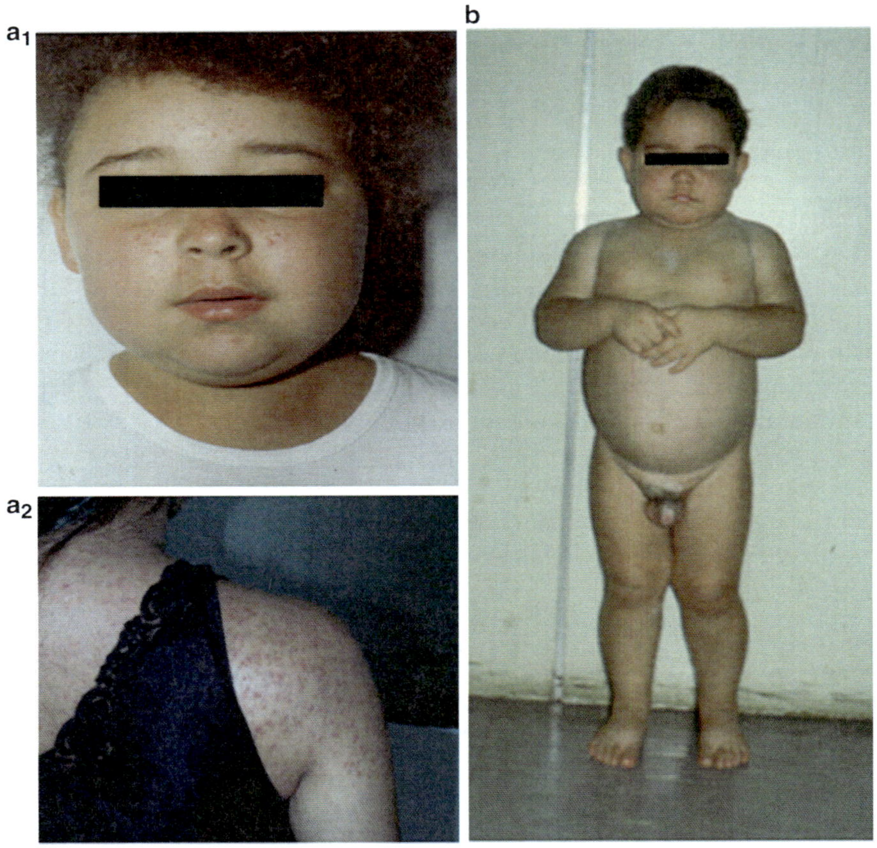

Fig. 1. (**a***1*, **a***2*) A 9-year-old girl presenting mixed syndrome with signs of Cushing's syndrome (moon face, obesity, abdominal striae) and virilization (acne) due to an adrenocortical carcinoma. The tumor was classified Weiss score 7 and MacFarlane standing II (weight 220 g, diameter 9 cm). She had a fatal outcome, 1 year and 4 months, after radical surgery (nefrectomy and adrenalectomy) although she has been using mitotane during this time. (**b**) A 2.5-year-old boy also presenting mixed syndrome with signs of Cushing syndrome (moon face, obesity) and pseudoprecocious-puberty isosexual (pubic hair stage III, penis enlargement, and prepubertal testis) due to an adrenocortical carcinoma. The tumor was classified Weiss score 5 and MacFarlane standing IV (weight 250 g, diameter 20 cm). A fatal outcome occurred 8 months after surgery.

Androgen secreting tumors induce virilization in women and isosexual or heterosexual pseudoprecocious puberty in children *(13, 14)*. The most common manifestations of virilization syndrome in adult females are deepening of voice, male pattern baldness, hirsutism, alopecia, acne, clitoral hypertrophy, oligomenorrhea, and infertility. In men the manifestations of androgen excess are less noticeable. In the pediatric group, the main signs are related to pseudoprecocious puberty as aggressive behavior, pubic hair development, facial acne, axillary sweating, penis enlargement without concomitant testicular enlargement, clitoral hypertrophy, and increased growth velocity with advanced bone age (Fig. 1) *(15–17)*.

Estrogen-secreting adrenal tumors are rare. In males, they may lead to gynecomastia, testicular atrophy, and decreased libido, and are almost invariably malignant *(18, 19)*. In our cohort, we have only one such case: a 17-year-old male whose tumor was deemed malignant on histopathological examination but without tumor recurrence in 7 years of follow-up. Feminizing tumors in women can

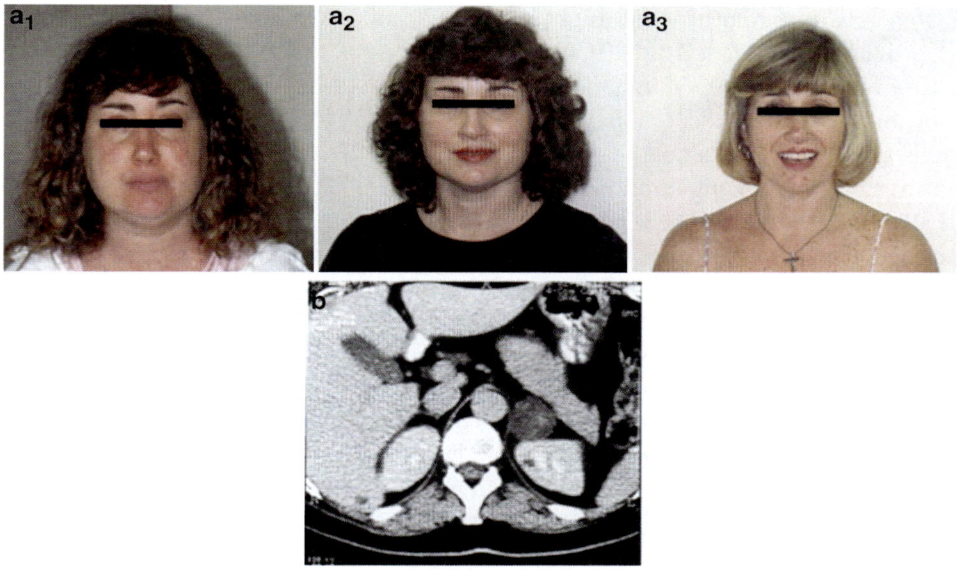

Fig. 2. (**a***1*) A 36-year-old woman with a mild CS due to an adrenocortical adenoma. (**a***2*, **a***3*) 1 and 5 years after adrenalectomy respectively. (**b**) Contrast-enhanced CT scan image (late phase) showed a homogeneous, encapsulated, ovoid and well-defined low attenuation mass at the left adrenal topography. The CT attenuation value was 5 HU, indicating the presence of intracellular lipid, a characteristic feature of benign adenomas. She underwent a left adrenalectomy (Weiss score 1 and McFarlane II, weight 15 g, diameter 6 cm).

cause breast tenderness and dysfunctional uterine bleeding. Prepubertal girls with feminizing tumors experience early breast and uterine development and early onset of menarche *(15, 20)*.

The diagnosis of malignancy in nonmetastatic tumors relies on careful presurgical assessment of clinical, biological, and radiological features and detailed pathological examination of the excised tumor (see below).

Adrenocortical adenomas are benign tumors of the adrenal cortex, usually small and unilateral. Most of these tumors cause endocrine symptoms due to ACTH-independent steroid secretion. Benign adrenocortical tumors usually secrete a single class of steroid. The excessive production of cortisol, aldosterone or, rarely, androgens or estrogens may occur. Co-secretion of androgens and cortisol is not frequent in benign adrenocortical tumor but can occur *(3, 21)*.

Symptoms and signs of CS result from chronic exposure to excessive glucocorticoid. The Cushing's syndrome is associated with considerable morbidity and increased mortality. In a population-based study of CS, mortality was increased in the first year after diagnosis, even in those patients without concurrent cancer, and some of the deaths occurred before treatment could be initiated.

Several laboratory analyses are useful in establishing or confirming excessive glucocorticoid secretion and in monitoring these patients. No single laboratory test is perfect, though. The three most commonly used tests used for the diagnosis of Cushing's syndrome are the determination of 24-h urinary free cortisol, the measurement of midnight plasma cortisol or late-night salivary cortisol, and the low-dose dexamethasone (1 mg overnight) suppression test *(22)*.

Adrenocortical carcinomas are rare tumors and more than a half of these tumors produce hormonal and metabolic syndromes that lead to their discovery. The remaining cases are silent and are usually discovered either through metastatic manifestation or when the primary tumor becomes large enough to produce abdominal symptoms *(1, 6)*. Although adrenal incidentalomas are rarely ACC, a growing number of cases are currently being diagnosed during the evaluation of incidentalomas *(11, 12, 23)*.

This circumstance is important since it might be a way to diagnose an ACC at an earlier stage and to improve the prognosis *(24, 25)*. The ACC may also be associated with complex genetic syndromes such as the Li–Fraumeni and Wiedemann–Beckwith syndromes *(24, 26, 27)*.

The proportion of ACC that secrete hormone varies from 25 to 75% in the literature. The ACC can secrete various types of steroids and co-secretion of androgens and cortisol is the most frequent and highly suggestive of a malignant adrenocortical tumor *(9, 21)*. The ACC can also secrete mineralocorticoids and steroid precursors *(14, 21, 28)*.

Detection of steroid excess is important for establishing the adrenocortical origin of the tumor and for follow-up. Probably, less than a third of ACCs is "nonhypersecretory" after careful hormonal investigations. In these cases, one should be cautious not to under diagnose a tumor in the adrenal area as an ACC. These nonhypersecretory ACCs can be diagnosed following the investigation of adrenal incidentalomas or discovered by the manifestations of the tumor growth or extension: local symptoms (pain, palpation of a mass, venous thrombosis, etc.) or distant metastases (liver, lung, and bones) *(28)*. Fever may occur due to tumor necrosis. The general condition of the patient is most often preserved until very late stages, resulting in a delay in the diagnosis of nonhypersecretory ACCs *(29)*.

DIAGNOSIS

Several laboratorial analyses are useful in establishing or confirming excessive glucocorticoid secretion and in monitoring these patients. The three most commonly used tests for the diagnosis of Cushing's syndrome are the determination of 24-h urinary free cortisol, the measurement of midnight plasma cortisol or late-night salivary cortisol, and the low-dose dexamethasone (1 mg overnight) suppression test. No single test is perfect, therefore is prudent to use at least two tests to confirm Cushing's syndrome diagnosis.

Hormonal Findings

Hormonal evaluation is mandatory in all patients with a suspected adrenocortical tumor. Unfortunately, hormone determinations are usually of limited help in predicting malignancy. However, in the presence of an adrenal lesion, extremely elevated serum dehydroepiandrosterone sulphate (DHEAS) levels suggest an ACC, as benign adrenocortical tumors often exhibit low serum DHEAS levels *(3, 9, 14, 21)*. A high testosterone level was the most common finding in adults and children with virilization followed by high DHEAS, androstenedione, and dehydroepiandrosterone. High 11-deoxycortisol levels were frequently associated with tumor recurrence. Cortisol suppression after dexamethasone was altered in 93% of patients with virilization and no clinical features, suggesting autonomous cortisol secretion *(13)*. The diagnosis of ACTH-independent cortisol hypersecretion is established by undetectable plasma ACTH levels concomitantly to increased urinary cortisol excretion that is not suppressed by high doses of dexamethasone (see "Dynamic Tests" section). Serum and salivary midnight cortisol and low-dose dexamethasone suppression test (DST) can confirm CS.

Virilizing tumors are usually characterized by exhibiting high serum levels of testosterone, androstenedione, and DHEAS, whereas patients with feminizing tumors have high serum estradiol levels. Some of these tumors produce intermediate products of the steroid biosynthetic pathway, such as progesterone, 11-deoxycortisol, DOC, androstenedione, and estradiol. Secretion of aldosterone by ACC is not frequent and can be detected by plasma aldosterone and renin assays. An unusual hormone secretion by ACC was demonstrated in a 30-year-old male who had selective FSH suppression due to inhibin B and estrogen tumor secretion *(30)*.

It is important to determine the level of the adrenal steroids prior to surgical resection of the tumor because they can be used as biochemical markers in the postoperative follow-up *(1)*.

DYNAMIC TESTS

24-h Urinary Free Cortisol Level

Hypercortisolism is best established by the determination 24-h excretion of urinary free cortisol. In this test, cortisol levels should be determined in at least two or three 24-h urine samples. The upper limit of normality varies in different laboratories, according to the measurement technique used.

More than 90% of patients with the CS present high levels of 24-h excretion of cortisol urinary free (three to four times above the limit of assay) *(31)*.

Midnight Plasma Cortisol and Late-Night Salivary Cortisol Measurements

Cortisol production is normally suppressed at night, but in CS this suppression does not occur. Therefore, if the serum or salivary cortisol is elevated during the night, CS should be suspected. Sampling of midnight serum cortisol generally requires a 48-h hospital admission in order to avoid falsely elevated serum cortisol levels due to stress. However, a late-night or bedtime salivary sample can be obtained at home, and then tested to determine the free cortisol levels. Diagnostic ranges vary, depending on the measurement technique used. The overnight single-low-dose (1 mg) dexametasone suppression test is a useful screening test for CS. Serum cortisol levels at 8:00 a.m. higher than 1.8 µg/dL (50 nmol/L) indicate failure of suppression. In addition, a low plasma ACTH levels concomitant to elevate serum cortisol levels indicate autonomous activity of the adrenal glands *(3, 28, 32)*.

Dexamethasone Suppression Test

Two modalities of DST are widely used: overnight and 48 h. For the overnight test, 1 mg of dexamethasone is given at midnight and serum cortisol levels are measured on the following morning at 8:00–9:00 a.m. For the 48-h test, 0.5 mg of dexamethasone is given every 6 h for 2 days at 9:00, 15:00, 21:00, and 3:00 h, and cortisol levels are measured in the serum at 8:00 h at the beginning and at the end of the test. To exclude Cushing's syndrome, serum cortisol levels should be of 50 nmol/L (1.8 µg/dL) or less after either test. Due to its simplicity, the 1-mg DST probably is still the most frequently used screening tool to rule out Cushing's syndrome *(22)*. The 48-h test may also be used as a screening test but it is more often used as a confirmatory test. Although more cumbersome than the overnight test, it is more specific and with adequate regular instructions can be done by outpatients. For both tests, potential malabsorption of dexametasone must be ruled out as well as the use of drugs that increase the hepatic clearance of dexamethasone, such as carbamazepine, phenytoin, phenobarbital, rifampicin, meprobamate, aminoglutethimide, methaqualone, and troglitazone *(32)*.

RADIOLOGICAL INVESTIGATION

In patients with ACTH-independent Cushing's syndrome due to an adrenal lesion, the most common diagnostic dilemma is distinguishing an adrenal adenoma from carcinoma. A variety of imaging procedures can be useful to discriminate the benign from malignant characteristics of an adrenal cortical neoplasm (Table 2). In a series of 210 patients with an incidental finding of an adrenal mass, a cutoff diameter of 5 cm yielded 93% sensitivity and 63% specificity for the diagnosis of carcinoma *(33)*. The most commonly used procedures are computed tomography scans (CT scans) and chemical-shift magnetic resonance imaging (MRI) (Fig. 2). Both techniques rely on the presence of intracellular lipids to characterize adenomas *(34)* (see also Chap. 8).

The CT scans are very informative for the diagnosis of adrenocortical tumors. The ACC carcinomas will most commonly be identified as large unilateral masses (above 5–6 cm, typically 10 cm

Table 2
Nonspecific Findings of Anatomical Imaging that May Help in Differentiating Benign from Malignant Adrenal Masses

Features	*Benign mass*	*Malignant tumor*[a]
Size	<4 cm	>4 cm
Shape/margins	Round/smooth	Thick/irregular
Homogeneity CT or MRI	Homogeneous	Heterogenous
Lipid content	High (except lipid-poor adenomas)	Low
Growth rate	Slow	Rapid
CT density	<10 HU (lipid-rich adenomas)	
>10 HU (lipid-poor adenomas)	>10 HU	
CT enhancement after contrast administration	Early enhancement and early washout	Variable enhancement with slow washout
% Absolute enhancement washout (AEW)	>60%	<60%
% Relative enhancement washout (REW)	>40%	<40%
MRI signal on T2-weighted sequences	Low	High

[a]Primary adrenal carcinoma or metastasis

and above), compressing the kidney. Besides the size of the tumor, other features may suggest malignancy such as the lack of homogeneity with foci of necrosis and irregular margins; spontaneous high density before injection of contrast media [above 10 Hounsfield units (HU)], indicating a low fat content in opposition to the high fat content often found in adrenal adenomas. The threshold value of 10 HU is associated with 71% specificity and 98% specificity for the diagnosis of carcinoma. This is comparable to results obtained with chemical shift MRI (Fig. 3). For the identification of lipid-depleted poor adenomas, delayed contrast-enhanced CT is more accurate. Threshold attenuation values of 30–40 HU or the washout after contrast media injection during CT scan below 50% at 15 min are equally efficacious to distinguish typical ACC enhancement washout of 60% at 15 min. The combination of attenuation values and percentage of washout correctly characterized 96% of adenomas in a recent report *(35)*. On MRI, tumors are often hypointense in comparison to the liver on T1-weighted images and hyperintense on T2-weighted images. Superior identification of blood vessels and the multiplanar capability of MRI make it the imaging modality of choice for evaluating the extent of disease and planning surgical excision. The distinction between benign and malignant masses on the basis of the presence of lipid can also be determined by chemical shift MRI, with 81% sensitivity and 100% specificity *(36)*. Lipid-rich adenomas show a 34% change in relative signal intensity between in-phase and out-of-phase imaging, whereas nonadenomas do not change. The CT scan and MRI are also employed for the detection of local invasion, distant metastases (lung), liver nodules, venous invasion, and potentially involved lymph nodes *(35)* (Fig. 3). Defining metastatic extension is crucial for staging the disease and planning treatment. Adrenal scintigraphy with iodocholesterol is not routinely necessary, although it might occasionally help since adrenocortical adenomas tend to uptake the radionuclide *(37)*. By contrast, ACC – especially

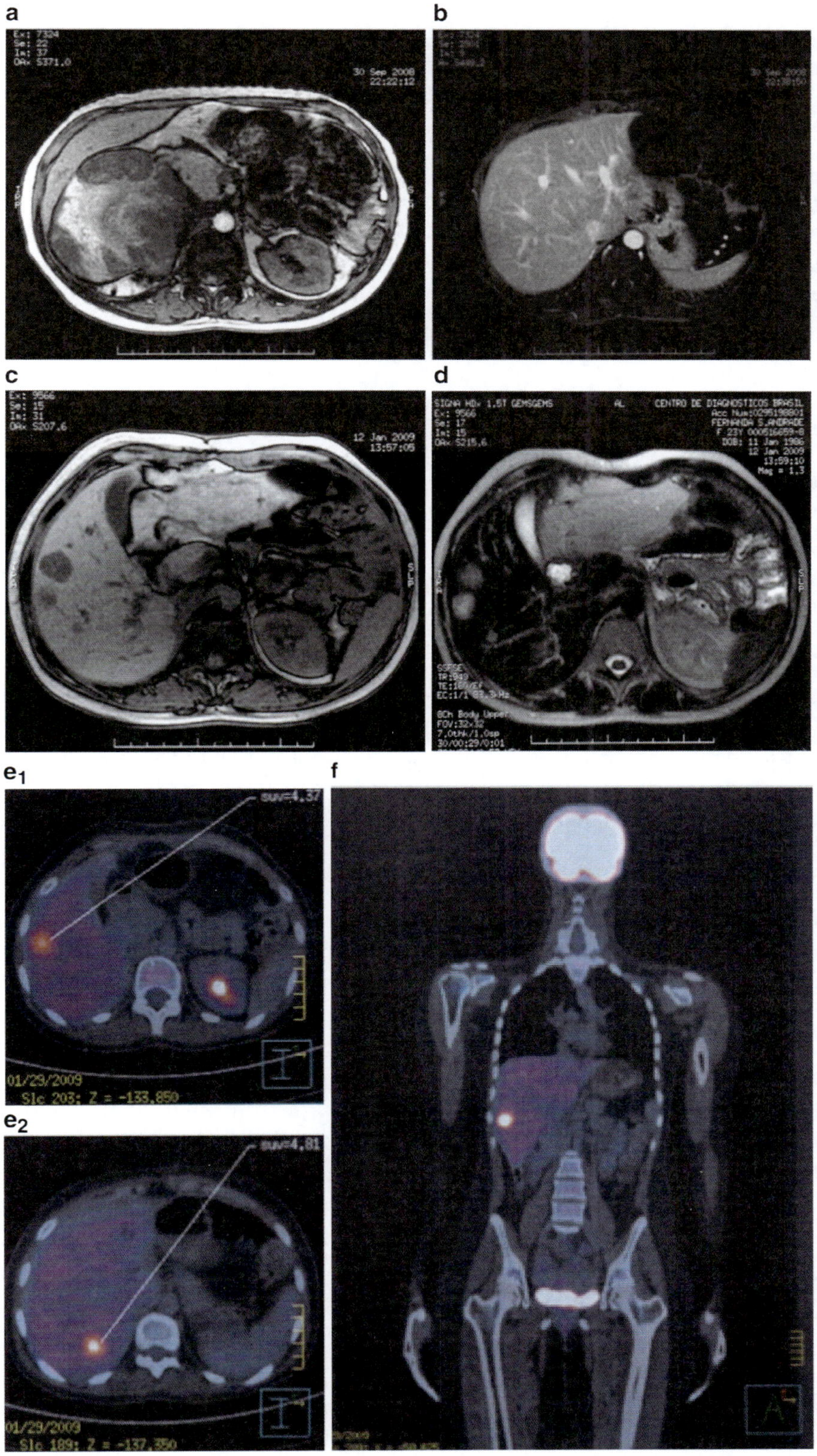

Fig. 3. (**a**) A 23-year-old woman with mild CS due to an adrenocortical carcinoma. An axial T1-weighted in-phase MR image showed a large ($10.9 \times 9.5 \times 11.5$ cm^3), heterogeneous mass in the left adrenal gland, containing high-signal

nonsecreting tumors – often do not uptake the radionucleotide. Bone scintigraphy may help to evaluate bone metastases. However, in patients with CS, bone remodeling and/or fracture can induce false positive results of bone scintigraphy *(38)*. More recently, studies have demonstrated that ACCs almost invariably have a high uptake of 18-fluorodesoxyglucose (18)-FDG *(39)*. Thus, (18)-FDG positron emission tomography (PET) scan appears to distinguish between benign and malignant adrenal tumors *(40, 41)* (Fig. 3). This simple, nontraumatic imaging procedure can also be used for the extension workup. PET using C-labeled metomidate is a tissue-specific imaging procedure that has been demonstrated to detect both adrenal adenomas and ACC *(42)*. Its use in the extension workup of ACC needs to be investigated.

HISTOPATHOLOGICAL EVALUATION

Adrenocortical tumors may arise from any of three cortical layers: glomerulosa, fasciculate, and reticularis. They have classically been considered as epithelial tumors and therefore are classified as carcinoma or adenoma, however even after surgical removal this distinction may remain difficult *(43)*. A number of diagnostic protocols have been published, some of them attributing different numerical weighting to a combination of clinical, biochemical, and morphologic features. A score corresponding to sum of these criteria defines the tumor as adenoma, carcinoma, or of uncertain malignant potential *(44, 45)*. In the pediatric group, tumor staging is more reliable than Weiss criteria (see below) *(16)*.

Adult group: The classification of adrenocortical tumors is also based on their size assessed by imaging. The tumor weight is important as well, since most of them weigh between 20 and 50 g, while most malignant cortical tumors weigh more than 100 g. The histopathological examination should be performed by an experienced pathologist *(46)* Differentiation between benign and malignant adrenal lesions is based on macroscopic features (tumor weight, hemorrhage, breached, or intact tumor capsule) and microscopic assessment using the Weiss score, the most widely used tool *(44, 45)*. Weiss criteria was based on nine features and the presence of any three of these indicated malignant potential in adult patients *(16)* (Table 3). Nuclear atypia, atypical and frequent mitoses (more than five per 50 high-power fields), vascular and capsular invasion, and necrosis are suggestive of malignancy. In addition, broad fibrous bands are a characteristic feature differentiating ACC from benign tumors. This system is widely used by pathologists and is reported to have 96% specificity, 100% sensitivity, and good correlation of the overall score (r - 0.94) in adults *(16)*. Immunohistochemistry provides important additional information. Several studies have demonstrated the value of Ki67 staining in differentiating benign from malignant lesions *(47)*. In addition, Ki67 expression may be of prognostic relevance as high expression has been associated with poor survival *(47)*. Other markers like D11, inhibin, melan-A, and chromogranin A are helpful to

Fig. 3. (continued) intensity areas within the mass, suggesting hemorrhage. A full contact surface of the tumor mass and the liver is noted and a clear cleavage line between these structures was not evident. (**b**) An axial fast spin echo T2-weighted MR image did not identify liver metastases before surgery. (**c**) Axial T1-weighted out-of-phase image showed multiple liver metastases (four solid nodules). (**d**) Axial T2-weighted out-of-phase image showed no loss of signal intensity within the nodules in the liver metastases. The patient was in use of mitotane and chemotherapy at day 92 postsurgery. (**e**) The image obtained with [18F]-fluorodopamine (FDA) positron emission tomography-computed tomography fusion (PET-CT) of the same patient showed a high homogeneous uptake in the abdominal projection, corresponding to two nodules in liver (V and VI segments). (**f**) [18F] FDA-PET showed no uptake in chest.

Table 3
Histological Features to Be Assessed to Determine Malignant Potential

Weiss score
1. Diffuse architecture
2. Clear cells – 25% of total
3. Significant nuclear pleomorphism
4. Confluent necrosis
5. Mitotic count – 6 per 50 high-power fields
6. Atypical mitoses
7. Capsular invasion
8. Sinusoidal invasion
9. Venous invasion

Adrenocortical tumors with Weiss score 3 are classified as malignant tumors in adult group *(44, 45)*

confirm the adrenocortical origin of the tumor. Finally, several new markers (LOH at 17p13, IGF-II overexpression, cyclin E) have been proposed to distinguish between benign and malignant adrenal lesions *(48, 49)*.

Pediatric group: The pathologic classification of pediatric adrenocortical tumors is troublesome. Clinical manifestation and biologic behavior of these lesions can be quite distinct from their histological equivalents in the adult population *(48)*, meaning that pathological criteria (Weiss score) alone are not reliable for distinguishing benign from malignant tumors *(48)*. A retrospective study of 83 adrenal cortical neoplasms investigate if adult clinical and histological features can be applied to pediatric patients, using an outcome-based analysis *(16)*. Most of the patients (50 girls and 33 boys) presented with hormone-related symptoms for a mean of 6.8 months. The tumors ranged in size from 2 to 20 cm (mean 8.8 cm). Histological parameters examined included capsular and/or vascular invasion, extra adrenal soft tissue extension, growth pattern, cellularity, necrosis, cytoplasmic eosinophilia, nuclear pleomorphism, nuclear-to-cytoplasmic ratio, prominent nucleoli, mitotic figures, atypical mitotic figures, bands of fibrosis, and calcifications. Immunophenotypically, there was reactivity with inhibin, vimentin, CK5, and focally with p53 and Ki-67. All patients underwent adrenalectomy, and 20 patients received adjuvant therapy. All patients with tumors classified as adenomas ($n = 9$) were alive, without evidence of disease (mean 14.7 years), whereas 21 patients with carcinomas had died with disease (mean 2.4 years). Only 31% of histologically malignant tumors behaved in a clinically malignant fashion. Features associated with an increased probability of a malignant clinical behavior included tumor weight (>400 g), tumor size (>10.5 cm), vena cava invasion, capsular and/or vascular invasion, extension into periadrenal soft tissue, confluent necrosis, severe nuclear atypia, >15 mitotic figures/20 high power fields, and the presence of atypical mitotic figures. Vena cava invasion, necrosis, and increased mitotic activity (>15 mitotic figures/20 high power fields) independently suggested malignant clinical behavior in multivariate analysis *(16)*. The clinical manifestations and biologic behavior of adrenal cortical neoplasms in pediatric population can be quite distinct from their histologically similar counterparts in the adult population, making classical pathologic criteria for distinguishing benign from malignant tumors equivocal. In general, the presence of most of these markers and molecular changes becomes more frequent as the tumoral malignancy grade increases. Some of the genetic changes described are uncovered in the late stages of the disease, and it is likely that a better understanding of early events may lead to a more effective control of the process of tumorigenesis.

STAGING

Staging of Adrenocortical Tumor

A variety of staging systems have been used for adrenocortical cancer *(51)* and most investigators use a surgical staging system based on the size of the primary tumor and regional or distant tumor extension, as described by MacFarlane (1958) and modified by Sullivan (1978) *(50, 52)*.

The system is most frequently used to predict the prognosis *(50, 52)*. However, the proposed modifications are plausible, as they may reflect the natural history of the disease in a better way and correlate closely with other staging systems used for solid tumors *(53, 54)*. Accordingly, the new "Union International Contre Cancer" (UICC) staging system published by the World Health Organization in 2004 is based on this classification *(55)*. Stages I and II comprise localized tumors with 5 cm or smaller and larger than 5 cm, respectively. Locally invasive tumors or tumors with regional lymph node metastases are classified as stage III, whereas stage IV consists of tumors invading adjacent organs or presenting with distant metastases. In the majority of patients with stages I–III, complete tumor removal may be achievable, whereas this is highly unlikely in the presence of distant metastasis (stage IV). While in older series *(10)*, most patients were diagnosed in advanced stages of disease (stage IV), some more recent studies have reported the highest percentage of patients in stage II *(56, 57)* probably reflecting improved and more widely available imaging technology. Distant metastases affect most often liver and lungs, with prevalence ranging from 44 to 93% and 46 to 79%, respectively, according to different series *(51, 58)*.

Recently, Fassnacht et al. *(51)* proposed a new staging classification for ACC on the basis of results obtained from German ACC Registry comprising 492 patients. These patients were diagnosed between 1986 and 2007 with detailed information on primary diagnosis and a minimum follow-up of 6 months. Patients were assigned to UICC tumor stage, and disease-specific survival (DSS) was evaluated from the following staging system assessed (Table 4). Using their revised staging system [the European Network for the Study of Adrenal Tumors (ENSAT) classification] the 5-year DSS rate in this cohort was 82% for stage I, 61% for stage II, 50% for stage III, and 13% for stage IV. These data indicate improved outcome prediction in comparison to the 2004 UICC classification, as DSS differed considerably between stage II and III *(51)*.

Table 4
MacFarlane Classification Modified by Sullivan of Adrenal Cortical Carcinoma Based on Size and Extent of Disease

Stage	*Tumor size*	*Lymphadenopathy*	*Invasion*	*Metastases*	*TNM*
I	<5 cm	–	–	–	T1-N0-M0
II	>5 cm	–	–	–	T2-N0-M0
III	Any size	+	+	–	T1 or T2-N1-M0
IV	Any size	+	+	+	T1 or T2-N1-M1

TNM tumor-node-metastasis *(48, 50)*

THERAPY

Surgery

In stages I–III, complete tumor resection continues to be the treatment of choice for ACC *(57)*. It is best performed by an experienced surgeon using a transabdominal or even a thoraco-abdominal approach *(57, 59)*. Intact tumor capsule and a margin-free resection (R0 resection) are associated with a superior prognosis and prediction of long-term survival *(54, 58)*. Invasion by or adherence of the carcinoma into adjacent organs often requires en bloc excision of the kidney, the spleen, partial hepatectomy, or pancreatectomy *(56)*. In addition, lymphadenectomy has often to be performed. The presence of a tumor thrombus in the renal vein or the inferior vena cava does not preclude a complete resection, although cardiac bypass technique may be necessary for successful removal of tumor tissue extending into the inferior vena cava or even the right atrium *(54, 59)*. The role of tumor debulking in the presence of metastatic disease is a matter of debate. Incomplete resection of the primary tumor or metastatic disease not amenable to surgery is associated with a particular poor prognosis. In most studies, the median survival is below 12 months *(60, 61)*. However, tumor debulking may help to control hormonal excess and may in individual cases facilitate other therapeutic options.

Local recurrence and metastatic disease during follow-up is common especially in adult patients even if complete resection has been achieved. Risk factors include McFarlane stage III tumors; a tumor diameter or weight above 12 cm and 200 g, respectively; a high mitotic index and intratumoral hemorrhage to both pediatric and adult groups *(62)*. Since its introduction in 1992, minimal invasive laparoscopic adrenalectomy has become the treatment of choice for benign adrenal lesions with a diameter of less than 6 cm because of less postoperative pain and a shorter hospital stay (see Chap.11). At present, there is a consensus that open adrenalectomy remains the operation of choice for ACC with invasion of adjacent organs, enlarged regional lymph nodes, or tumors larger than 10–12 cm in size *(46, 53)*. In addition, a definitive margin-free resection is potentially difficult to be performed through laparoscopic resection *(63–65)*. Cobb et al. *(66)* identified 25 cases of ACC removed by laparoscopic resection and local recurrence was observed in 40% of these patients. High local recurrence after laparoscopic adrenalectomy was also observed in a recent series reported by Gonzalez et al. *(67)*.

Surgical resection of recurrent disease is an important therapeutic option associated with prolonged survival *(68, 69)*, although cure is seldom achieved. Surgery for recurrent disease includes locoregional recurrence as well as isolated hepatic and pulmonary metastases. The most frequent indication for reoperation is locoregional disease *(68, 69)*. Surgery-related mortality has improved but remains significant *(70)* particularly for MacFarlane stage III disease with invasion of adjacent organs. Recently, successful thermo-ablation for recurrent or metastatic ACC has also been reported *(71)*.

Radiation Therapy

There are very few data in the medical literature documenting efficacy of radiation therapy, therefore its role in ACC is not been well defined. However, palliative radiotherapy for metastatic disease has been effective in a significant percentage of patients *(72)* and is the treatment choice for bone metastases (30–40 Gy). More importantly, radiotherapy may have a role as adjuvant postoperative radiation therapy in patients at high risk for local recurrence. In a small series of patients with stage III disease, the survival was higher than expected from historical series *(73)*. Postoperative radiation of the tumor bed (50–60 Gy) may therefore improve the long-term outcome in stage III ACC or high-risk stage II patients (tumor diameter >12 cm, high mitotic index, violation of the tumor capsule, or frank evidence of tumor spillage during surgery). The risk–benefit ratio for radiotherapy in patients with ACC should be individually assessed.

Radiofrequency Thermal Ablation

Image-guided local tumor ablation with radiofrequency current may offer a minimally invasive and safe treatment option for patients who have had multiple recurrent surgeries, who are not ideal surgical candidates, or for whom the proven benefits of surgery do not outweigh the risks. Thermal ablation makes local tissue destruction possible in a rapid, predictable, and inexpensive manner with minimal morbidity and a short recovery time. There is evidence that this method may be an alternative to surgery in some patients with metastatic ACC and lesions less than 5 cm in size, but its utility and value remain to be proven, and potential benefits have to be weighed against complications *(71)*. Long-term follow-up will need to be performed and appropriate patient selection criteria will need to be determined in future randomized trials.

MEDICAL THERAPY

Medical therapy aims to control hormonal hypersecretion and – more importantly – to maintain partial or complete remission of disease.

Mitotane Adjuvant Therapy

More than 40 years ago the successful use of *o,p′*-DDD (mitotane) in patients with metastatic ACC was reported for the first time. Mitotane [1,1 dichloro-2(*o*-chlorophenyl)-2-(*p*-chloro-phenyl) ethane] is an isomer of the insecticide *p,p′*-DDD and a chemical congener of the insecticide DDT. It is an adrenolytic compound that acts specifically on the adrenal cortex *(74)*. Mitotane belongs to a class of drugs that require intraadrenal transformation into active metabolites for therapeutic action. Mitotane is hydroxylated in the mitochondria at the β-carbon and further transformed into an acylchloride. It has been reported that the active metabolites cause toxicity by oxygen activation with superoxide formation or by covalent binding to specific proteins *(74)*.

The role of mitotane in adjuvant therapy after complete surgical removal of ACC remains a matter of debate *(75, 76)*. Due to the high rate of locoregional or metastatic recurrence after seemingly curative resection, adjuvant treatment options are clearly needed. It is important to notice that its impact on survival of patients with ACC cannot be properly assessed without prospective randomized trials with a sufficient number of patients and in the absence of those, the value of adjuvant therapy with mitotane remains uncertain *(77)*. Mitotane is either given as tablets (Lysodren®, Bristol Myers Squibb, Princeton, USA) in doses >3 g/day or as capsules of micronized compound mixed with cellulose acetylphthalate, which have a lower absorption rate, but possibly, a better gastrointestinal tolerance (usually higher doses up to 12 g/day are required) *(9, 78, 79)*. Drug monitoring is important and the serum mitotane levels between 14 and 20 mg/L are required in order to induce tumor regression. An objective response in metastatic disease was found in 31% of patients who maintained this level, whereas no response was seen in patients with lower serum concentrations *(79)*.

Since side effects are more frequently observed when serum levels exceed 20 mg/L and serum levels are not closely correlated to oral dosage *(78)*, drug monitoring may also improve quality of life during mitotane treatment by avoiding overtreatment. Due to its long half-life, higher levels are achieved only after several months of therapy *(79)*. Accordingly, in our experience, mitotane-induced side effects may become more pronounced with ongoing treatment on a constant dose as drug levels gradually increase. Side effects of mitotane occur frequently and are often dose limiting mainly involving the gastrointestinal tract (diarrhea, nausea, anorexia) or concern the central nervous system (lethargy, somnolence, ataxia, dizziness, confusion). Patients rarely tolerate doses >6 g/day in the long term and since its action is more therapeutically pronounced in fasciculata cells, glucocorticoid deficiency precedes mineralocorticoid deficiency. Inadequately treated adrenal insufficiency enhances mitotane-induced side effects and reduces its tolerance *(79)*. High-dose glucocorticoid replacement may be needed due to increased metabolic clearance of glucocorticoids (e.g., dexamethasone). Hydrocortisone is the treatment of choice and the replacement therapy is best monitored by careful clinical assessment and regular measurements of plasma ACTH levels, which should not be elevated *(80)*. A daily dose of 50-mg hydrocortisone (20–20–10 mg) or cortisone acetate (25–12.5 mg) may be needed. It may be necessary to add fludrocortisone depending on blood pressure, serum potassium levels, and plasma renin activity.

Contraceptive methods should be indicated in all patients with menacme age and maintained at least 1 year after the end of therapy, since mitotane remains stored in fat tissue for at least 7 months after withdrawal of the drug. Nonclinical data on the general toxicity of mitotane are limited. There are not studies of reproductive toxicity with mitotane. However, DDT and other similar biphenyl polychlorinated are recognized as exerting adverse effects on fertility, pregnancy, and fetal development, estimating that the mitotane presents the same properties. It was not yet investigated on the genotoxic and carcinogenic potential of mitotane.

Increases in hepatic gamma glutamyl transferase levels are frequent *(9, 81)* and in most cases do not require drug withdrawal. However, severe hepatotoxicity has been described. Mitotane increases serum cholesterol mainly by increasing low-density lipoprotein (LDL) cholesterol. In addition, mitotane can prolong the bleeding time by changing platelet aggregation response *(82)*. Of particular importance are mitotane-induced endocrine abnormalities. Mitotane strongly increases hormone-binding globulins (e.g., cortisol-binding globulin and sex hormone-binding globulin) and therefore measurement of total hormone concentrations may give normal results in the presence of clearly impaired bioavailability of free hormones *(83)*. Additionally, total thyroxine levels may be reduced as mitotane competes with endogenous thyroxin for thyroxine binding globulin (TBG) binding sites. In some patients, free thyroid hormone concentrations decrease and thyroxin replacement may also become necessary.

For the management of nausea, 5-hydroxytryptamine (5-HT) blockers may be useful. In case of significant neuropsychiatric side effects, drug treatment should be interrupted for a minimum of 1 week and restarted with a lower dose. Adequate serum concentrations of mitotane may persist for weeks to months after cessation of therapy due to its long half-life.

Systemic chemotherapy most often results in solely temporary improvement. Chemotherapeutic agents used in the treatment of metastatic adrenal carcinoma include doxorubicin hydrochloride, cisplatin, etoposide, paclitaxel, 5-fluorouracil, vincristine sulfate, cyclophosphamide, and suramin sodium. Several series have shown that systemic chemotherapy is not very effective when given at stage IV; however, several factors complicate the comparison of treatment outcomes. These include a relatively small number of patients per series, variability of treatment between and within series, lack of definition of the extent of disease at the time of treatment, and variable grades of malignancy. Some series include patients with low-grade malignancy as well as patients with high-grade malignancy. Further studies that complicate comparisons between treatments are the lack of a uniform definition of response, the duration of response is not being always clearly stated, the fact that patients within a series frequently receive multiple drugs in a variable sequence, and the occasional combination of radiotherapy with chemotherapy *(3)*.

Treatment of Hormone Excess

Hypersecretion of hormonal steroids in ACC frequently contributes to the disease burden and can severely affect quality of life. In particular, CS often induces hypokalemia, muscle wasting, osteoporotic fractures, and infectious complications. Due to its slow onset of action and its dose-limiting toxicity, mitotane treatment alone is frequently insufficient to rapidly control hypersecretion in all patients. Adrenostatic drugs like ketoconazole, metyrapone, aminoglutethimide, and etomidate have been successfully used to block steroidogenic enzymes and to lower circulating cortisol levels into the normal range *(84)* (seeChap.13).

Some of these drugs also possess antiproliferative activity in vitro *(83)*, and occasional tumor responses has been reported *(85)*. Ketoconazole (400–1,200 mg/day) is most often used and can be combined with mitotane, in which case liver enzymes should be frequently monitored due to ketoconazole hepatotoxicity.

Intravenous etomidate (e.g., 80 mg/day as continuous infusion) potently reduces circulating cortisol levels and can be used in emergencies (e.g., glucocorticoid-induced psychosis) *(84, 86)*. Close monitoring by is mandatory to keep cortisol in the target range and to avoid adrenal insufficiency with use of all adrenostatic drugs. Patients on mitotane with hypokalemia may be treated preferentially with amiloride, as the use of spironolactone may impair the antitumor activity of mitotane *(87)*.

FUTURE DIRECTIONS

The prognosis of patients with adrenal cortical carcinoma is poor, but the life expectancy of these patients can be significantly increased by surgical proceed in stages I, II, and by oncologic surgical resection and mitotane in stage III. For patients presenting at stage IV, a combination of surgical procedures and systemic cytotoxic chemotherapy may be the best option. There are individual cases in which curative resection has been possible and others in which metastatic lesions have regressed on chemotherapy. Early diagnosis is possible in patients with functioning neoplasms, in whom the metabolic manifestations of hormone excess can lead to the discovery of tumors in stages I and II. In contrast, the prognosis of patients in stage IV is dismal. The difficulty in assessing the effectiveness of published treatment protocols stems from the fact that most series are limited in the number of patients studied. There is great variability in the drugs used, the stage and extent of the tumor, and the grade of malignancy. Because adrenal cancer is rare, collaborative, worldwide, multicenter controlled studies will be necessary in order to reach consensus on the efficacy and safety of treatment protocols. More effective therapy is needed for ACC, and it is likely to be achieved once there is a better understanding of tumor biology, including the tumorigenic processes that induce early mutations and that drive progression with growth and dissemination of an established tumor. The identification of specific gene mutations in ACC may be helpful in determining not only the diagnosis, but also the malignant grade and prognosis of these patients individually, based on blocking or reversing the biologic mechanisms of tumorigenesis. The First International Randomized Trial in Locally Advanced and Metastatic Adrenocortical Carcinoma Treatment (FIRM-ACT) is currently under way to compare the results of the two treatments as proposed at the Ann Arbor International Consensus Conference on ACC (2008), etoposide, doxorubicin, and cisplatin in combination with mitotane or streptozotocin plus mitotane. To date, about 190 patients (of a total of 300 planned) have been enrolled *(3)*. New researches concerning ACC treatment have demonstrated that the selective IGF-IR kinase inhibitor had antitumor effects in adult and pediatric adrenocortical tumor cell lines, suggesting that IGF-IR inhibitors represent a promising therapy for human adrenocortical carcinoma *(88, 89)*. Because adrenal cancer is rare, collaborative worldwide multicenter controlled studies will be necessary in order to reach consensus on the efficacy and safety of treatment protocols.

REFERENCES

1. Newell-Price J, Bertagna X, Grossman AB, Nieman LK. Cushing's syndrome. Lancet 2006;367:1605–1617.
2. Stratakis CA, Kirschner LS. Clinical and genetic analysis of primary bilateral adrenal diseases (micro- and macronodular disease) leading to Cushing syndrome. Horm Metab Res 1998;30:456–463.
3. Allolio B, Fassnacht M. Clinical review: adrenocortical carcinoma: clinical update. J Clin Endocrinol Metab 2006;91: 2027–2037.
4. Pinto EM, Billerbeck AE, Fragoso MC, Mendonca BB, Latronico AC. Deletion mapping of chromosome 17 in benign and malignant adrenocortical tumors associated with the Arg337His mutation of the p53 tumor suppressor protein. J Clin Endocrinol Metab 2005;90:2976–2981.
5. Michalkiewicz E, Sandrini R, Figueiredo B, et al. Clinical and outcome characteristics of children with adrenocortical tumors: a report from the International Pediatric Adrenocortical Tumor Registry. J Clin Oncol 2004;22:838–845.
6. Ng L, Libertino JM. Adrenocortical carcinoma: diagnosis, evaluation and treatment. J Urol 2003;169:5–11.
7. Latronico AC, Chrousos GP. Neoplasms of the adrenal cortex. Clinical and basic aspects. Cancer Treat Res 1997;89:217–237.
8. Barzilay JI, Pazianos AG. Adrenocortical carcinoma. Urol Clin North Am 1989;16:457–468.
9. Luton JP, Cerdas S, Billaud L, et al. Clinical features of adrenocortical carcinoma, prognostic factors, and the effect of mitotane therapy. N Engl J Med 1990;322:1195–1201.
10. Wooten MD, King DK. Adrenal cortical carcinoma. Epidemiology and treatment with mitotane and a review of the literature. Cancer 1993;72:3145–3155.
11. Tabarin A, Bardet S, Bertherat J, et al. Exploration and management of adrenal incidentalomas. French Society of Endocrinology Consensus. Ann Endocrinol (Paris) 2008;69:487–500.
12. Mantero F, Terzolo M, Arnaldi G, et al. A survey on adrenal incidentaloma in Italy. Study Group on Adrenal Tumors of the Italian Society of Endocrinology. J Clin Endocrinol Metab 2000;85:637–644.
13. Mendonca BB, Lucon AM, Menezes CA, et al. Clinical, hormonal and pathological findings in a comparative study of adrenocortical neoplasms in childhood and adulthood. J Urol 1995;154:2004–2009.
14. Wajchenberg BL, Albergaria Pereira MA, Medonca BB, et al. Adrenocortical carcinoma: clinical and laboratory observations. Cancer 2000;88:711–736.
15. Pereira RM, Michalkiewicz E, Sandrini F, et al. [Childhood adrenocortical tumors]. Arq Bras Endocrinol Metabol 2004;48:651–658.
16. Wieneke JA, Thompson LD, Heffess CS. Adrenal cortical neoplasms in the pediatric population: a clinicopathologic and immunophenotypic analysis of 83 patients. Am J Surg Pathol 2003;27:867–881.
17. Sandrini R, Ribeiro RC, DeLacerda L. Childhood adrenocortical tumors. J Clin Endocrinol Metab 1997;82:2027–2031.
18. Fukai N, Hirono Y, Yoshimoto T, et al. A case of estrogen-secreting adrenocortical carcinoma with subclinical Cushing's syndrome. Endocr J 2006;53:237–245.
19. Moreno S, Guillermo M, Decoulx M, Dewailly D, Bresson R, Proye C. Feminizing adreno-cortical carcinomas in male adults. A dire prognosis. Three cases in a series of 801 adrenalectomies and review of the literature. Ann Endocrinol (Paris) 2006;67:32–38.
20. Ribeiro RC, Michalkiewicz EL, Figueiredo BC, et al. Adrenocortical tumors in children. Braz J Med Biol Res 2000;33: 1225–1234.
21. Abiven G, Coste J, Groussin L, et al. Clinical and biological features in the prognosis of adrenocortical cancer: poor outcome of cortisol-secreting tumors in a series of 202 consecutive patients. J Clin Endocrinol Metab 2006;91:2650–2655.
22. Findling JW, Raff H, Aron DC. The low-dose dexamethasone suppression test: a reevaluation in patients with Cushing's syndrome. J Clin Endocrinol Metab 2004;89:1222–1226.
23. Luton JP, Martinez M, Coste J, Bertherat J. Outcome in patients with adrenal incidentaloma selected for surgery: an analysis of 88 cases investigated in a single clinical center. Eur J Endocrinol 2000;143:111–117.
24. Lin MT, Shieh JJ, Chang JH, Chang SW, Chen TC, Hsu WH. Early detection of adrenocortical carcinoma in a child with Li–Fraumeni syndrome. Pediatr Blood Cancer 2009;52:541–544.
25. Kebebew E, Reiff E, Duh QY, Clark OH, McMillan A. Extent of disease at presentation and outcome for adrenocortical carcinoma: have we made progress? World J Surg 2006;30:872–878.
26. Koch CA, Pacak K, Chrousos GP. The molecular pathogenesis of hereditary and sporadic adrenocortical and adrenomedullary tumors. J Clin Endocrinol Metab 2002;87:5367–5384.

27. Libe R, Bertherat J. Molecular genetics of adrenocortical tumours, from familial to sporadic diseases. Eur J Endocrinol 2005;153:477–487.
28. Allolio B, Hahner S, Weismann D, Fassnacht M. Management of adrenocortical carcinoma. Clin Endocrinol (Oxf) 2004;60:273–287.
29. Morioka M, Tanaka H, Ohashi Y, Jin TX, Watanabe H, Furihata M. Nonfunctioning adrenal cortical cancer and analysis of the steroidogenic activity of the tumor: a case report. Int J Urol 1998;5:170–173.
30. Fragoso MC, Kohek MB, Martin RM, et al. An inhibin B and estrogen-secreting adrenocortical carcinoma leading to selective FSH suppression. Horm Res 2007;67:7–11.
31. Kikuchi E, Yanaihara H, Nakashima J, et al. Urinary steroid profile in adrenocortical tumors. Biomed Pharmacother 2000;54(Suppl 1):194s–197s.
32. Patalano A, Brancato V, Mantero F. Adrenocortical cancer treatment. Horm Res 2009;71(Suppl 1):99–104.
33. Terzolo M, Ali A, Osella G, Mazza E. Prevalence of adrenal carcinoma among incidentally discovered adrenal masses. A retrospective study from 1989 to 1994. Gruppo Piemontese Incidentalomi Surrenalici. Arch Surg 1997;132:914–919.
34. Yoh T, Hosono M, Komeya Y, et al. Quantitative evaluation of norcholesterol scintigraphy, CT attenuation value, and chemical-shift MR imaging for characterizing adrenal adenomas. Ann Nucl Med 2008;22:513–519.
35. Rockall AG, Babar SA, Sohaib SA, et al. CT and MR imaging of the adrenal glands in ACTH-independent Cushing syndrome. Radiographics 2004;24:435–452.
36. Dunnick NR, Korobkin M. Imaging of adrenal incidentalomas: current status. AJR Am J Roentgenol 2002;179:559–568.
37. Fagour C, Bardet S, Rohmer V, et al. Usefulness of adrenal scintigraphy in the follow-up of adrenocortical incidentalomas: a prospective multicenter study. Eur J Endocrinol 2009;160:257–264.
38. Gross MD, Avram A, Fig LM, Rubello D. Contemporary adrenal scintigraphy. Eur J Nucl Med Mol Imaging 2007;34: 547–557.
39. Gross MD, Avram A, Fig LM, Fanti S, Al-Nahhas A, Rubello D. PET in the diagnostic evaluation of adrenal tumors. Q J Nucl Med Mol Imaging 2007;51:272–283.
40. Leboulleux S, Dromain C, Bonniaud G, et al. Diagnostic and prognostic value of 18-fluorodeoxyglucose positron emission tomography in adrenocortical carcinoma: a prospective comparison with computed tomography. J Clin Endocrinol Metab 2006;91:920–925.
41. Mackie GC, Shulkin BL, Ribeiro RC, et al. Use of [18F]fluorodeoxyglucose positron emission tomography in evaluating locally recurrent and metastatic adrenocortical carcinoma. J Clin Endocrinol Metab 2006;91:2665–2671.
42. Hennings J, Lindhe O, Bergstrom M, Langstrom B, Sundin A, Hellman P. [11C]metomidate positron emission tomography of adrenocortical tumors in correlation with histopathological findings. J Clin Endocrinol Metab 2006;91:1410–1414.
43. Libe R, Fratticci A, Bertherat J. Adrenocortical cancer: pathophysiology and clinical management. Endocr Relat Cancer 2007;14:13–28.
44. Weiss, LM. Comparative histologic study of 43 metastasizing and nonmetastasizing adrenocortical tumors. Am J Surg Pathol 1984 8(3):163–169.
45. Weiss, LM, Medeiros LJ, Vickery AL, Jr. Pathologic features of prognostic significance in adrenocortical carcinoma. Am J Surg Pathol 1989;13(3):202–206.
46. Saeger W. Histopathological classification of adrenal tumours. Eur J Clin Invest 2000;30(Suppl 3):58–62.
47. Morimoto R, Satoh F, Murakami O, et al. Immunohistochemistry of a proliferation marker Ki67/MIB1 in adrenocortical carcinomas: Ki67/MIB1 labeling index is a predictor for recurrence of adrenocortical carcinomas. Endocr J 2008;55:49–55.
48. Stojadinovic A, Brennan MF, Hoos A, et al. Adrenocortical adenoma and carcinoma: histopathological and molecular comparative analysis. Mod Pathol 2003;16:742–751.
49. Tissier F, Louvel A, Grabar S, et al. Cyclin E correlates with malignancy and adverse prognosis in adrenocortical tumors. Eur J Endocrinol 2004;150:809–817.
50. Macfarlane DA. Cancer of the adrenal cortex: the natural history, prognosis and treatment in a study of fifty-five cases. Ann R C Surg Engl 1958;23:155–186.
51. Fassnacht, M. Limited prognostic value of the 2004 International Union Against Cancer staging classification for adrenocortical carcinoma: proposal for a revised TNM Classification. Cancer 2009;115(2):243–250.
52. Sullivan M. Adrenal cortical carcinoma. J Urol 1978;120:660–665.
53. Icard P, Louvel A, Chapuis Y. Survival rates and prognostic factors in adrenocortical carcinoma. World J Surg 1992;16:753–758.
54. Lee JE, Berger DH, el-Naggar AK, et al. Surgical management, DNA content, and patient survival in adrenal cortical carcinoma. Surgery 1995;118:1090–1098.

55. DeLellis RA, Lloyd RV, Heitz PU, Eng C. eds World Health Organization: Pathology and Genetics of Tumors of Endocrine Organs. France, IARC 2004.
56. Icard P, Goudet P, Charpenay C, et al. Adrenocortical carcinomas: surgical trends and results of a 253-patient series from the French Association of Endocrine Surgeons study group. World J Surg 2001;25:891–897.
57. Kendrick ML, Lloyd R, Erickson L, et al. Adrenocortical carcinoma: surgical progress or status quo? Arch Surg 2001;136:543–549.
58. Assie G, Antoni G, Tissier F, et al. Prognostic parameters of metastatic adrenocortical carcinoma. J Clin Endocrinol Metab 2007;92:148–154.
59. Dackiw AP, Lee JE, Gagel RF, Evans DB. Adrenal cortical carcinoma. World J Surg 2001;25:914–926.
60. Khorram-Manesh A, Ahlman H, Jansson S, et al. Adrenocortical carcinoma: surgery and mitotane for treatment and steroid profiles for follow-up. World J Surg 1998;22:605–611; discussion 11–12.
61. Zografos GC, Driscoll D, Karakousis C, Rao U, Huben R. Staging and grading in the survival of adrenal carcinomas. Eur J Surg Oncol 1994;20:449–453.
62. Zografos GC, Driscoll DL, Karakousis CP, Huben RP. Adrenal adenocarcinoma: a review of 53 cases. J Surg Oncol 1994;55:160–164.
63. Jensen JC, Pass HI, Sindelar WF, Norton JA. Recurrent or metastatic disease in select patients with adrenocortical carcinoma. Aggressive resection vs chemotherapy. Arch Surg 1991;126:457–461.
64. Saunders BD, Doherty GM. Laparoscopic adrenalectomy for malignant disease. Lancet Oncol 2004;5:718–726.
65. Iino K, Oki Y, Sasano H. A case of adrenocortical carcinoma associated with recurrence after laparoscopic surgery. Clin Endocrinol (Oxf) 2000;53:243–248.
66. Cobb WS, Kercher KW, Sing RF, Heniford BT. Laparoscopic adrenalectomy for malignancy. Am J Surg 2005;189:405–411.
67. Gonzalez RJ, Shapiro S, Sarlis N, et al. Laparoscopic resection of adrenal cortical carcinoma: a cautionary note. Surgery 2005;138:1078–1085; discussion 85–86.
68. Bellantone R, Ferrante A, Boscherini M, et al. Role of reoperation in recurrence of adrenal cortical carcinoma: results from 188 cases collected in the Italian National Registry for Adrenal Cortical Carcinoma. Surgery 1997;122:1212–1218.
69. Schulick RD, Brennan MF. Long-term survival after complete resection and repeat resection in patients with adrenocortical carcinoma. Ann Surg Oncol 1999;6:719–726.
70. Ohwada S, Izumi M, Kawate S, et al. Surgical outcome of stage III and IV adrenocortical carcinoma. Jpn J Clin Oncol 2007;37:108–113.
71. Wood BJ, Abraham J, Hvizda JL, Alexander HR, Fojo T. Radiofrequency ablation of adrenal tumors and adrenocortical carcinoma metastases. Cancer 2003;97:554–560.
72. Markoe AM, Serber W, Micaily B, Brady LW. Radiation therapy for adjunctive treatment of adrenal cortical carcinoma. Am J Clin Oncol 1991;14:170–174.
73. Didolkar MS, Bescher RA, Elias EG, Moore RH. Natural history of adrenal cortical carcinoma: a clinicopathologic study of 42 patients. Cancer 1981;47:2153–2161.
74. Schteingart DE. Conventional and novel strategies in the treatment of adrenocortical cancer. Braz J Med Biol Res 2000;33:1197–1200.
75. Terzolo M, Angeli A, Fassnacht M, et al. Adjuvant mitotane treatment for adrenocortical carcinoma. N Engl J Med 2007;356:2372–2380.
76. Bertherat J, Coste J, Bertagna X. Adjuvant mitotane in a-drenocortical carcinoma. N Engl J Med 2007;357:1256–1257; author reply 9.
77. Ahlman H, Khorram-Manesh A, Jansson S, et al. Cytotoxic treatment of adrenocortical carcinoma. World J Surg 2001;25:927–933.
78. Baudin E, Pellegriti G, Bonnay M, et al. Impact of monitoring plasma 1,1-dichlorodiphenildichloroethane (o,p'DDD) levels on the treatment of patients with adrenocortical carcinoma. Cancer 2001;92:1385–1392.
79. Terzolo M, Pia A, Berruti A, et al. Low-dose monitored mitotane treatment achieves the therapeutic range with manageable side effects in patients with adrenocortical cancer. J Clin Endocrinol Metab 2000;85:2234–2238.
80. Kasperlik-Zaluska AA. Clinical results of the use of mitotane for adrenocortical carcinoma. Braz J Med Biol Res 2000;33:1191–1196.
81. Neuman O, Bruckert E, Chadarevian R, Jacob N, Turpin G. [Hepatotoxicity of a synthetic cortisol antagonist: OP'DDD (mitotane)]. Therapie 2001;56:793–797.
82. Haak HR, Caekebeke-Peerlinck KM, van Seters AP, Briet E. Prolonged bleeding time due to mitotane therapy. Eur J Cancer 1991;27:638–641.

83. van Seters AP, Moolenaar AJ. Mitotane increases the blood levels of hormone-binding proteins. Acta Endocrinol (Copenh) 1991;124:526–533.
84. Miller JW, Crapo L. The medical treatment of Cushing's syndrome. Endocr Rev 1993;14:443–458.
85. Fassnacht M, Hahner S, Beuschlein F, Klink A, Reincke M, Allolio B. New mechanisms of adrenostatic compounds in a human adrenocortical cancer cell line. Eur J Clin Invest 2000;30(Suppl 3):76–82, 84.
86. Allolio B, Schulte HM, Kaulen D, Reincke M, Jaursch-Hancke C, Winkelmann W. Nonhypnotic low-dose etomidate for rapid correction of hypercortisolaemia in Cushing's syndrome. Klin Wochenschr 1988;66:361–364.
87. Wortsman J, Soler NG. Mitotane. Spironolactone antagonism in Cushing's syndrome. JAMA 1977;238:2527.
88. Almeida MQ, Fragoso MC, Lotfi CF, Santos MG, Nishi MY, Costa MH, Lerario AM, Maciel CC, Mattos GE, Jorge AA, Mendonca BB, Latronico AC Expression of insulin-like growth factor-II and its receptor in pediatric and adult adrenocortical tumors. J Clin Endocrinol Metab 2008;93(9):3524–3531.
89. Barlaskar FM, Spalding AC, Heaton JH, Kuick R, Kim AC, Thomas DG, Giordano TJ, Ben-Josef E, Hammer GD. Preclinical targeting of the type I insulin-like growth factor receptor in adrenocortical carcinoma. J Clin Endocrinol Metab 2009;94(1):204–212.

17 ACTH-Independent Cushing's Syndrome: Bilateral Macronodular Hyperplasia

Isabelle Bourdeau, Antoine Lampron, Tânia Longo Mazzuco, and André Lacroix

CONTENTS

SUMMARY

ACTH-independent macronodular adrenal hyperplasia (AIMAH) is an infrequent cause of Cushing's syndrome. AIMAH presents as incidental radiological finding or with subclinical or overt Cushing's syndrome, occasionally with secretion of mineralocorticoids or sex steroids. The pathophysiology of this entity is heterogeneous. The aberrant adrenal expression and function of one or several G-protein coupled receptors can lead to cell proliferation and abnormal regulation of steroidogenesis. In familial cases of AIMAH, specific aberrant hormone receptors may be functional in the adrenal of affected members. Somatic genetic events related to cell cycle regulation, adhesion, and transcription factors occur in addition in the various nodules. Other mechanisms such as Gsp or ACTH receptor mutations and paracrine adrenal hormonal secretions have been rarely identified in other cases of AIMAH. The identification of aberrant receptors can offer specific pharmacological approach to prevent disease progression and control abnormal steroidogenesis alternatively to the usual unilateral or bilateral adrenalectomy.

Key Words: ACTH-independent macronodular adrenal hyperplasia (AIMAH), aberrant adrenal G-protein coupled receptors, Cushing's syndrome

From: *Contemporary Endocrinology: Cushing's Syndrome: Pathophysiology, Diagnosis and Treatment*
Edited by: M.D. Bronstein (ed.), DOI 10.1007/978-1-60327-449-4_17,

INTRODUCTION

ACTH-independent macronodular adrenal hyperplasia (AIMAH) represents less than 1% of endogenous Cushing's syndrome (CS); however, as 10% of incidentally found adrenal lesions are bilateral, AIMAH with subclinical cortisol secretion is increasingly recognized *(1)*. AIMAH was first described in 1964 *(2)* and 30 years later, only 24 similar cases had been published *(3)*. A variety of terms have been used to report larger number of cases including "massive macronodular adrenocortical disease," "autonomous macronodular adrenal hyperplasia," "ACTH-independent massive bilateral adrenal disease," "giant or huge macronodular adrenal hyperplasia," and "macronodular adrenal dysplasia" *(4–7)*.

The AIMAH should not be confused with bilateral diffuse nodular adrenals following chronic stimulation by ACTH in Cushing's disease or ectopic ACTH secretion; this can rarely generate relatively autonomous nodules that secrete sufficient cortisol to partially suppress ACTH *(8)*.

EPIDEMIOLOGY

The AIMAH presents a bimodal age distribution, with a rare subset presenting in the first years of life particularly with the McCune–Albright syndrome (MAS) *(9)*. Most AIMAH patients present in the fifth and sixth decades, a later age of onset compared with unilateral adenomas, primary pigmented nodular adrenocortical disease (PPNAD), or Cushing's disease *(3, 4, 8, 10)*. In contrast to the predominant female distribution in most cases of CS, AIMAH is equally distributed between genders *(1, 3, 4, 7)*. One report suggested an increased frequency in males *(11)*, while an increased occurrence of gastric inhibitory polypetide (GIP)-dependent AIMAH was found in women *(1)*.

GENETIC CAUSES OF AIMAH

In the majority of cases, AIMAH appeared to be sporadic. Several reports of familial clustering have been published suggesting an autosomal dominant pattern of transmission *(12–19)*. The prevalence of familial forms of AIMAH is not known yet, as systematic familial screening was not conducted. In recently studied families with AIMAH, aberrant hormone receptors have been identified in their adrenal tissues (see later section), but the genes implicated have not been identified yet *(12–14, 18)*. Bilateral adrenal enlargement was found in up to 21% of MEN 1 patients, but no sporadic somatic mutation of the *Menin* gene have been identified in adrenocortical tissue in AIMAH *(20, 21)*. Bilateral adrenal nodules have also been found in patients with familial adenomatous polyposis, but a somatic point mutation of the adenomatous polyposis coli (*APC* gene) was not found *(22, 23)*. In one report, AIMAH was identified in a patient with hereditary leiomyomatosis and renal cell cancer disorder due to a mutation in the fumarate hydratase gene (*FH*) *(24)*.

CLINICAL AND LABORATORY FEATURES

Patients with AIMAH are identified either following an incidental radiological finding or the investigation of an adrenal oversecretion syndrome *(1, 3–7, 25–27)*. The most common clinical presentation is subclinical, followed by clinical CS, which may be present for a number of years. In one series, the diagnosis of CS was delayed by a mean of 7.8 years *(5)*. Plasma ACTH becomes progressively suppressed when cortisol production becomes elevated; when ACTH is fully suppressed, dexamethasone administration fails to suppress cortisol production *(3, 5, 25, 26, 28)*. The occurrence of subclinical CS is defined as the absence of clinical signs of CS, slightly elevated midnight plasma or salivary cortisol, subnormal suppression following the 1-mg overnight dexamethasone suppression test (>50 nmol/L or >1.8 μg/dL), a partially suppressed ACTH, and normal 24-h urinary free cortisol production *(27)*. In cases with subclinical CS, ACTH can be incompletely suppressed and increase following administration of CRH *(25, 26, 28)*. The natural history of AIMAH causing subclinical CS is largely unknown. Ohashi et al. *(28)* reported a 7-year follow-up during which a patient with subclinical CS developed overt CS. Concurrent secretion of cortisol and mineralocorticoids *(26, 29)*, estrone *(30)*, or pure androgen production have been described in patients with AIMAH *(31)*.

Although adrenal proliferation in AIMAH occurs in the absence of ACTH, its melanocortin-2 receptor (*MC2R*) is still expressed, albeit at lower level than in normal adrenal gland *(32)*. Patients with AIMAH respond to ACTH with large increase of cortisol that helps to distinguish it from other causes of bilaterally enlarged adrenals such as metastatic or infiltrative diseases *(33)*. The hormone secretion in AIMAH results from an increase in the number of adrenocortical cells rather than an augmented synthesis per cell. There is a relatively inefficient hormonal synthesis in AIMAH with decreased expression of several steroidogenic enzymes and higher levels of certain precursors such as plasma 17-OH-progesterone or urinary 17-OH corticosteroids *(25, 34)*. This was confirmed by various immunohistochemical steroidogenic enzymes studies *(11, 32, 34, 35)*. This inefficient steroidogenesis may explain the discrepancy between some subclinical cortisol hypersecretion despite massive adrenal enlargement.

IMAGING IN AIMAH

On CT scan, bilateral adrenal nodules measuring up to 5 cm, of soft tissue density, distort the normal adrenal glands *(6, 36, 37)*. In some cases, the adrenal glands appear diffusely enlarged but lack distinct nodules (Fig. 1). On MRI, T1-weighted images are hypointense relative to the liver and

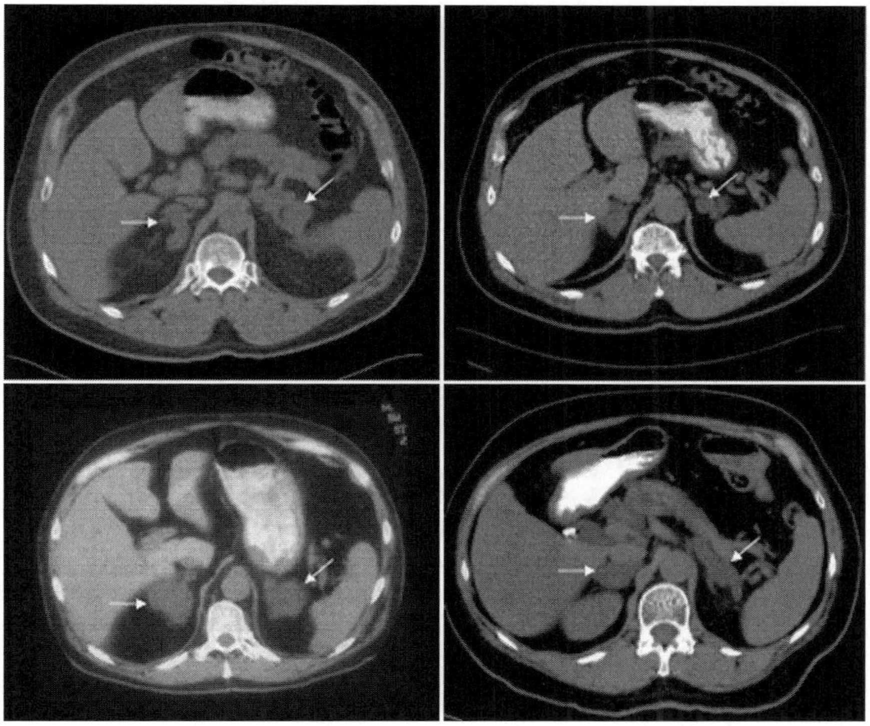

Fig. 1. CT scan from three patients with AIMAH and Cushing's syndrome. The *left* and *right upper panels* are from the same patient and illustrate the variable nature of nodular hyperplasia of both adrenals on sequential slices of CT scan. The *white arrows* are pointed towards the adrenal glands.

isointense relative to muscle. T2-weighted images tend to be hyperintense relative to the liver *(36, 37)*. In contrast, the nodules of patients with chronic ACTH stimulation appear isointense relative to the liver on T2-weighted MR images *(6, 36, 37)*. Occasionally, there is an asymmetric development of nodules in AIMAH, leading to the erroneous diagnosis of unilateral disease *(38)*. Iodine 131–6-β-iodomethyl-19-norcholesterol (NP-59) scintigraphy usually shows bilateral uptake *(6)*.

PATHOLOGY

The combined adrenal weight is usually above 60 g and can reach 200 g per gland. The mean combined weight in one series was 132 g *(36)*. In patients with Cushing's disease, it was 22.9 g in a series of 30 patients *(39)*. On cut sections, the nodules are yellow due to their high lipid content *(11)*. The nodules are composed of two cell types either with clear cytoplasm (lipid rich) that form cordon nest-like structures or with compact cytoplasm (lipid poor) that form nest or island-like structures *(11, 34)*. The status of internodular cortex is controversial in AIMAH; diffuse hyperplasia is present in several cases while internodular atrophy has been described in other cases *(9, 11, 35, 40)*. The AIMAH is a benign process that has never been shown to acquire a malignant potential or to metastasize.

PATHOPHYSIOLOGY OF AIMAH

Evidence for a primary adrenal alteration was provided by initial in vitro cell cultures from AIMAH tissues with a high rate of growth and cortisol production *(41)*. Constitutive ACTH receptor (*MC2R*) mutations is not a common cause of adrenal hyperplasia or tumor formation *(42, 43)*. In one patient with AIMAH, a C-terminal *MC2R* mutation (F278C) led to impaired desensitization and internalization of the receptor and elevated basal camp *(44)*. In a patient with hypersensitivity to ACTH, two mutations (C21R or S247G) were found in the same *MC2R* allele; a single mutation produced an inactive receptor but combined mutations led to constitutive receptor activity *(45)*.

In the MAS, activating mutations of the Gsα subunit occur in a mosaic pattern in the adrenal during early embryogenesis resulting in constitutive activation of the cAMP pathway *(46)*. The association of MAS with bilateral nodular adrenal hyperplasia and CS has been described *(9, 46–50)*. Two different *gsp* mutations at codon Arg^{201} were found in adrenal tissues of three of five patients with CS due to AIMAH and who exhibited no signs of the MAS *(51)*.

Aberrant Hormone Adrenal Receptors in Adrenal CS

The mechanism by which cortisol production is stimulated in AIMAH despite suppressed ACTH was previously unknown and referred to as an "autonomous" process. Work by several groups has demonstrated that cortisol secretion in most patients with AIMAH and a large proportion of unilateral adrenal adenomas with clinical or subclinical CS are regulated by hormones other than ACTH via the aberrant expression of several membrane-bound hormone receptors *(1, 25, 33, 52–54)*. The aberrant stimulation of steroidogenesis can be driven by the expression of ectopic receptors such as those for glucose-dependent insulinotropic peptide (GIPR), catecholamines (β-adrenergic receptors, vasopressin (V_2-V_3-vasopressin receptor), serotonin (5-HT_7 receptor), and probably angiotensin II receptor (AT1R) and glucagon. It can also result from increased expression or altered activity of eutopic receptors such as those for vasopressin (V_1-vasopressin receptor), luteinizing hormone/human chorionic gonadotropin (LH/hCGR), serotonin (5-HT_4 receptor), and leptin receptor *(1, 25, 33, 52–54)*. Analysis of the second messengers involved indicates that these aberrant G-protein coupled receptors (GPCRs) regulate steroidogenesis by mimicking the cellular events that are triggered normally by ACTH receptor (Fig. 2) *(1, 25, 33, 52–54)*.

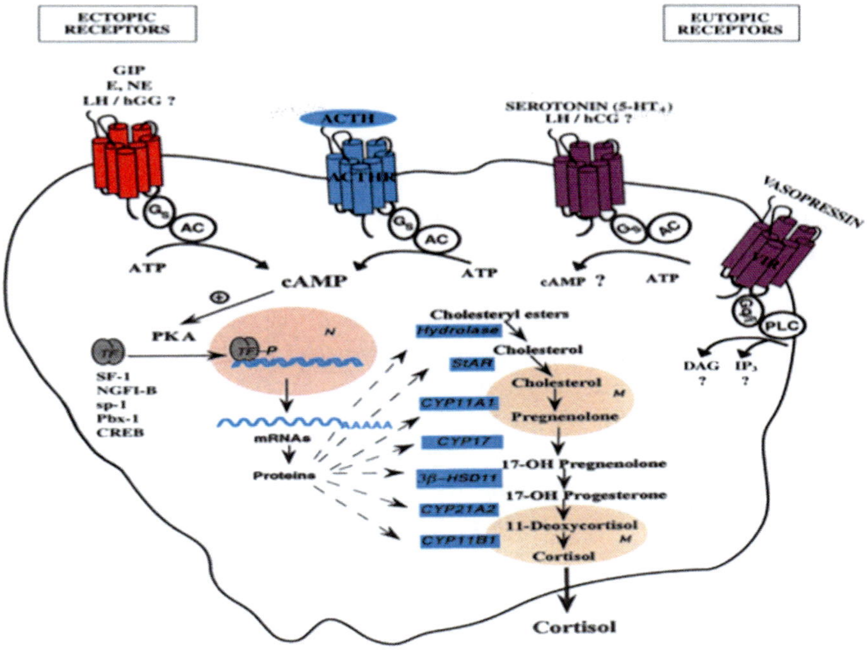

Fig. 2. Regulation of steroidogenesis by aberrant hormone receptors in adrenal cortex. In this model, the ectopic or eutopic receptors regulate steroidogenesis by mimicking the cellular events triggered by ACTH receptors activation. Reproduced with permission from *Trends Endocrinol Metab*, 2004 *(54)*.

GIP-Dependent AIMAH

GIP-dependent CS can occur in patients with AIMAH *(1, 33, 38, 55–59)* and with unilateral adenomas *(1, 38, 57–62)*. Patients with CS can present low fasting plasma cortisol levels, which increase following meals, despite suppression of ACTH. Cortisol increased following physiological increase in plasma level of GIP after meals, as a result of the ectopic expression of nonmutated GIP receptor in zona fasciculata-type cells in AIMAH or unilateral adenomas. To date, more than 30 such cases have been reported in whom adrenal hormonal hypersecretion including clinical or subclinical CS *(1, 38, 57–62)* or androgen secretion resulting in hirsutism *(63)* was correlated to GIP stimulation. The adrenal nodules in rare patients with GIP-dependent AIMAH can progress asynchronously, first in one adrenal, later in the other *(38)*; the larger nodules were the result of secondary clonal proliferation events in addition to GIP receptor overexpression *(64)*. In some patients there was combined expression of GIP receptor with other receptors such as LH/hCG receptor *(65)*. This may explain why cortisol levels may not always be suppressed during fasting if more than one receptor is functional in the same tissue.

The GIP increases cAMP production and DNA synthesis in GIP-dependent cortisol-secreting tissue suggesting that GIP can be implicated both in steroidogenesis and cellular proliferation *(57)*. The molecular mechanisms involved in the aberrant expression of this receptor remain unclear. It was suggested that chronic stimulation by ACTH could result in increased *GIPR* expression, but other studies did not confirm *GIPR* overexpression in the adrenal glands of patients with Cushing's disease or ectopic ACTH syndrome *(60, 62, 66, 67)*. Interestingly, the expression of the GIP receptor can be detected in the early phases of adrenal hyperplasia *(38, 64)*. The demonstration that bovine adrenal cells transfected with the GIP receptor and injected under the renal capsule in mice leads to the development of hyperplastic adrenals and hypercortisolism further supports the initiation role of the ectopic receptor expression in the pathophysiology of AIMAH *(68)*.

Vasopressin-Responsive CS

A number of patients with either AIMAH or unilateral adenomas with CS and completely suppressed ACTH have been described in whom exogenous vasopressin or physiological stimuli of vasopressin secretion such as upright posture stimulate the secretion of cortisol *(12, 13, 18, 19, 25, 33, 69–76)*. Fluctuations of endogenous physiological levels of vasopressin (water and hypertonic sodium loading) resulted in parallel changes of plasma cortisol levels. The action of vasopressin was mediated via nonmutated V1-vasopressin receptors that are expressed at higher or similar levels compared with controls *(69, 70, 73–75)*. As the V1 receptor is normally expressed in the adrenal cortex and its activation leads to a modest in vitro increase in steroidogenesis, the observed exaggerated steroidogenic response represents an aberrant response of a eutopic receptor. An abnormal adrenal stimulation of cortisol by vasopressin can also occur in patients with subclinical AIMAH *(12, 25)*. The ectopic expression of V2 and V3-vasopressin receptors has been documented in vitro in adrenal tissue from patients with AIMAH; the significance of this finding is unclear, because a cortisol response was not observed when dDAVP, a preferential V2-vasopressin receptor agonist, was administered to some of these patients *(12–18)*.

Catecholamine-Responsive AIMAH

The ectopic expression of β-adrenergic receptors was first reported in vitro in adrenal tumors causing CS *(1)*. In vivo, aberrant responses of cortisol following elevations of endogenous catecholamines induced by upright posture, insulin-induced hypoglycemia, or exercise were documented in patients with AIMAH and CS *(13, 14, 33, 77–79)*. Isoproterenol infusion stimulated cortisol and aldosterone secretion in these patients but failed to do so in normal subjects. Aberrant cortisol responses mediated by β-adrenergic agonists were also found in families with AIMAH and were present in patients with subclinical stages of the disease *(13, 14)*. These aberrant responses were reduced by pretreatment with propranolol, a β-adrenergic antagonist *(14, 77, 79)*. High affinity binding sites compatible with β-1- or β-2-adrenergic receptors were efficiently coupled to steroidogenesis in the adrenal tissues in these patients, but not in controls, indicating the ectopic nature of this receptor *(77, 78)*. The combined presence of adrenal β-adrenergic receptor and V1-vasopressin receptor has been observed in some patients with AIMAH *(13, 33, 78)*.

LH/hCG-Responsive AIMAH

Hypercortisolism due to aberrant LH/hCG receptors was first identified in a woman with transient Cushing's syndrome during sequential pregnancies; persistent Cushing's syndrome and AIMAH developed only after the postmenopausal sustained increase of LH secretion *(80)*. In this patient, cortisol secretion was stimulated by the exogenous administration of GnRH, hCG, or recombinant LH. Administration of the long-acting GnRH agonist, leuprolide acetate, resulted in suppression of endogenous LH and normalization of cortisol production *(80)*. A virilized woman with androgen-secreting AIMAH regulated by hCG was shown to express the LH/hCG receptor in one resected adrenal; suppression of endogenous LH with leuprolide acetate normalized androgen secretion from the contralateral adrenal, avoiding bilateral adrenalectomy *(31)*. Other cases of aberrant receptors for LH/hCG either alone or in combination with serotonin 5HT4 or GIP receptors have been reported *(65, 80, 81)*. The aberrant response to LH/hCG was also found in patients with subclinical production of cortisol and incidentally found AIMAH *(25)*.

Serotonin-Responsive AIMAH

In the normal adrenal gland, 5-HT4 receptor agonists are potent stimulators of aldosterone secretion but only weakly affect cortisol secretion in vitro *(1, 82–84)*. In vivo, they normally do not produce an increase in plasma cortisol *(1, 82–84)*. In the first patient described above with LH/hCG responsive AIMAH, serotonin 5-HT4 receptor agonists, cisapride and metoclopramide, also stimulated plasma cortisol *(80)*. In six cases of CS and AIMAH with aberrant responses to cisapride or metoclopramide, adrenal overexpression of the 5HT-4 receptor was found in the adrenal glands of four of these patients *(82)*. Another patient with cisapride-responsive CS and AIMAH was shown to have adrenal overexpression of the 5-HT4 receptor *(84)*. The aberrant response to 5-HT4R agonists was also found in patients with familial AIMAH, subclinical production of cortisol, and incidentally found AIMAH *(12, 25)*. The ectopic expression of 5-HT-7 receptors has also been demonstrated in a patient with AIMAH and CS *(83)*.

Angiotensin-Responsive AIMAH

Adrenal hypersensitivity to angiotensin II was suggested in a patient with AIMAH and CS in whom a large increase in plasma aldosterone and cortisol was noted during upright posture *(85)*. The short-term oral administration of candesartan, an AT-1 receptor antagonist, eliminated the stimulation of these adrenal hormones. An angiotensin infusion was not performed nor was a trial of long-term pharmacotherapy with an AT-1 receptor blockers attempted. In vitro stimulation of cortisol secretion by angiotensin-II was also found in other patients with AIMAH and CS who had increases in cortisol levels with upright posture, but the presence of the AT-1 receptor has not been studied directly *(65)*.

Other Abnormal Responses in AIMAH

In a patient with AIMAH and CS, GIP and leptin were shown to aberrantly increase cortisol production in vitro *(86)*. In two patients with AIMAH and CS, insulin-induced hypoglycemia stimulated cortisol production while ACTH levels remained undetectable *(87, 88)*; in vitro, adrenal cortisol secretion was not stimulated by insulin, catecholamine, vasopressin, or angiotensin II. An increase in cortisol following in vivo administration of glucagon was found in two patients with CS and unilateral adenoma; glucagon receptor and glucagon were found in the tumor tissue, suggesting combined ectopic receptor and paracrine ligand production *(89)*.

Aberrant Hormone Receptors in Familial Forms of AIMAH

In the familial cases of AIMAH without other diseases, the potential presence of aberrant receptors was evaluated only in the recently studied families. Some aberrant receptors that have been identified so far were as follows: V1-vasopressin and β-adrenergic in one family *(13)*; β-adrenergic in two families *(14, 90)*; V1–V2 and V3-vasopressin in another two families *(18, 19)*, and combined $5HT_4$ and V1–V2-vasopressin in other one *(12)*. A systematic clinical screening of a family with cortisol-secreting β-adrenergic responsive AIMAH revealed unsuspected subclinical CS with aberrant β-adrenergic regulation of cortisol in approximately 50% of the studied members of the kindred *(14)*.

Molecular Mechanisms of Aberrant Hormone Receptors

The development and function of the adrenal cortex requires tissue-specific expression of the appropriate hormone receptors and regulatory mechanisms for these receptors, involving *cis*-acting regulatory elements (promoters) and *trans*-acting factors (transcription factors, co-activators and co-repressors). The GIPR has been the most extensively characterized ectopic receptor in AIMAH. *GIPR* gene sequence analysis did not reveal mutations of coding or putative promoters regions in adrenals of patients with GIP-dependent CS and the analysis of transcription factors (Sp1 and Sp3) necessary to *GIPR* expression also did not show any specific abnormalities *(62, 66, 91)*. Expression profiling of AIMAH using microarrays have been utilized to identify genes and signaling pathways potentially involved in this adrenal disease. In eight AIMAH samples, 82 and 31 genes were found to be consistently up- (those implicating in transcription, cell cycle, and adhesion) and down-regulated (genes involved in immune responses and insulin signaling) compared with normal adrenal glands *(92)*. In another study, the entire transcriptome profile of ten cases of cortisol-producing adrenocortical hyperplasias [half were ACTH dependent (Cushing's disease) and half were GIP dependent] was compared in order to reveal the genes with expression profiles related to the presence of aberrant GIP receptor. A list of 723 probesets was reported, their levels of expression were able to segregate both types of hyperplasias independently. Functional clustering of these probesets identified a number of molecular mechanisms including metabolism-related processes, cellular proliferation, molecular signaling mechanisms, immunity-related genes, and cellular adhesion *(64)*. Both studies reported the presence of a number of probesets related to the WNT pathway of cellular proliferation and adhesion.

It was unclear whether aberrant hormone receptors are a primary phenomenon responsible for the pathogenesis of AIMAH or adenomas, or an epiphenomenon resulting from cell proliferation and dedifferentiation; there are now several evidences in favor of the former hypothesis. The reversal of hyperplasia between pregnancies in LH/hCG-dependent CS favors the first hypothesis *(80)*. The germline transmission of the same aberrant receptors in all affected family members in familial AIMAH is another strong indication in favor of an initiating role of the aberrant receptor *(12, 14, 18)*. The demonstration that bovine adrenocortical cells transfected with the *GIPR* or LH/hCGR and injected under the renal capsule in immunodeficient mice lead to the development of hyperplastic adrenals and hypercortisolism further supports the initiation role of the ectopic receptor in pathophysiology of AIMAH *(68, 93)*.

The presence of aberrant receptors in unilateral lesions could arise from a monoclonal somatic mutation. In patients with AIMAH, the mutation can occur either from germline transmission (familial forms) or somatically at an early stage of embryogenesis to involve both adrenal cortices. Our hypothesis is that the aberrant adrenocortical expression of a receptor is a primary phenomenon which initiates bilateral diffuse hyperplasias and CS. In addition to the initiating effect of aberrant receptor on hyperplasia formation, other somatic genetic events occur in time, as demonstrated by microarray data *(64)*, generating diverse monoclonal nodule formation resulting in the AIMAH phenotype (Fig. 3).

Although *PRKAR1A* mutations were not found in AIMAH, somatic losses of the 17q22–24 region, PKA subunit, and enzymatic activity changes show that PKA signaling is altered in AIMAH in a very similar way to other adrenal tumors *(94)*. Recently, one of the two familial AIMAH cases was a carrier of a variation (R867G) in the gene (*PDE11A*) that codified the phosphodiesterase 11A4 implicated in the regulation of cyclic nucleotide levels *(95)*.

Paracrine Mechanisms in AIMAH

In addition to the aberrant hormone receptors, other paracrine regulatory mechanisms were proposed in some AIMAH cases after the demonstration of increased adrenocortical expression of pro-opiomelanocortin/ACTH, serotonin, vasopressin, or glucagon in some affected adrenal tissues *(65, 74, 83, 89, 96)*.

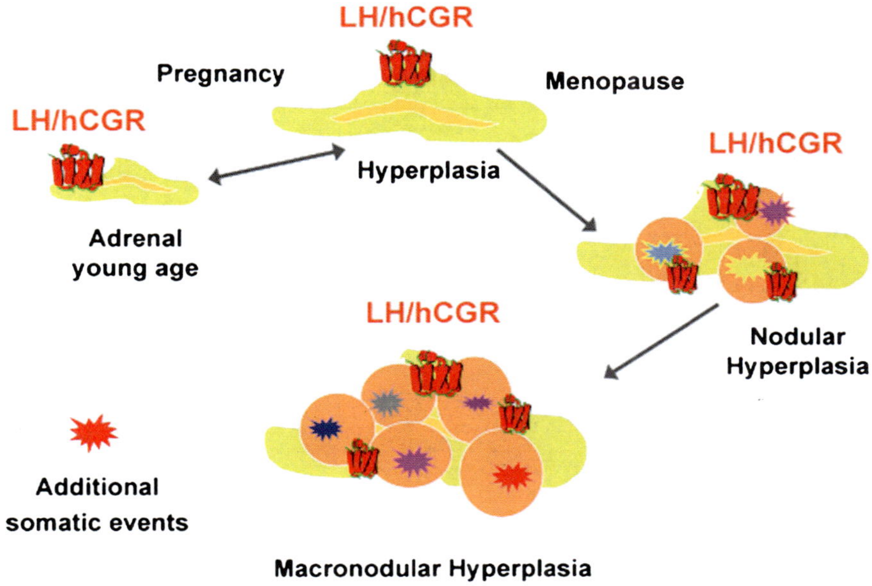

Fig. 3. Hypothesis of sequential genetic events leading to AIMAH. The initial event is the aberrant expression of the LH/hCG receptor in the adrenal cortex during early embryonic life. Upon stimulation of this receptor, as during pregnancy (activation by hCG), diffuse adrenal hyperplasia (polyclonal) and transient CS occurs, but this is still reversible when hCG and LH levels are reduced following delivery. After menopause, the constant elevation of LH causes diffuse hyperplasia and CS. Other (second, third) somatic events occur progressively with time in a small number of cells; the monoclonal proliferation of these cells leads to appearance of several nodules which have maintained the expression of aberrant LH/hCGR. The inhibition of LH levels is able to control the excess production of steroids; this may be able to induce regression of adrenal growth at the stage of hyperplasia, but it may become insufficient to cause tumor regression when other oncogenic events have provided additional growth advantage to these cells. Reproduced with permission from *Trends Endocrinol Metab*, 2004 *(54)*.

Investigation Protocol for Aberrant Receptors

Investigative protocols have been developed to screen patients with adrenal CS to identify the regulation of steroid production by one or several aberrant receptor *(97, 98)*. The strategy consists of modulating the plasma levels of diverse hormone (endogenous or exogenous) ligands for the potential aberrant receptors, while monitoring plasma levels of cortisol, other steroid hormones, and ACTH. All tests are performed following an overnight fast and in a supine position for at least 1 h. For patients with subclinical CS, the studies are conducted under suppression with 1-mg dexamethasone every 6 h, beginning 48 h before the tests in order to avoid any effect of ACTH on steroidogenesis. The initial screening (Table 1) is performed in 3 days and involves during the first day a posture test to screen for receptors to angiotensin II, vasopressin, or catecholamines; a standard mixed meal to assess the presence of GIP or other gastrointestinal hormone receptors; and cosyntropin test (ACTH 250 μg i.v.) *(97)*. During the second day, the administration of GnRH 100 μg i.v. evaluates responses to GnRH, LH, and FSH; TRH 200 μg i.v. screens for modulation by TRH, TSH, or prolactin. On the last day, the protocol is completed with the sequential administration of glucagon 1 mg i.m., vasopressin 10 UI i.m., and 10-mg metoclopramide orally as a serotonin 5-HT_4 agonist. Serial measurements of ACTH, cortisol, and other steroid hormones are performed at 30–60 min intervals during 2–3 h following the intervention. The increment of 25–49% from the baseline of the steroid levels in the absence of an increase in ACTH level is defined as a partial response and an increase more than 50% or greater is considered a positive response; the test should be repeated to confirm the response

Table 1
In Vivo Screening Protocol to Detect the Presence of Aberrant Adrenal Hormone Receptors in Adrenal Cushing's Syndrome

Time (min)	*Day 1*	*Day 2*	*Day 3*
−60	Fasting supine	Fasting supine	Fasting supine
−15	[a]	[a]	[a]
0	Upright[a]	GnRH 100 μg i.v.[a]	Glucagon 1 mg i.v.[a]
+30	Upright[a]	[a]	[a]
+60	Upright[a]	[a]	[a]
+90	Upright[a]	[a]	[a]
+120	Upright[a]	[a]	[a]
+150	Supine[a]	(meal)	
+180	Mixed meal[a]		Vasopressin 10 IU i.m.[a]
+210	[a]		[a]
+240	[a]		[a]
+270	[a]	[a]	[a]
+300	[a]	TRH 200 μg i.v.[a]	[a]
+330		[a]	
+360	ACTH 1–24 250 μg i.v.[a]	[a]	Metoclopramide 10 mg orally[a]
+390	[a]	[a]	[a]
+420	[a]	[a]	[a]
+450	[a]		[a]
+480	[a]		[a]

Modified with permission from the *Endocrinologist* 9:9–15, 1999 *(97)*
[a]Blood samples for determination of cortisol, ACTH, other hormones, and vital signs

to the specific ligand and its reproducibility. Fluctuations of the putative ligand hormones of interest are also measured to better characterize the modulator of the response. When a positive response following this initial screening is confirmed, further stimulatory test should be undertaken to precisely define the hormone and the specific receptor type implicated (Fig. 4).

TREATMENT OF AIMAH

Bilateral adrenalectomy by overt or laparoscopic approach has been the most utilized treatment in patients with AIMAH and hormonal hypersecretion *(3–5, 7)*. However, in patients with moderately increased hormonal production, unilateral adrenalectomy has been proposed as a safe and effective alternative; it is expected that, as the cell mass increases in the contralateral adrenal, a second adrenalectomy may be further necessary *(90, 99, 100)*. In patients with subclinical AIMAH, the decision for therapy should consider the manifestation of cortisol excess, such as hypertension, diabetes, osteoporosis, apparent brain atrophy, or neuropsychological manifestations. Medical treatment with adrenal enzyme inhibitors could be helpful to control cortisol secretion before surgery. AIMAH is a

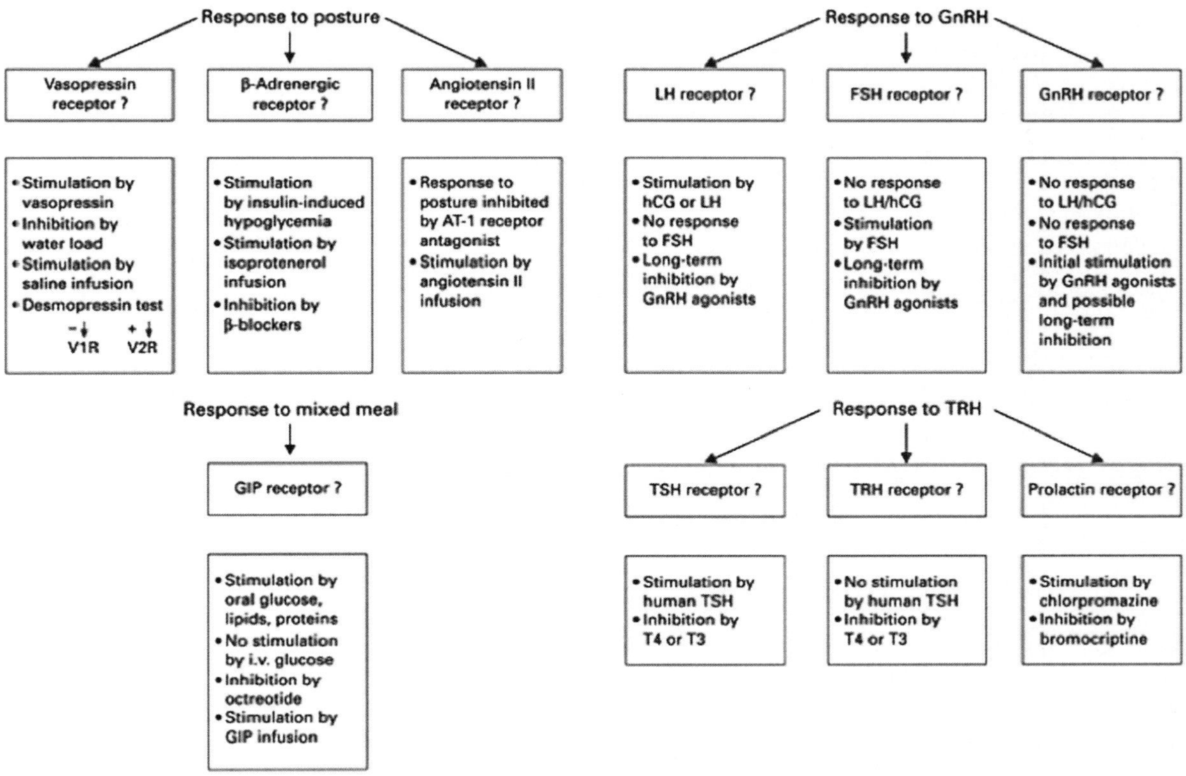

Fig. 4. Further in vivo characterization of aberrant adrenal hormone receptors following the initial screening protocol. Adapted from the *Endocrinologist* 1999 *(97)*.

benign process that has never been shown to become malignant; in subclinical CS with AIMAH, follow-up with annual CT scan and biochemical assessment is sufficient.

The identification of aberrant adrenal hormone receptors in AIMAH provides new opportunities for specific pharmacological therapies as alternative to adrenalectomy (Table 2). Pharmacological blockade of postprandial release of GIP using octreotide led to clinical and biochemical improvement of CS, although the benefit lasted only a few months, probably as the result of eventual desensitization of somatostatin receptors in GIP-secreting duodenal K cells *(56, 101)*. In catecholamine-dependent CS in AIMAH, β-adrenergic receptor antagonists were efficient in the long-term control of hormonal hypersecretion *(14, 77)*. In LH/hCG-dependent AIMAH and CS or androgen excess, suppression of endogenous LH levels with long-acting leuprolide acetate controlled steroid secretion and avoided bilateral adrenalectomy *(56, 101)*. It is possible that tumor regression might not occur, despite complete blockade of the aberrant receptors, because other genetic events (other than aberrant receptors) inducing proliferation can appear over time (Fig. 3) *(54, 64)*.

CONCLUSION

In recent years, several new findings have contributed to a better understanding of the heterogeneity of pathogenesis in AIMAH. Aberrantly expressed GPCRs in the adrenal cortex appear to play a central role in the hormonal hypersecretion and cell proliferation in this disease. However, other

Table 2
Medical Treatment Options for Identified Aberrant Adrenal Hormone Receptors Using an In Vivo Screening Protocol in AIMAH

Aberrant receptor	*In vivo screening protocol*	*Medical treatment options*
GIP receptor	Mixed meal; oral glucose	Octreotide; GIPR antagonist
Vasopressin receptor	Upright posture	VP receptor antagonist
(V1, V2, V3)	Administration of arginine-vasopressin or desmopressin	
β-adrenergic receptor	Upright posture, isoproterenol infusion	β-blockers
LH/hCG receptor	GnRH administration; hCG, recombinant LH	Long-acting GnRH agonist
5-HT4 receptor	Administration of 5-HT4 receptor agonists	5-HT4 receptor antagonist
AT-1 receptor	Upright posture, angiotensin infusion	AT-1 receptor antagonist

molecular mechanisms, as *Gsp* or ACTH receptor mutations, and adrenal paracrine hormonal secretion can also be implicated in this disease. Together, these studies have contributed to a more precise evaluation of patients with AIMAH, improving earlier diagnosis and offering new therapeutic and potentially preventive strategies.

ACKNOWLEDGMENTS

This work was supported by grant MT-13–189 from Canadian Institutes of Health Research.

REFERENCES

1. Lacroix A, N'Diaye N, Tremblay J, et al. Ectopic and abnormal hormone receptors in adrenal Cushing's syndrome. Endocr Rev 2001;22:75–110.
2. Kirschner MA, Powell RD, Jr, Lipsett MB. Cushing's syndrome: Nodular cortical hyperplasia of adrenal glands with clinical and pathological features suggesting adrenocortical tumor. J Clin Endocrinol Metab 1964;24:947–955.
3. Lieberman SA, Eccleshall TR, Feldman D. ACTH-independent massive bilateral adrenal disease (AIMBAD): a subtype of Cushing's syndrome with major diagnostic and therapeutic implications. Eur J Endocrinol 1994;131:67–73.
4. Stratakis CA, Kirschner LS. Clinical and genetic analysis of primary bilateral adrenal diseases (micro- and macronodular disease) leading to Cushing syndrome. Horm Metab Res 1998;30:456–463.
5. Swain JM, Grant CS, Schlinkert RT, et al. Corticotropin-independent macronodular adrenal hyperplasia: a clinicopathologic correlation. Arch Surg 1998;133, 541–545;discussion 545–546.
6. Doppman JL, Chrousos GP, Papanicolaou DA, et al. Adrenocorticotropin-independent macronodular adrenal hyperplasia: an uncommon cause of primary adrenal hypercortisolism. Radiology 2000;216:797–802.
7. Malchoff CD, MacGillivray D, Malchoff DM. Adrenocorticotropic hormone-independent adrenal hyperplasia. Endocrinologist 1996;6:79–85.
8. Newell-Price J, Bertagna X, Grossman AB, et al. Cushing's syndrome. Lancet 2006;367:1605–1617.
9. Kirk JM, Brain CE, Carson DJ, et al. Cushing's syndrome caused by nodular adrenal hyperplasia in children with McCune–Albright syndrome. J Pediatr 1999;134:789–792.
10. Zeiger MA, Nieman LK, Cutler GB, et al. Primary bilateral adrenocortical causes of Cushing's syndrome. Surgery 1991;110:1106–1115.

11. Aiba M, Hirayama A, Iri H, et al. Adrenocorticotropic hormone-independent bilateral adrenocortical macronodular hyperplasia as a distinct subtype of Cushing's syndrome. Enzyme histochemical and ultrastructural study of four cases with a review of the literature. Am J Clin Pathol 1991;96:334–340.
12. Vezzosi D, Cartier D, Regnier C, et al. Familial adrenocorticotropin-independent macronodular adrenal hyperplasia with aberrant serotonin and vasopressin adrenal receptors. Eur J Endocrinol 2007;156:21–31.
13. Miyamura N, Taguchi T, Murata Y, et al. Inherited adrenocorticotropin-independent macronodular adrenal hyperplasia with abnormal cortisol secretion by vasopressin and catecholamines: detection of the aberrant hormone receptors on adrenal gland. Endocrine 2002;19:319–326.
14. Bourdeau I, Boisselle A, Rioux D, et al. Systematic clinical screening of members of a family with hereditary cortisol-secreting B-adrenergic responsive ACTH-Independent Macronodular Adrenal Hyperplasia (AIMAH) reveals unsuspected subclinical Cushing's Syndrome (CS) and aberrant B-adrenergic regulation of cortisol secretion. In: Program of the 89th Annual Meeting of the Endocrine Society, Toronto, CA, 2007: p. 148: Abstract OR154–142.
15. Minami S, Sugihara H, Sato J, et al. ACTH independent Cushing's syndrome occurring in siblings. Clin Endocrinol (Oxf) 1996;44:483–488.
16. Nies C, Bartsch DK, Ehlenz K, et al. Familial ACTH-independent Cushing's syndrome with bilateral macronodular adrenal hyperplasia clinically affecting only female family members. Exp Clin Endocrinol Diabetes 2002;110:277–283.
17. Findlay JC, Sheeler LR, Engeland WC, et al. Familial adrenocorticotropin-independent Cushing's syndrome with bilateral macronodular adrenal hyperplasia. J Clin Endocrinol Metab 1993;76:189–191.
18. Lee S, Hwang R, Lee J, et al. Ectopic expression of vasopressin V1b and V2 receptors in the adrenal glands of familial ACTH-independent macronodular adrenal hyperplasia. Clin Endocrinol (Oxf) 2005;63:625–630.
19. Gagliardi L, Hotu C, Casey G, et al. Familial vasopressin-sensitive ACTH-independent macronodular adrenal hyperplasia (VPs-AIMAH): clinical studies of three kindreds. Clin Endocrinol (Oxf) 2009;70:883–891.
20. Burgess JR, Harle RA, Tucker P, et al. Adrenal lesions in a large kindred with multiple endocrine neoplasia type 1. Arch Surg 1996;131:699–702.
21. Skogseid B, Larsson C, Lindgren PG, et al. Clinical and genetic features of adrenocortical lesions in multiple endocrine neoplasia type 1. J Clin Endocrinol Metab 1992;75:76–81.
22. Yamakita N, Murai T, Ito Y, et al. Adrenocorticotropin-independent macronodular adrenocortical hyperplasia associated with multiple colon adenomas/carcinomas which showed a point mutation in the APC gene. Intern Med 1997;36: 536–542.
23. Marchesa P, Fazio VW, Church JM, et al. Adrenal masses in patients with familial adenomatous polyposis. Dis Colon Rectum 1997;40:1023–1028.
24. Matyakhina L, Freedman RJ, Bourdeau I, et al. Hereditary leiomyomatosis associated with bilateral, massive, macronodular adrenocortical disease and atypical Cushing syndrome: a clinical and molecular genetic investigation. J Clin Endocrinol Metab 2005;90:3773–3779.
25. Bourdeau I, D'Amour P, Hamet P, et al. Aberrant membrane hormone receptors in incidentally discovered bilateral macronodular adrenal hyperplasia with subclinical Cushing's syndrome. J Clin Endocrinol Metab 2001;86:5534–5540.
26. Yamada Y, Sakaguchi K, Inoue T, et al. Preclinical Cushing's syndrome due to adrenocorticotropin-independent bilateral adrenocortical macronodular hyperplasia with concurrent excess of gluco- and mineralocorticoids. Intern Med 1997;36: 628–632.
27. Mazzuco TL, Bourdeau I, Lacroix A. Adrenal incidentalomas and subclinical Cushing's syndrome – diagnosis and treatment. Curr Opin Endocrinol Diabetes Obes 2009;16(3):203–210.
28. Ohashi A, Yamada Y, Sakaguchi K, et al. A natural history of adrenocorticotropin-independent bilateral adrenal macronodular hyperplasia (AIMAH) from preclinical to clinically overt Cushing's syndrome. Endocr J 2001;48:677–683.
29. Hayashi Y, Takeda Y, Kaneko K, et al. A case of Cushing's syndrome due to ACTH-independent bilateral macronodular hyperplasia associated with excessive secretion of mineralocorticoids. Endocr J 1998;45:485–491.
30. Malchoff CD, Rosa J, DeBold CR, et al. Adrenocorticotropin-independent bilateral macronodular adrenal hyperplasia: an unusual cause of Cushing's syndrome. J Clin Endocrinol Metab 1989;68:855–860.
31. Goodarzi MO, Dawson DW, Li X, et al. Virilization in bilateral macronodular adrenal hyperplasia controlled by luteinizing hormone. J Clin Endocrinol Metab 2003;88:73–77.
32. Antonini SR, Baldacchino V, Tremblay J, et al. Expression of ACTH receptor pathway genes in glucose-dependent insulinotrophic peptide (GIP)-dependent Cushing's syndrome. Clin Endocrinol (Oxf) 2006;64:29–36.
33. Mircescu H, Jilwan J, N'Diaye N, et al. Are ectopic or abnormal membrane hormone receptors frequently present in adrenal Cushing's syndrome? J Clin Endocrinol Metab 2000;85:3531–3536.
34. Sasano H, Suzuki T, Nagura H. ACTH-independent macronodular adrenocortical hyperplasia: immunohistochemical and in situ hybridization studies of steroidogenic enzymes. Mod Pathol 1994;7:215–219.

35. Aiba M, Kawakami M, Ito Y, et al. Bilateral adrenocortical adenomas causing Cushing's syndrome. Report of two cases with enzyme histochemical and ultrastructural studies and a review of the literature. Arch Pathol Lab Med 1992;115:146–150.
36. Doppman JL, Nieman LK, Travis WD, et al. CT and MR imaging of massive macronodular adrenocortical disease: a rare cause of autonomous primary adrenal hypercortisolism. J Comput Assist Tomogr 1991;15:773–779.
37. Rockall AG, Babar SA, Sohaib SA, et al. CT and MR imaging of the adrenal glands in ACTH-independent Cushing syndrome. Radiographics 2004;24:435–452.
38. N'Diaye N, Hamet P, Tremblay J, et al. Asynchronous development of bilateral nodular adrenal hyperplasia in gastric inhibitory polypeptide-dependent Cushing's syndrome. J Clin Endocrinol Metab 1999;84:2616–2622.
39. Smals AG, Pieters GF, van Haelst UJ, et al. Macronodular adrenocortical hyperplasia in long-standing Cushing's disease. J Clin Endocrinol Metab 1984;58:25–31.
40. Cugini P, Battisti P, Di Palma L, et al. "GIANT" macronodular adrenal hyperplasia causing Cushing's syndrome: case report and review of the literature on a clinical distinction of adrenocortical nodular pathology associated with hypercortisolism. Endocrinol Jpn 1989;36:101–116.
41. Cheitlin RA, Westphal M, Cabrera CM, et al. Cushing's syndrome due to bilateral adrenal macronodular hyperplasia with undetectable ACTH: cell culture of adenoma cells on extracellular matrix. Horm Res 1988;29:162–167.
42. Light K, Jenkins PJ, Weber A, et al. Are activating mutations of the adrenocorticotropin receptor involved in adrenal cortical neoplasia? Life Sci 1995;56:1523–1527.
43. Latronico AC, Reincke M, Mendonca BB, et al. No evidence for oncogenic mutations in the adrenocorticotropin receptor gene in human adrenocortical neoplasms. J Clin Endocrinol Metab 1995;80:875–877.
44. Swords FM, Baig A, Malchoff DM, et al. Impaired desensitization of a mutant adrenocorticotropin receptor associated with apparent constitutive activity. Mol Endocrinol 2002;16:2746–2753.
45. Swords FM, Noon LA, King PJ, et al. Constitutive activation of the human ACTH receptor resulting from a synergistic interaction between two naturally occurring missense mutations in the MC2R gene. Mol Cell Endocrinol 2004;213:149–154.
46. Mauras N, Blizzard RM. The McCune–Albright syndrome. Acta Endocrinol Suppl (Copenh) 1986;279:207–217.
47. Aarskog D, Tveteraas E. McCune–Albright's syndrome following adrenalectomy for Cushing's syndrome in infancy. J Pediatr 1968;73:89–96.
48. Benjamin DR, McRoberts JW. Polyostotic fibrous dysplasia associated with Cushing syndrome. Arch Pathol 1973;96:175–178.
49. MacMahon HE. Albright's syndrome – thirty years later. (Polyostotic fibrous dysplasia). Pathol Annu 1971;6:81–146.
50. Danon M, Robboy SJ, Kim S, et al. Cushing syndrome, sexual precocity, and polyostotic fibrous dysplasia (Albright syndrome) in infancy. J Pediatr 1975;87:917–921.
51. Fragoso MC, Domenice S, Latronico AC, et al. Cushing's syndrome secondary to adrenocorticotropin-independent macronodular adrenocortical hyperplasia due to activating mutations of GNAS1 gene. J Clin Endocrinol Metab 2003;88:2147–2151.
52. Bertagna X, Groussin L, Luton JP, et al. Aberrant receptor-mediated Cushing's syndrome. Horm Res 2003;59(Suppl 1):99–103.
53. Schorr I, Ney RL. Abnormal hormone responses of an adrenocortical cancer adenyl cyclase. J Clin Invest 1971;50:1295–1300.
54. Lacroix A, Baldacchino V, Bourdeau I, et al. Cushing's syndrome variants secondary to aberrant hormone receptors. Trends Endocrinol Metab 2004;15:375–382.
55. Lacroix A, Bolte E, Tremblay J, et al. Gastric inhibitory polypeptide-dependent cortisol hypersecretion – a new cause of Cushing's syndrome. N Engl J Med 1992;327:974–980.
56. Reznik Y, Allali-Zerah V, Chayvialle JA, et al. Food-dependent Cushing's syndrome mediated by aberrant adrenal sensitivity to gastric inhibitory polypeptide. N Engl J Med 1992;327:981–986.
57. Lebrethon MC, Avallet O, Reznik Y, et al. Food-dependent Cushing's syndrome: characterization and functional role of gastric inhibitory polypeptide receptor in the adrenals of three patients. J Clin Endocrinol Metab 1998;83:4514–4519.
58. Groussin L, Perlemoine K, Contesse V, et al. The ectopic expression of the gastric inhibitory polypeptide receptor is frequent in adrenocorticotropin-independent bilateral macronodular adrenal hyperplasia, but rare in unilateral tumors. J Clin Endocrinol Metab 2002;87:1980–1985.
59. Croughs RJ, Zelissen PM, Van Vroonhoven TJ, et al. GIP-dependent adrenal Cushing's syndrome with incomplete suppression of ACTH. Clin Endocrinol (Oxf) 2000;52:235–240.
60. Chabre O, Liakos P, Vivier J, et al. Cushing's syndrome due to a gastric inhibitory polypeptide-dependent adrenal adenoma: insights into hormonal control of adrenocortical tumorigenesis. J Clin Endocrinol Metab 1998;83:3134–3143.

61. de Herder WW, Hofland LJ, Usdin TB, et al. Food-dependent Cushing's syndrome resulting from abundant expression of gastric inhibitory polypeptide receptors in adrenal adenoma cells. J Clin Endocrinol Metab 1996;81:3168–3172.
62. N'Diaye N, Tremblay J, Hamet P, et al. Adrenocortical overexpression of gastric inhibitory polypeptide receptor underlies food-dependent Cushing's syndrome. J Clin Endocrinol Metab 1998;83:2781–2785.
63. Tsagarakis S, Tsigos C, Vassiliou V, et al. Food-dependent androgen and cortisol secretion by a gastric inhibitory polypeptide-receptor expressive adrenocortical adenoma leading to hirsutism and subclinical Cushing's syndrome: in vivo and in vitro studies. J Clin Endocrinol Metab 2001;86:583–589.
64. Lampron A, Bourdeau I, Hamet P, et al. Whole genome expression profiling of glucose-dependent insulinotropic peptide (GIP)- and adrenocorticotropin-dependent adrenal hyperplasias reveals novel targets for the study of GIP-dependent Cushing's syndrome. J Clin Endocrinol Metab 2006;91:3611–3618.
65. Bertherat J, Contesse V, Louiset E, et al. In vivo and in vitro screening for illegitimate receptors in adrenocorticotropin-independent macronodular adrenal hyperplasia causing Cushing's syndrome: identification of two cases of gonadotropin/gastric inhibitory polypeptide-dependent hypercortisolism. J Clin Endocrinol Metab 2005;90:1302–1310.
66. Baldacchino V, Oble S, Decarie PO, et al. The Sp transcription factors are involved in the cellular expression of the human glucose-dependent insulinotropic polypeptide receptor gene and overexpressed in adrenals of patients with Cushing's syndrome. J Mol Endocrinol 2005;35:61–71.
67. Swords FM, Aylwin S, Perry L, et al. The aberrant expression of the gastric inhibitory polypeptide (GIP) receptor in adrenal hyperplasia: does chronic adrenocorticotropin exposure stimulate up-regulation of GIP receptors in Cushing's disease? J Clin Endocrinol Metab 2005;90:3009–3016.
68. Mazzuco TL, Chabre O, Feige JJ, et al. Aberrant expression of human luteinizing hormone receptor by adrenocortical cells is sufficient to provoke both hyperplasia and Cushing's syndrome features. J Clin Endocrinol Metab 2006;91: 196–203.
69. Arnaldi G, Gasc JM, de Keyzer Y, et al. Variable expression of the V1 vasopressin receptor modulates the phenotypic response of steroid-secreting adrenocortical tumors. J Clin Endocrinol Metab 1998;83:2029–2035.
70. Daidoh H, Morita H, Hanafusa J, et al. In vivo and in vitro effects of AVP and V1a receptor antagonist on Cushing's syndrome due to ACTH-independent bilateral macronodular adrenocortical hyperplasia. Clin Endocrinol (Oxf) 1998;49:403–409.
71. Horiba N, Suda T, Aiba M, et al. Lysine vasopressin stimulation of cortisol secretion in patients with adrenocorticotropin-independent macronodular adrenal hyperplasia. J Clin Endocrinol Metab 1995;80:2336–2341.
72. Iida K, Kaji H, Matsumoto H, et al. Adrenocorticotrophin-independent macronodular adrenal hyperplasia in a patient with lysine vasopressin responsiveness but insensitivity to gastric inhibitory polypeptide. Clin Endocrinol (Oxf) 1997;47:739–745.
73. Lacroix A, Tremblay J, Touyz RM, et al. Abnormal adrenal and vascular responses to vasopressin mediated by a V1-vasopressin receptor in a patient with adrenocorticotropin-independent macronodular adrenal hyperplasia, Cushing's syndrome, and orthostatic hypotension. J Clin Endocrinol Metab 1997;82:2414–2422.
74. Louiset E, Contesse V, Groussin L, et al. Expression of vasopressin receptors in ACTH-independent macronodular bilateral adrenal hyperplasia causing Cushing's syndrome: molecular, immunohistochemical and pharmacological correlates. J Endocrinol 2008;196:1–9.
75. Mune T, Murase H, Yamakita N, et al. Eutopic overexpression of vasopressin V1a receptor in adrenocorticotropin-independent macronodular adrenal hyperplasia. J Clin Endocrinol Metab 2002;87:5706–5713.
76. Perraudin V, Delarue C, de Keyzer Y, et al. Vasopressin-responsive adrenocortical tumor in a mild Cushing's syndrome: in vivo and in vitro studies. J Clin Endocrinol Metab 1995;80:2661–2667.
77. Lacroix A, Tremblay J, Rousseau G, et al. Propranolol therapy for ectopic beta-adrenergic receptors in adrenal Cushing's syndrome. N Engl J Med 1997;337:1429–1434.
78. Miyamura N, Tsutsumi A, Senokuchi H, et al. A case of ACTH-independent macronodular adrenal hyperplasia: simultaneous expression of several aberrant hormone receptors in the adrenal gland. Endocr J 2003;50:333–340.
79. Mazzuco TL, Thomas M, Martinie M, et al. Cellular and molecular abnormalities of a macronodular adrenal hyperplasia causing beta-blocker-sensitive Cushing's syndrome. Arq Bras Endocrinol Metabol. 2007;51:1452–62.
80. Lacroix A, Hamet P, Boutin JM. Leuprolide acetate therapy in luteinizing hormone-dependent Cushing's syndrome. N Engl J Med 1999;341:1577–1581.
81. Feelders RA, Lamberts SW, Hofland LJ, et al. Luteinizing hormone (LH)-responsive Cushing's syndrome: the demonstration of LH receptor messenger ribonucleic acid in hyperplastic adrenal cells, which respond to chorionic gonadotropin and serotonin agonists in vitro. J Clin Endocrinol Metab 2003;88:230–237.
82. Cartier D, Lihrmann I, Parmentier F, et al. Overexpression of serotonin4 receptors in cisapride-responsive adrenocorticotropin-independent bilateral macronodular adrenal hyperplasia causing Cushing's syndrome. J Clin Endocrinol Metab 2003;88:248–254.

83. Louiset E, Contesse V, Groussin L, et al. Expression of serotonin7 receptor and coupling of ectopic receptors to protein kinase A and ionic currents in adrenocorticotropin-independent macronodular adrenal hyperplasia causing Cushing's syndrome. J Clin Endocrinol Metab 2006;91:4578–4586.
84. Mannelli M, Ferruzzi P, Luciani P, et al. Cushing's syndrome in a patient with bilateral macronodular adrenal hyperplasia responding to cisapride: an in vivo and in vitro study. J Clin Endocrinol Metab 2003;88:4616–4622.
85. Nakamura Y, Son Y, Kohno Y, et al. Case of adrenocorticotropic hormone-independent macronodular adrenal hyperplasia with possible adrenal hypersensitivity to angiotensin II. Endocrine 2001;15:57–61.
86. Pralong FP, Gomez F, Guillou L, et al. Food-dependent Cushing's syndrome: possible involvement of leptin in cortisol hypersecretion. J Clin Endocrinol Metab 1999;84:3817–3822.
87. Makino S, Hashimoto K, Sugiyama M, et al. Cushing's syndrome due to huge nodular adrenocortical hyperplasia with fluctuation of urinary 17-OHCS excretion. Endocrinol Jpn 1989;36, 655–663.
88. Hashimoto K, Kawada Y, Murakami K, et al. Cortisol responsiveness to insulin-induced hypoglycemia in Cushing's syndrome with huge nodular adrenocortical hyperplasia. Endocrinol Jpn 1986;33:479–487.
89. Louiset E, Duparc C, Groussin L, et al. Abnormal sensitivity of cortisol secretion to glucagon in primary adrenal Cushing's syndrome. In: XIII Adrenal Cortex Conference, San Francisco, CA, 2008: p. 52: Abstract 33.
90. Imohl M, Koditz R, Stachon A, et al. [Catecholamine-dependent hereditary Cushing's syndrome – follow-up after unilateral adrenalectomy]. Med Klin (Munich) 2002;97:747–753.
91. Antonini SR, N'Diaye N, Baldacchino V, et al. Analysis of the putative regulatory region of the gastric inhibitory polypeptide receptor gene in food-dependent Cushing's syndrome. J Steroid Biochem Mol Biol 2004;91:171–177.
92. Bourdeau I, Antonini SR, Lacroix A, et al. Gene array analysis of macronodular adrenal hyperplasia confirms clinical heterogeneity and identifies several candidate genes as molecular mediators. Oncogene 2004;23:1575–1585.
93. Mazzuco TL, Chabre O, Sturm N, et al. Ectopic expression of the gastric inhibitory polypeptide receptor gene is a sufficient genetic event to induce benign adrenocortical tumor in a xenotransplantation model. Endocrinology 2006;147:782–790.
94. Bourdeau I, Matyakhina L, Stergiopoulos SG, et al. 17q22–24 chromosomal losses and alterations of protein kinase a subunit expression and activity in adrenocorticotropin-independent macronodular adrenal hyperplasia. J Clin Endocrinol Metab 2006;91:3626–3632.
95. Hsiao HP, Kirschner LS, Bourdeau I, et al. Clinical and genetic heterogeneity, overlap with other tumor syndromes, and atypical glucocorticoid hormone secretion in ACTH-independent macronodular adrenal hyperplasia compared to other adrenocortical tumors. J Clin Endocrinol Metab 2009;94:2930–37.
96. Lefebvre H, Duparc C, Chartrel N, et al. Intraadrenal adrenocorticotropin production in a case of bilateral macronodular adrenal hyperplasia causing Cushing's syndrome. J Clin Endocrinol Metab 2003;88:3035–3042.
97. Lacroix AM, H Hammet P. Clinical evaluation of the presence of abnormal hormone receptors in adrenal Cushing's syndrome. Endocrinologist 1999;9:9–15.
98. Reznik Y, Lefebvre H, Rohmer V, et al. Aberrant adrenal sensitivity to multiple ligands in unilateral incidentaloma with subclinical autonomous cortisol hypersecretion: a prospective clinical study. Clin Endocrinol (Oxf) 2004;61:311–319.
99. Boronat M, Lucas T, Barcelo B, et al. Cushing's syndrome due to autonomous macronodular adrenal hyperplasia: long-term follow-up after unilateral adrenalectomy. Postgrad Med J 1996;72:614–616.
100. Lamas C, Alfaro JJ, Lucas T, et al. Is unilateral adrenalectomy an alternative treatment for ACTH-independent macronodular adrenal hyperplasia? Long-term follow-up of four cases. Eur J Endocrinol 2002;146:237–240.
101. Herder WW, Hofland LJ, Usdin TB, et al. Food-dependent Cushing's syndrome resulting from abundant expression of gastric inhibitory polypeptide receptors in adrenal adenoma cells. J Clin Endocrinol Metab 1996;81:3168–3172.

18 ACTH-Independent Cushing's Syndrome: Primary Pigmented Nodular Adrenal Disease in the Context of Carney's Complex

Constantine Stratakis

Contents

Summary

In this chapter, we discuss clinical and molecular findings of micronodular adrenal hyperplasias (MAHs) that lead to ACTH-independent Cushing syndrome. We focus on the role of genetic defects in cyclic AMP (cAMP) signaling-related molecules, namely *PRKAR1A*, *GNAS*, *PDE11A*, and *PDE8B*; molecular defects in the phosphodiesterases (PDE) family are the most recently discovered genetic defects predisposing to adrenocortical tumor formation. The prototype of these disorders was Carney complex (CNC) in the context of which the first MAH was described: primary pigmented nodular adrenocortical disease or PPNAD. PPNAD is due to defects in *PRKAR1A*, the gene that functions as a receptor for the cAMP. In contrast to *GNAS* and *PRKAR1A*, defects in PDE genes are associated more frequently with incomplete penetrance. Identifying low-penetrance mutations in more than one *PDE* in patients with MAHs is suggestive for a complementary role of the different PDEs in the adrenal gland, and possible involvement of other members of this gene family in adrenocortical tumors and ACTH-independent Cushing syndrome.

Key Words: Adrenocortical tumors, cAMP signaling, phosphodiesterases, PKA

From: *Contemporary Endocrinology: Cushing's Syndrome: Pathophysiology, Diagnosis and Treatment*
Edited by: M.D. Bronstein (ed.), DOI 10.1007/978-1-60327-449-4_18,

INTRODUCTION

Embryologically, the adrenal cortex is derived from the mesoderm, and is composed of three layers: in the outer region *zona glomerulosa*, in the middle *zona fasciculata*, and in the inner part of the gland *zona reticularis*. Adrenocortical lesions include hyperplasia (which may be diffuse or nodular), adenomas, and carcinomas. The frequency of benign adrenocortical lesions is high, and it has been estimated that more than one in ten adults has at least one adrenocortical nodule up to 1 cm on autopsy; these benign tumors may contribute to metabolic syndrome, hypertension, obesity, and abnormalities of the hypothalamic-pituitary-adrenal axis that can be linked to other serious disorders such as osteoporosis, depression, and late-onset diabetes mellitus *(1)*. In contrast, adrenocortical cancer is a very rare disease (with an incidence of less than one per million per year), which, unless identified at an early stage, is almost invariably fatal. Clonal composition analyses and comparative genomic hybridization experiments have established that adrenocortical tumorigenesis is a multistep process resulting from sequential genetic alterations that lead to progression from normal to adenomatous and, eventually, malignant phenotypes *(2, 3)*. Despite intensive investigations, the remarkable discrepancy between the frequencies of benign and malignant tumor formation in this tissue remains obscure. Better understanding of the molecular processes that underlie the benign and malignant adrenocortical transformation is expected to provide clues not only for diagnosis, but also for improved treatment and prevention.

Here we discuss all forms of micronodular bilateral adrenocortical hyperplasias (BAHs) and review current concepts on the genetic factors involved in its predisposition and progress.

ADRENOCORTICAL HYPERPLASIAS: NOMENCLATURE AND FEATURES

A recent article reviews and classifies the types of benign and malignant adrenocortical lesions, and it also proposes a nomenclature to be used in both scientific and clinical applications *(4)*. In brief, corticotrophin-independent BAH can be classified as macro- and micronodular on the basis of the size of their nodules (>1 cm or <1 cm in diameter, respectively). Nodules less than 1 cm in diameter can be seen in macronodular adrenocortical disease, especially in the form associated with McCune–Albright syndrome (MAS), and single large nodules can be associated with primary pigmented nodular adrenocortical disease (PPNAD) in older individuals; however, the vast majority of patients with BAH present with either a macronodular or a micronodular form. Micronodular adrenocortical hyperplasia (MAH), which is in the focus of this chapter, can be further subdivided in three groups: PPNAD as part of Carney Complex (CNC) – a multiple endocrine neoplasia syndrome (CNC-PPNAD or c-PPNAD), isolated micronodular adrenocortical disease (i-MAD), and its pigmented variant, isolated PPNAD (i-PPNAD) *(4–6)*. These forms are indistinguishable on computed tomography (CT) or other imaging (Fig. 1). Two additional criteria are used in the classification of MAHs: the status of the internodular cortex – hyperplastic or atrophic and the presence of pigment, most often lipofuscin. Lipofucsin is thought to be derived from lysosomal residual bodies containing end products of oxidative damage to lipid molecules *(7)*. In PPNAD (and other cortisol-producing tumors), lipofuscin appears microscopically as light to brown dark, or, sometimes, black stained spots. Lipofuscin accumulates also with age in both human and other mammalian adrenocortical tissue *(6–8)*. Histology of PPNAD (Fig. 2) and other forms of MAHs (Fig. 3) can vary and often these lesions are hard to distinguish although the cases shown in Figs. 2 and 3 show clearly different features.

The PPNAD has a bimodal age of presentation – but in most cases, and, particularly the ones associated with CNC, the disease is diagnosed in the second and third decade of life: a group of patients presents during early childhood (2–3 years) *(5)*. Nonpigmented, early onset BAH, or iMAD may be a distinct entity, which, although very similar to PPNAD, displays some specific features especially with regards to the presence or absence of hyperplasia in the surrounding cortex *(5, 9)*. Patients with

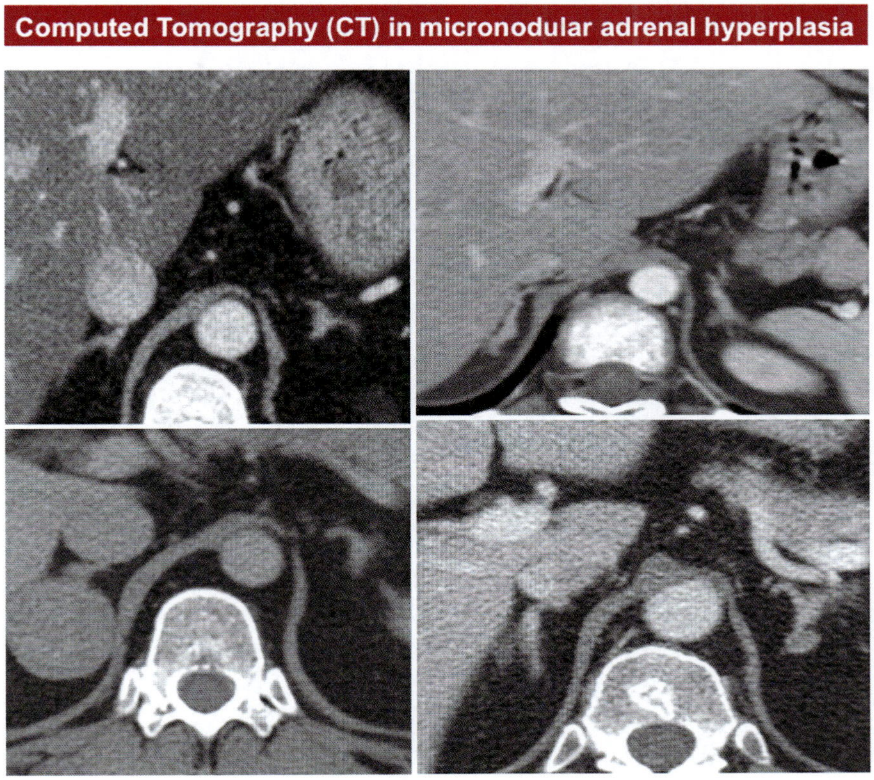

Fig. 1. Computed tomography from four patients with PPNAD and other forms of MAH; the picture of the adrenals ranges from almost completely normal to characteristic micronodularity and a "beads-on-a-string" appearance.

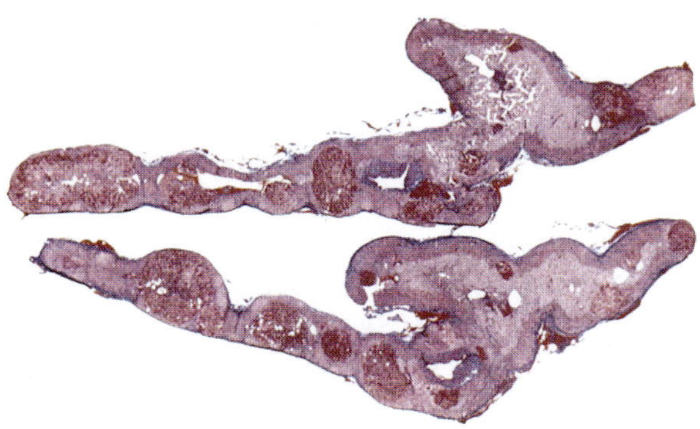

Fig. 2. Adrenal glands affected by PPNAD (slide courtesy of Dr. Carney, Mayo Clinic).

iMAD may present with classical Cushing's syndrome (CS), as well as with a variant, called "atypical" (ACS) *(10)*. The ACS is characterized by an asthenic, rather than obese, body habitus that is caused by severe osteoporosis, short stature, and severe muscle and skin wasting. Patients with ACS tend to have normal or near-normal 24-h urinary free cortisol (UFC) production, with, however, disturbed circadian rhythmicity *(11, 12)*. Occasionally, normal cortisol production is interrupted by days or weeks of hypercortisolism that gives rise to a yet another variant called "periodic CS" (PCS). The PCS is frequently found in children and adolescents with PPNAD *(12)*. In both ACS and PCS, as well as in classic CS, caused by PPNAD, paradoxical increase of UFC and/or 17-hydroxy-corticosteroids

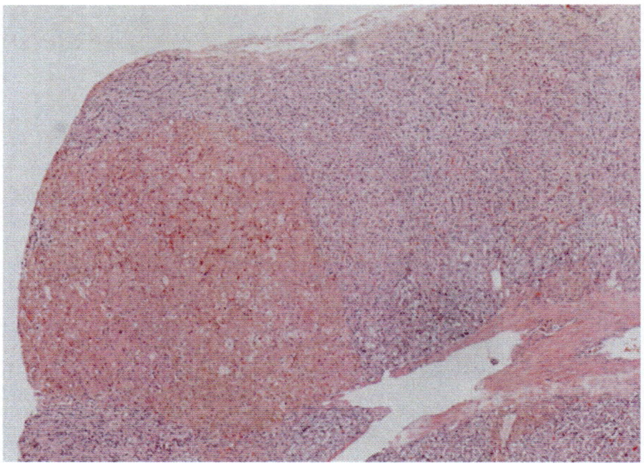

Fig. 3. An adrenal gland affected by MAH that is not due to *PRKAR1A* mutations (from the National Institutes of Health database).

is seen during the second phase (high dose dexamethasone administration) of the Liddle's test *(13)*. This feature may be useful diagnostically for PPNAD, iMAD, and related abnormalities of the adrenal cortex; it probably reflects a tendency that these nodules have for increased responsiveness to other steroids *(14)*.

GENETICS OF MICRONODULAR ADRENOCORTICAL DISEASE

Primary Pigmented Nodular Adrenocortical Disease Associated with Carney Complex

Most commonly PPNAD is seen in the context of CNC – c-PPNAD accounts for more than 90% of all reported cases *(15, 16)*. CNC is associated with several other lesions, including cardiac myxomas and other cutaneous tumors, breast myxomatosis, spotty skin pigmentation and other lesions, pituitary adenomas and acromegaly, large-cell calcifying Sertoli cell tumors (among the rarest of testicular neoplasms), adrenocortical lesions, and Leydig cell tumors, psammomatous melanotic schwannoma, epithelioid blue nevus, and ductal adenoma of the breast and thyroid follicular neoplasms, both benign and malignant *(17)*. PPNAD is the most frequent endocrine manifestation of CNC *(6)*.

The CNC is transmitted as an autosomal dominant trait, and a genome-wide screen of CNC families was able to demonstrate linkage to genetic loci at chromosomes 2p16 and 17q22–24 *(18–20)*. Further studies have led to the identification of the responsible gene on 17q22–24: *PRKAR1A*, the gene that encodes the type 1α regulatory subunit (RIα) of cAMP-dependent protein kinase A (PKA) *(21)*. To date, more than 60% of CNC patients are identified to harbor pathogenic *PRKAR1A* mutations *(21–24)*. The gene on chromosome 2p16 is yet to be revealed.

The PKA plays a major role in eukaryotic cell signaling. In its inactive state, the holoenzyme consists of a tetramer of two homo- or heterodimers of regulatory subunits (*PRKAR1A*, *PRKAR1B*, *PRKAR2A*, *PRKAR2B*) and two catalytic subunits (*PRKACA*, *PRKACB*) *(25, 26)*. Each regulatory monomer contains a dimerization/docking domain at the amino terminal, two tandem binding domains for adenosine 3′,5′-cyclic monophosphate (cAMP) at the carboxyl terminus (cAMP:A and cAMP:B), and a linker region that contains the main docking site for the C subunit *(25, 26)*. Elevation in the cellular cAMP levels, and, consequently, binding of cAMP molecules to the regulatory subunits leads to activation of the regulatory subunits, dissolution of the holoenzyme, and release of the catalytic subunits *(26)*. The free catalytic subunits, which are serine-threonine kinases, can then go or to phosphorylate a series of targets that regulate downstream effector enzymes, ion channels, and transcription of specific genes that mediate cell growth and differentiation *(26)*. Thus, functionally, inactivation of *PRKAR1A* is associated with excess PKA signaling in affected tissues *(27, 28)*.

PRKAR1A extends to a total genomic length of approximately 21 kb and is composed of 11 exons with a coding region of 1,143 bp, starting from exon 2. Since the identification of *PRKAR1A* mutations in CNC, more than 100 disease-causing pathogenic sequence changes have been reported; they are spread all over the coding length of the gene, without a preference for a region or exon *(24)*. Most of the mutations are unique, that is they are identified in single families only. Only two mutations [c.491_492delTG/p.Val164fsX4, and c.709 (-7-2) del6(ttttta)] in the gene have been seen so far in more than three unrelated CNC families *(22, 29)*.

The vast majority of the mutations consist of base substitutions, small deletions and insertions, or combined rearrangements, involving up to 15 bp *(21)*; although rare, large *PRKAR1A* deletions have been reported *(30)*. In the majority of the cases, the sequence change results in a premature stop codon; this leads to degradation of mutant mRNAs by nonsense mediated mRNA decay and, consequentially, the absence of the predicted mutant protein product *(22)*. Loss of the normal 17q22-23 allele in CNC lesions (loss-of-heterozygosity, LOH) has also been noted, indicating that *PRKAR1A* may act as a tumor-suppressor gene *(21, 31)*: oncogenesis in CNC tumors was due to the complete lack of a functional PRKAR1A *(5)*. A strong genotype–phenotype correlation appears to be absent in premature stop codon-generating mutations, since nonsense-mediated mRNA decay (NMD) leads to *PRKAR1A* haploinsufficiency for all these mutations.

Rarely, mutations that escape NMD and lead to the expression of an abnormal, defective PRKAR1A protein have been identified *(29, 30, 32)*: these "expressed" mutations appear to lead to different phenotypes. A splice-site variant that eliminates "in frame" exon 7 is seen mostly with isolated PPNAD, presumably due to adrenal-specific regulation of expression or partial splicing defect and an increased sensitivity of the adrenal gland to even subtle alterations in cAMP signaling *(29)*. In contrast, germline "in frame" deletion of exon 3 results in severe expression of the majority of the CNC manifestations – this phenotype likely reflects the importance of exon 3, linking the dimerization/docking domain and the first cAMP binding domain for the overall functional conformation of PRKAR1A *(30)*.

Important clues on the function of the different PRKAR1A domains are provided by a recent study that investigates the in vitro effect of naturally occurring expressed mutations in the gene *(32)*. The study examined six expressed variants resulting from missense substitutions in the coding region for the functional domains of the protein (Ser9Asn, Arg74Cys, Arg146Ser, Asp183Tyr, Ala213Asp, Gly289Trp), together with the previously reported exon 3-skipping expressed *PRKAR1A* isoform *(30, 32)*. Transfection studies with mutant constructs bearing the expressed mutations showed increased PKA activity, which was attributed to decreased binding to cAMP and/or the catalytic subunit. A correlation between the localization of the mutation, domain function, and in vitro effects was observed. Three of the investigated mutations (Asp183Tyr, Ala213Asp, and Gly289Trp) were located in the cAMP-binding domains of PRKAR1A. These domains contain the phosphate binding cassettes (PBCs), where the residues essential for cAMP binding are positioned; these regions are the most conserved portions of these domains *(25, 33)*. Significant decrease in the cAMP binding ability was measured for all three mutations, consistent with their proximity to or placement in a PBC and suggesting their possible importance for normal PKA conformation and function *(25)*. Furthermore, in contrast to previous studies reporting only partial kinase activation for PRKAR1A subunits defective in cAMP binding domains, this study showed increased PKA activity, PKA specific activation, and pCREB/CREB ratios for these three naturally occurring mutations.

Perhaps even more interesting results were revealed by mutations that affect the catalytic subunit binding sites. In the absence of cAMP, the two regulatory subunits bind the two catalytic subunits, rendering the PKA holoenzyme inactive. Experimental data have shown that binding of the regulatory to the catalytic subunit requires at least two sites to achieve high affinity binding. The exon 3 skipping mutation, which lacks residues 60–117, spans the primary site (residues 94–98, the inhibitor sequence), while the Arg146Ser mutation disrupts the secondary site (residues 138–148, 232–247) *(33)*. Increased PKA specific activation and extremely high PKA activity even without cAMP were measured for these mutations due to the inability of the mutated PRKAR1A to bind the catalytic subunit, as supported by co-immunoprecipitation studies *(33)*. As expected, levels of unbound cAMP declined even as cAMP binding affinity fell; since the catalytic subunit is coupled to both the inhibitor sequence and cAMP binding domain, it is not surprising that a mutation that affects the catalytic subunit binding would also affect cAMP binding, likely by altering the arrangement of amino acids important for these functions.

The remaining two expressed mutations (Ser9Asn and Arg74Cys) were located in the dimerization/docking domain, and in the linker region, outside of any known functional domain, respectively; it has been hypothesized that they likely affect higher order protein structure and/or RIα interaction with partner proteins outside of the PKA tetramer *(33, 34)*. Indeed, increased PKA activity and PKA-specific activation and decreased binding of both cAMP and Cα were observed *(33)*. These studies support previous suggestions that alteration of PRKAR1A function alone (not only its complete loss) can lead to increased PKA activity leading to tumorogenic changes in the adrenal cortex and other cAMP-sensitive tissues, and to CNC.

Isolated Primary Pigmented Nodular Adrenocortical Disease

Although rare, familial cases of isolated PPNAD have also been reported *(29)*. Like CNC, PPNAD is inherited in an autosomal dominant manner. By definition, no other clinical features associated with CNC are seen in these families; however, subtle disease manifestations may have been missed *(35, 36)*. Isolated, non-familial PPNAD has been very rarely reported, and, in most of the cases, like in familial PPNAD, the genetic defect is a germline mutation in PRKAR1A *(29)*.

Isolated Micronodular Adrenocortical Disease

The genetic basis of isolated corticotropin-independent MAD is supported by its invariably bilateral appearance and very early disease onset. In a recent study, employing a genome-wide screen of ten kindreds negative for *PRKAR1A* mutations, a strong association between the disease and inactivating mutations in phosphodiesterase 11A (*PDE11A*), was identified *(37, 38)*. Most of the individuals included in this study presented with an overall normal adrenoglandular size and weight; adrenocortical samples from these patients featured multiple small yellow-to-brown nodules surrounded by a cortex with a uniform appearance. Microscopy showed moderate diffuse cortical hyperplasia with multiple capsular deficits and massive circumscribed and infiltrating extra-adrenal cortical excrescences with micronodules; in other patients, histology was indistinguishable from that in PPNAD.

PDE11A is located on chromosome 2q31.2 and belongs to the large family of human PDEs comprised of 21 so far identified genes that are classified in 11 different subfamilies based on structural similarity such as sequence homology, protein domains, and enzymatic properties including substrate specificity, kinetic properties, and sensitivity to endogenous regulators and inhibitors *(39, 40)*. All PDE genes are transcribed in multiple splice isoforms that have mostly unique tissue-expression patterns, kinetic properties, regulation, subcellular localization, and interaction with associated proteins. PDE11A is a dual specificity PDE that degrades both second messengers cAMP and cGMP. PDE11A is expressed in several endocrine tissues, including the adrenal cortex *(41, 42)*. It contains one active catalytic domain end two N-terminal phosphorylation sites for PKA and PKG are identified. The gene spans approximately 0.5 MB and is composed of 23 exons which by alternative splicing results in the expression of four different isoforms *PDE11A1*, *PDE11A2*, *PDE11A3*, and *PDE11A4 (39)*. Of the four, only the full length (*PDE11A4*, ~2.8 kb) shows high adrenal specific expression.

Five different *PDE11A* mutations were identified so far among the patients with isolated PPNAD – three of them resulted in premature stop codon generation; the remaining two were single base substitutions in the catalytic domain of the protein and were shown to significantly affect the ability of PDE11A to degrade cAMP in vitro *(37, 38)*. Cyclic AMP (cAMP) and cGMP levels in adrenocortical tumors from individuals with inactivating *PDE11A* mutations were significantly elevated compared to control samples. This observation suggested that the pathophysiological mechanism by which mutations in *PDE11A* predispose to adrenocortical tumor formation seems to be linked to activation or abnormal cAMP signaling. Investigation of the different PDE11A isoforms showed adrenal expression of only one of the four known splice variants – *PDE11A4*. Decreased PDE11A4 mRNA and protein expression levels were measured in adrenocortical tumors of patients carrying inactivating mutations in the gene *(37)*. Further, fluorescent in situ hybridization analysis indicated LOH, with retention of the mutant allele in some of these patients with inactivating *PDE11A* mutations *(37)*.

The above described genome-wide association study suggested a number of other chromosomal loci as potentially linked to the development of iMAD; the second most favored such locus was 5q13 containing the gene for a cAMP-specific PDE, *PDE8B (37)*. *PDE8B* was also shown to have significantly higher expression in the adrenal gland compared to all other cAMP-specific PDEs *(37)*. Sequencing of the *PDE8B*-coding regions identified a single base substitution (c.914A > T, p.H305P) in a young girl with CS; the patient inherited the mutation from her father, who presented with very mild to indistinguishable adrenocortical phenotype *(43)*. The substitution affects an evolutionary conserved residue (H305) and was not seen among extended cohorts of healthy unrelated control subjects. In vitro studies indicated an impaired ability of the protein to degrade cAMP *(43)*.

Adrenocortical Hyperplasia Associated with McCune–Albright Syndrome

Another type of BAH leading to Cushing syndrome – macronodular adrenocortical hyperplasia – is associated with somatic mutations in the stimulatory (Gsα) gene of the G protein cascade (*GNAS*) in MAS *(44)*. The members of the G protein family of signal transducers form heterotrimers (subunits α, β, γ), most clearly distinguished by their different alpha chains. The α-stimulating subunit encoded by *GNAS*, located on chromosome 20q13.3 *(45)* has intrinsic GTPase activity and after activation stimulates the adenylyl cyclase-mediated cAMP production and interacts with other cell-specific intracellular effectors *(45)*.

Expressed Genes and Pathways in Primary Pigmented Nodular Adrenocortical Disease

Serial Analysis of Gene Expression (SAGE) of a human adrenal affected by PPNAD was completed to compare gene expression with that of a normal adrenal and previous studies in macronodular hyperplasias *(46, 47)*. An interesting finding was the involvement of the Wnt signaling pathway in both types of hyperplasia: the expression levels of several members of this pathway were found elevated. Genes such as catenin (cadherin-associated protein)-like 1 (*CTNNAL1*), disheveled, dsh homolog 2 (Drosophila; *DVL2*), casein kinase 1 (*CSNK1E*), axin 1 (*AXIN1*), catenin-b1 (*CTNNB1*), WNT1-inducible signaling pathway protein 2 (*WISP2*), and glycogen synthase kinase-3b (*GSK3B*) were all overexpressed. The Wnt-signaling pathway regulates many important cellular and developmental processes, including proliferation, cell-to-cell adhesion, cell fate decisions, and differentiation. The involvement of this pathway in other adrenocortical tumors was recently supported by the finding of somatic activating mutations in β-catenin in as high as approximately 30% of adrenal adenomas and carcinomas *(48)*. Another finding in common for the two hyperplasias was increased expression of *PRKAR2B*, one of the other PKA subunits that seem to counteract PRKAR1A actions *(21, 49)* in human tissues bearing *PRKAR1A* inactivating mutations, as well as in Prkar1a-deficient mice *(50–52)*. An important group of genes that were found inversely regulated in PPNAD and macronodular hyperplasia were those involved in steroidogenesis, and particularly, in cortisol production. In PPNAD, as expected from a high cortisol-producing tissue, *CYP11B1*, *CYP17A1*, *CYP21A2*, and *HSD3B2* were overexpressed; in contrast, in macronodular hyperplasia, expression levels of *CYP11B1*, *CYP17A1*, and *CYP21A2* were decreased *(53)*, a finding that reflects the relatively low efficiency with which macronodular cells produce cortisol compared to the volume of the tissue and the degree of their hypertrophy *(54)*.

CONCLUSION

Defects in several key molecules of the cAMP pathway predispose to nodular adrenocortical disease: *GNAS*, *PRKAR1A*, *PDE11A*, and *PDE8B*. PDE-inactivating mutations appear to be a novel cause of inherited predisposition to mostly micronodular forms of hyperplasia. Incomplete penetrance of functionally harmful sequence variations in these genes requires further investigation. In the adrenal cortex, factors that affect tumorigenicity are likely to be developmental, hormonal, and possibly gender-related. Adrenocortical tumors and CS are generally more frequent in females *(37, 38, 43)*; on the other hand, in all cases where inheritance of a *PDE11A* mutation could be shown, the asymptomatic carrier was the father *(37, 38, 43)*. The presence of allelic losses of the corresponding normal allele in adrenal tissues seems to be a determining factor in the development of an adrenal tumor as it is suggested by the *PDE11A*-associated tumor genetic studies *(37)*. Although the cause of all forms of nodular adrenocortical disease studied to date seems to be linked to increased cAMP signaling, the histopathological changes in the adrenal glands of patients with the various mutations or functional abnormalities of this pathway differ significantly and overlap only partially *(55)*. *PRKAR1A* mutations are associated with PPNAD *(24)*, whereas *GNAS* mutations are associated with the mostly macronodular and clearly nonpigmented form of BAH that one sees in MAS. *PDE11A* and *PDE8B* mutations seem to predispose to a variety of lesions from isolated (without any other associated tumors) PPNAD to nonpigmented iMAD and other forms of BAH. The importance of PDEs for normal adrenocortical function is currently being explored.

ACKNOWLEDGMENTS

This work was supported by the Intramural Program of the *Eunice Kennedy Shriver* National Institutes of Child Health & Human Development (NICHD), National Institutes of Health (NIH), Bethesda, MD; funds for this project are provided by the NICHD, NIH intramural project Z01-HD-000642-04 to Dr. C. A. Stratakis.

REFERENCES

1. Stratakis CA. Adrenocortical tumors, primary pigmented adrenocortical disease (PPNAD)/Carney complex, and other bilateral hyperplasias: the NIH studies. Horm Metab Res 2007;39:467–473.
2. Beuschlein F, Reincke M, Karl M, et al. Clonal composition of human adrenocortical neoplasms. Cancer Res 1994;54:4927–4932.

3. Gicquel C, Leblond-Francillard M, Bertagna X, et al. Clonal analysis of human adrenocortical carcinomas and secreting adenomas. Clin Endocrinol (Oxf) 1994;40:465–477.
4. Stratakis CA, Boikos SA. Genetics of adrenal tumors associated with Cushing's syndrome: a new classification for bilateral adrenocortical hyperplasias. Nat Clin Pract Endocrinol Metab 2007;3:748–757.
5. Gunther DF, Bourdeau I, Matyakhina L, et al. Cushing syndrome presenting in infancy: an early form of primary pigmented nodular adrenocortical disease, or a new entity? J Clin Endocrinol Metab 2004;89:3173–3182.
6. Stratakis CA, Kirschner LS, Carney JA. Clinical and molecular features of the Carney complex: diagnostic criteria and recommendations for patient evaluation. J Clin Endocrinol Metab 2001;86:4041–4046.
7. Mochizuki Y, Park MK, Mori T, Kawashima S. The difference in autofluorescence features of lipofuscin between brain and adrenal. Zoolog Sci 1995;12:283–288.
8. Lack EE. Tumors of the adrenal gland and extra-adrenal paraganglia. In: Saenger W, et al., eds. Atlas of Tumor Pathology. 3rd series, fascicle 19. Washington, DC: Armed Forces Institute of Pathology, 1997:184–187.
9. Horvath A, Boikos S, Giatzakis C, et al. A genome-wide scan identifies mutations in the gene encoding phosphodiesterase 11A4 (*PDE11A*) in individuals with adrenocortical hyperplasia. Nat Genet 2006;38:794–800.
10. Mellinger RC, Smith RW Jr. Studies of the adrenal hyperfunction in 2 patients with atypical Cushing's syndrome. J Clin Endocrinol Metab 1956;16:350–366.
11. Sarlis NJ, Chrousos GP, Doppman JL, et al. Primary pigmented nodular adrenocortical disease: reevaluation of a patient with Carney complex 27 years after unilateral adrenalectomy. J Clin Endocrinol Metab 1997;82:1274–1278.
12. Gomez Muguruza MT, Chrousos GP. Periodic Cushing syndrome in a short boy: usefulness of the ovine corticotropin releasing hormone test. J Pediatr 1989;115:270–273.
13. Sarlis NJ, Papanicolaou DA, Chrousos GP, Stratakis CA. Paradoxical increase of urinary free cortisol and 17-hydroxysteroids to dexamethasone during Liddle's test: a diagnostic test for primary pigmented adrenocortical disease. [Abstract P2–76]. In: Proceedings of the 79th Annual Meeting of the Endocrine Society in Minneapolis, MN, Endocrine Society Press, 1997;303.
14. Caticha O, Odell WD, Wilson DE, et al. Estradiol stimulates cortisol production by adrenal cells in estrogen-dependent primary adrenocortical nodular dysplasia. J Clin Endocrinol Metab 1993;77:494–497.
15. Carney JA, Gordon H, Carpenter PC, et al. The complex of myxomas, spotty pigmentation, and endocrine overactivity. Medicine (Baltimore) 1985;64:270–283.
16. Kirschner LS, Taymans SE, Stratakis CA. Characterization of the adrenal gland pathology of Carney complex, and molecular genetics of the disease. Endocr Res 1998;24:863–864.
17. Stratakis CA, Courcoutsakis NA, Abati A, et al. Thyroid gland abnormalities in patients with the syndrome of spotty skin pigmentation, myxomas, endocrine overactivity, and schwannomas (Carney complex). J Clin Endocrinol Metab 1997;82:2037–2043.
18. Carney JA, Hruska LS, Beauchamp GD, Gordon H. Dominant inheritance of the complex of myxomas, spotty pigmentation, and endocrine overactivity. Mayo Clin Proc 1986;61:165–172.
19. Stratakis CA, Carney JA, Lin JP, et al. Carney complex, a familial multiple neoplasia and lentiginosis syndrome: analysis of 11 kindreds and linkage to the short arm of chromosome 2. J Clin Invest 1996;97:699–705.
20. Casey M, Mah C, Merliss AD, et al. Identification of novel genetic locus for familial cardiac myxomas and Carney complex. Circulation 1998;98:2560–2566.
21. Kirschner LS, Carney JA, Pack SD, et al. Mutations of the gene encoding the protein kinase A type I-α regulatory subunit in patients with the Carney complex. Nat Genet 2000;26:89–92.
22. Kirschner LS, Sandrini F, Monbo J, et al. Genetic heterogeneity and spectrum of mutations of the PRKAR1A gene in patients with the Carney complex. Hum Mol Genet 2000;9:3037–3046.
23. Casey M, Vaughan CJ, He J, et al. Mutations in the protein kinase A R1α regulatory subunit cause familial cardiac myxomas and Carney complex. J Clin Invest 2000;106:R31–R38.
24. Horvath A, Bertherat J, Groussin L, Grillaud-Bataille M, Tsang K, Cazabat L, Libé R, Remmers E, René-Corail F, Faucz FR, Clauser E, Calender A, Bertagna X, Carney JA, Stratakis CA. Mutations and polymorphisms in the gene encoding regulatory subunit type 1-alpha of protein kinase A(PRKAR1A): an update Hum Mutat. 2010;31:369–79.
25. Zawadski KM, Taylor S. cAMP-dependent protein kinase regulatory subunit type IIβ. J Biol Chem 2004;279: 7029–7036.
26. Shabb, JB. Physiological substrates of cAMP-dependent protein kinase. Chem Rev 2001;101:2381–2411.
27. Robinson-White A, Meoli E, Stergiopoulos S, et al. PRKAR1A mutations and protein kinase A interactions with other signaling pathways in the adrenal cortex. J Clin Endocrinol Metab 2006;91:2380–2388.
28. Bossis I, Stratakis CA. Minireview: PRKAR1A: normal and abnormal functions. Endocrinology 2004;145:5452–5258.
29. Groussin L, Horvath A, Jullian E, et al. PRKAR1A mutation associated with primary pigmented nodular adrenocortical disease in 12 kindreds. J Clin Endocrinol Metab 2006;91:1943–1949.

30. Horvath A, Bossis I, Giatzakis C, et al. Large deletions of the PRKAR1A gene in Carney complex. Clin Cancer Res 2008;14:388–395.
31. Boikos SA, Stratakis CA. Carney complex: the first 20 years. Curr Opin Oncol 2007;19:24–29.
32. Greene EL, Horvath AD, Nesterova M, et al. In vitro functional studies of naturally occurring pathogenic PRKAR1A mutations that are not subject to nonsense mRNA decay. Hum Mutat 2008;29(5):633–639.
33. Hamuro Y, Anand GS, Kim JS, et al. Mapping intersubunit interactions of the Regulatory Subunit (RIα) in the type I holoenzyme of protein kinase A by amide hydrogen/Deuterium Exchange Mass Spectrometry (DXMS). J Mol Biol 2004;340:1185–1196.
34. Veugelers M, Wilkes D, Burton K, et al. Comparative PRKAR1A genotype-phenotype analyses in humans with Carney complex and prkar1a haploinsufficient mice. Proc Natl Acad Sci U S A 2004;101:14222–14227.
35. Armstrong DK, Irvine AD, Handley JM, et al. Carney complex: report of a kindred with predominantly cutaneous manifestations. Br J Dermatol 1997;136:578–582.
36. Liebler GA, Magovern GJ, Park SB, et al. Familial myxomas in four siblings. J Thorac Cardiovasc Surg 1976;71:605–608.
37. Horvath A, Boikos S, Giatzakis C, et al. A genome-wide scan identifies mutations in the gene encoding phosphodiesterase 11A4 (PDE11A) in individuals with adrenocortical hyperplasia. Nat Genet 2006;38:794–800.
38. Horvath A, Giatzakis C, Robinson-White A, et al. Adrenal hyperplasia and adenomas are associated with inhibition of phosphodiesterase 11A in carriers of PDE11A sequence variants that are frequent in the population. Cancer Res 2006;66: 11571–11575.
39. Fawcett L, Baxendale R, Stacey P, et al. Molecular cloning and characterization of a distinct human phosphodiesterase gene family: PDE11A. Proc Natl Acad Sci U S A 2000;97:3702–3707.
40. Omori K, Kotera J. Overview of PDEs and their regulation. Circ Res 2007;100:309–327.
41. Conti M, Beavo J. Biochemistry and physiology of cyclic nucleotide phosphodiesterases: essential components in cyclic nucleotide signaling. Annu Rev Biochem 2007;76:481–511.
42. Bender AT, Beavo JA. Cyclic nucleotide phosphodiesterases: molecular regulation to clinical use. Pharmacol Rev 2006;58:488–520.
43. Horvath A, Mericq V, Stratakis CA. Mutation in PDE8B, a cyclic AMP-specific phosphodiesterase in adrenal hyperplasia. N Engl J Med 2008;358:750–752.
44. Weinstein LS, Shenker A, Gejman PV, et al. Activating mutations of the stimulatory G protein in the McCune–Albright syndrome. N Engl J Med 1991;325:1688–1695.
45. Gejman PV, Weinstein LS, Martinez M, et al. Genetic mapping of the Gs-alpha subunit gene (GNAS1) to the distal long arm of chromosome 20 using a polymorphism detected by denaturing gradient gel electrophoresis. Genomics 1991;9:782–783.
46. Bourdeau I, Antonini SR, Lacroix A, et al. Gene array analysis of macronodular adrenal hyperplasia confirms clinical heterogeneity and identifies several candidate genes as molecular mediators. Oncogene 2004;23:1575–1585.
47. Horvath A, Mathyakina L, Vong Q, et al. Serial analysis of gene expression in adrenocortical hyperplasia caused by a germline PRKAR1A mutation. J Clin Endocrinol Metab 2006;91:584–596.
48. Tissier F, Cavard C, Groussin L, et al. Mutations of beta-catenin in adrenocortical tumors: activation of the Wnt signaling pathway is a frequent event in both benign and malignant adrenocortical tumors. Cancer Res 2005;65:7622–7627.
49. Stratakis, C. Genetics of adrenocortical tumors: gatekeepers, landscapers and conductors in symphony. Trends Endocrinol Metab 2003;14:404–410.
50. Kirschner L, Kusewitt D, Matyakhina L, et al. A mouse model for the Carney complex tumor syndrome develops neoplasias in cyclic AMP-responsive tissues. Cancer Res 2005;65:4506–4514.
51. Griffin K, Kirschner L, Matyakhina L, et al. A transgenic mouse bearing an antisense construct of regulatory subunit type 1A of protein kinase A develops endocrine and other tumours: comparison with Carney complex and other PRKAR1A induced lesions. J Med Genet 2004;41:923–931.
52. Griffin K, Kirschner L, Matyakhina L, et al. Down-regulation of regulatory subunit type 1A of protein kinase A leads to endocrine and other tumors. Cancer Res 2004;64:8811–8815.
53. Bourdeau I, Stratakis, C. Cyclic AMP-dependent signaling aberrations in macronodular adrenal disease. Ann NY Acad Sci 2002;968:240–255.
54. Stratakis C, Kirschner L. Clinical and genetic analysis of primary bilateral adrenal diseases (micro- and macronodular disease) leading to Cushing syndrome. Horm Metab Res 1998;30:456–463.
55. Carney JA, Gaillard RC, Bertherat J, Stratakis CA. Familial micronodular adrenocortical disease, Cushing syndrome, and mutations of the gene encoding phosphodiesterase 11A4 (PDE11A). Am J Surg Pathol. 2010;34:547–55.

19 Glucocorticoid Resistance

Elisabeth F. C. van Rossum and Steven W. J. Lamberts

Contents

Summary

The syndrome of generalized glucocorticoid (GC) resistance is a familial disorder that is characterized by reduced cortisol effects, due to a GC receptor (GR) defect. This is compensated by increased activity of the hypothalamic-pituitary-adrenal (HPA)-axis, yielding elevated serum concentrations of cortisol, which does not result in the classical Cushingoid features related to cortisol overproduction. However, as a result of the increased levels of serum ACTH patients present with signs of adrenal overproduction of mineralocorticoids (hypertension and hypokalemic alkalosis) and, in females, of androgens (hirsutism, male pattern of baldness, menstrual irregularities). In some cases the underlying molecular basis has been elucidated, such as mutations in the gene coding for the GR, but in other patients the cause of GC resistance has not been revealed yet. We discuss the pathophysiology and provide tools for diagnosis and treatment of this rare hereditary syndrome.

Key Words: Glucocorticoid resistance, glucocorticoid receptor

From: *Contemporary Endocrinology: Cushing's Syndrome: Pathophysiology, Diagnosis and Treatment*
Edited by: M.D. Bronstein (ed.), DOI 10.1007/978-1-60327-449-4_19,

INTRODUCTION

The syndrome of familial GC resistance is rare and may frequently be undiagnosed since this syndrome is rather unknown and may result in several aspecific symptoms. At the tissue level, this disease is characterized by reduced cortisol action. As a result, a compensatory stimulation of ACTH secretion by the pituitary occurs, yielding elevated circulating levels of glucocorticoids (GCs), mineralocorticoids and androgens *(1, 2)*. This syndrome is inherited as an autosomal recessive or dominant disease.

In the last two decades a number of rare mutations of the *GR* gene have been reported, which explained dysfuntioning of the GR, resulting in clinical signs and symptoms of generalized cortisol resistance *(2)*. In healthy conditions the production of GCs is regulated by the hypothalamus, which responses to stimuli from the central nervous system *(3)*. In reaction to these stimuli the hypothalamus secretes corticotropin releasing hormone (CRH) and vasopressin *(4)*. Consequently, the pituitary is stimulated to secrete a large precursor protein, pro-opiomelanocortin (POMC), which is subsequently splitted into several hormones. One of these hormones is corticotropin (ACTH) *(5, 6)*. ACTH stimulates the adrenal glands to produce GCs (Fig. 1a). Because of GR defects, the normal effects of cortisol on target genes in the nucleus are impaired. Subsequently, the negative feedback of glucocorticoids at the level of the pituitary and the hypothalamus is diminished, ACTH levels rise, glucocorticoid production by the adrenals is elevated and cortisol binds with high affinity to the mineralocorticoid receptor (Fig. 1b). In addition, the elevated levels of ACTH stimulate adrenal

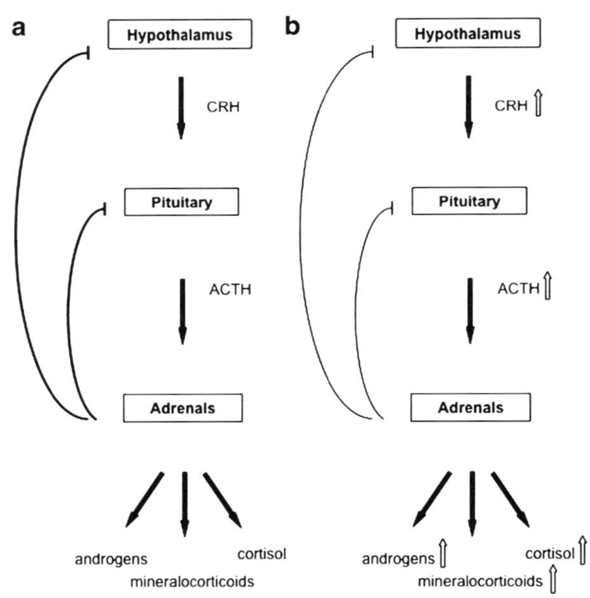

Fig. 1. Simplified scheme of the hypothalamic-pituitary-adrenal (HPA)-axis in the normal situation (**a**) and in conditions of the syndrome of Glucocorticoid (GC) resistance. (**b**) In healthy conditions, corticotrophin releasing hormone (CRH) is secreted by the hypothalamus, stimulating the pituitary to secrete adrenocorticotropin (ACTH). This latter hormone stimulates the adrenal glands to produce GCs (in humans mainly cortisol), mineralocorticoids and androgens. Cortisol exerts a negative feedback action on its own production, both at the pituitary level and at the hypothalamic level. In patients with GC resistance, the negative feedback mechanism, which is mediated by the glucocorticoid receptor (GR), is impaired. Consequently, the activation of the HPA-axis is increased and the production of the mentioned adrenal hormones is elevated, yielding symptoms of overproduction of mineralocorticoids and, important in women, androgens, but no signs of GC excess due to the defect GR.

production of androgens (dehydroepiandrosterone (DHEA), DHEA-sulfate and delta-4-androstenedione), as well as other adrenal corticosteroids with mineralocorticoid activity (corticosterone, and deoxycorticosterone).

CLINICAL FEATURES OF THE GLUCOCORTICOID RESISTANCE SYNDROME

The symptoms in patients with cortisol resistance result from the compensatory increased activation of the HPA-axis. Because of these elevated ACTH levels, patients experience symptoms related to an increased production of mineralocorticoids, leading to hypertension, hypokalemic alkalosis and fatigue. Female patients also suffer from symptoms of hyperandrogenism, such as hirsutism, male pattern of baldness and menstrual disturbances, because of increased production of androgens by the adrenals. In male patients the testicular production of androgens is much higher, and outweights the increased adrenal androgen production. In normal healthy conditions, organs in which mineralocorticoids have an important function (e.g. the kidneys) are protected from high cortisol levels by 11β-hydroxysteroid dehydrogenase type II. This enzyme converts intracellular cortisol into the inactive cortisone. In conditions of generalized cortisol resistance, cortisol levels exceed the capacity of this enzyme and can thereby contribute to increased mineralocorticoid effects. However, some patients with GC resistance are asymptomatic or complain only about chronic fatigue. The latter may be explained by a relative GC deficiency beacuse of insufficient compensation by the HPA-axis *(7)*.

PHYSIOLOGY OF THE GLUCOCORTICOID RECEPTOR

For mediating the effects of cortisol the glucocorticoid receptor (GR) is of crucial importance. This receptor is localized in the cytoplasm of virtually all cells in the human body. After binding of its ligand cortisol (or other glucocorticoids) a conformational change occurs, which leads to dissociation of the receptor from a large complex of proteins including heat shock protein 90 *(8, 9)*. This activated ligand-bound receptor translocates to the nucleus where it can act in several ways *(10)*. The GR can initiate transcription through binding to GC responsive elements of the target gene. The GR can also affect gene transcription through direct protein-protein interaction and can activate, as well as repress target gene expression *(11–13)*.

GLUCOCORTICOID RECEPTOR GENE MUTATIONS

In 1976 Vingerhoeds et al reported by the first patient with "spontaneous hypercortisolism without Cushing's syndrome" *(14)*. Further analysis showed a reduction in GR-ligand binding affinity in this patient. In his only mildly affected son and nephew a lesser reduction in affinity was measured. In a second stadium, the DNA sequence was analysed and an alteration of nucleotide 2054 was found. This mutation resulted in a substitution of valine for aspartic acid at amino acid residue 641 *(15)*. The finding that the index patient was homozygous for the mutation whereas the other family members carried only one mutated allele may explain the variability in clinical presentation within the family. Since this first patient, several other patients with GR mutations, leading to the GC resistance syndrome have been described (see Table 1 for overview of reported mutations and clinical presentation) *(15–24)*. Most mutations are located in the ligand binding domain *(25)*. These mutations in the GR yield decreased transactivating capacity *(17, 26)*, disturbances in ligand binding *(15, 27)*, diminished GR expression *(20)*, delayed nuclear translocation of the receptor, alterations in interaction with coactivators, alternative splicing or a combination of these changes in GR functioning *(16–26, 28)*. Previously, the molecular mechanisms of two previously reported mutants GRα R477H and GRα

Table 1
Overview of Mutations Resulting in Generalized Glucocorticoid Resistance (A Nonsuppressable Hypercortisolemia was Present in All Patients)

Domain in GR gene	*(non) coding region*	*Mutation*	*In vitro observations*	*Clinical phenotype*	*References*
DBD	Exon 4	R477H	Ligand affinity = Transactivating capacity ↓↓	Hypertension, hirsutism, fatigue, obesity	*(17, 26)*
DBD	Exon 5	I559N	Ligand affinity =, but binding sites by 50% ↓ Dominant-negative effect on the transactivating capacity of the wild-type GR Transrespressional capacity↓ mRNA GR copy number after EBV transformation ↓ Delayed nuclear translocation Abnormal interaction with the GR-interacting protein 1 coactivator	Hypertension,infertility, oligospermia, and secundary pituitary Cushing's disease	*(20, 24, 83, 84)*
DBD	Exon 5	V571A	Ligand affinity ↓ (6-fold) Transactivating capacity ↓ (10- to 50-fold less) Delayed nuclear translocation.	Hypertension, hypokaliemia, hyperandrogenism, female pseudohermaphroditism	*(21 84)*
LBD	Exon 6/ intron 6	4-Base deletion (2013del GAGT)	Transactivating capacity ↓ Removal of a donor splice site, expression of only one allele and a 50% decrease of GR protein on PBMLs and EBV transformed lymphoblasts	Hirsutism, menstrual irregularities, male-pattern baldness	*(19, 24)*
LBD	Exon 7	D641V	Ligand affinity ↓ (3-fold) Transactivating capacity ↓↓ Transrespressional capacity = Delayed nuclear translocation Abnormal interaction with the GR-interacting protein 1 coactivator mRNA GR copy number after EBV transformation ↓	Hypertension, hypokalemia	*(15, 24, 27, 81, 84)*

LBD	Exon 8	G679S	Ligand affinity ↓(2-fold) Transactivating capacity ↓	Asymptomatic, hypertension, hypokalemia hirsutism, fatigue	*(17, 26, 85)*
LBD	Intron 8	G → A, +81 bp exon 8 and C → G -9 bp exon 9	Transactivating capacity ↓ Transrespressional capacity = Expression of the GR-β splice variant↑(4-fold)	Despite low dose immunosuppressive medication 33 years after postmortem renal transplantation still uneventfull	*(24)*
LBD	Exon 9α	V729I	Ligand affinity ↓ Transactivating capacity ↓ (4-fold) Delayed nuclear translocation Abnormal interaction with the GR-interacting protein 1 coactivator	Isosexual precocious pseudopuberty in a boy, hyperandrogenism	*(16, 18, 84)*
LBD	Exon 9α	F737L	Ligand affinity ↓ (1.5-fold) Transactivating capacity ↓ Delayed nuclear translocation	Hypertension, hypokalemia	*(86)*
LBD	Exon 9α	I747M	Ligand affinity ↓ (2-fold) Transcriptional capacity ↓↓ (20- to 30-fold) Dominant negative effect on the wild-type GR Abnormal interaction with p160 coactivators due to an ineffective AF-2 domain	Asymptomatic, cystic acne, hirsutism, oligo-amenorrhea	*(22, 84)*
LBD	Exon 9α	N766N	Not tested	Hirsutism, fatigue, metabolic syndrome, dilated cardiomyopathy, gonadotropin and TSH insufficiency	*(17)*
LBD	Exon 9α	L773P	Ligand affinity ↓ (2.6-fold) Transactivating capacity ↓(2-fold) Delayed nuclear translocation Abnormal interaction with the GR-interacting protein 1 coactivator Dominant negative effect on the wild-type GR	Hypertension, chronic fatigue, anxiety, hyperandrogenism	*(23)*

DBD DNA binding domain; *EBV* Epstein–Barr virus; *GR* glucocorticoid receptor; *LBD* ligand binding domain; *PBML* peripheral blood mononuclear leukocytes; ↓ reduced; ↓↓ severely reduced; = unaltered

G679S, which both lead to systemic GC resistance, has been revealed by Charmandari et al. *(26)*. After the administration of dexamethasone the GRα G679S mutant showed a reduced capacity to stimulate transcription of the GC-responsive mouse mammary tumor virus promoter when compared with the wild-type GRα. The GRα R477H mutant displayed no transcriptional activity in these transient transfection assays. As demonstrated by dexamethasone binding assays Charmandari et al reported that the GRα G679S showed reduced ligand affinity, whereas the affinity of the GRα R477H was unaltered. The GRα R477H and G679S mutants displayed a slower translocation into the nucleus compared to the wild-type GRα. In contrast to the wild-type GRα and the GRα G679S, the GRα R477H mutant was not capable of binding to GC-response elements. Additionnally, it was shown that these mutant GRs interacted differentially with the GR-interacting protein 1 coactivator through its activation function (AF)-1 en AF-2.These studies show that a single nucleotide mutation in the GR can disturb various important events of the intracellular GC signaling pathway.

Recently, a male patient was reported, who underwent a postmortem renal transplantation 33 years ago for which he has been using only low-dose immunosuppressive medication (prednisone 7.5 mg/day, azathioprine 100 mg/day). Despite this minimal use of immunosuppressants he has been clinically well with only slightly impaired renal function today *(24)*, suggesting abnormal GC sensitivity. He did not suffer from Cushingoid side effects. DNA analysis revealed that this patient was heterozygous for two intronic *GR* gene mutations, of which one is close to the boundary of exon 9. This mutation resulted in an increased expression of the GR-β splice variant both in peripheral blood mononuclear leukocytes (PBMLs) and in in vitro EBV-transformed lymphoblasts. As has been extensively discussed in literature the GR-β is seems to be a dominant-negative inhibitor of the active GR-α and can thereby cause GC resistance, both an acquired as well as an inherited form of resistance *(24, 29, 30)*. Interestingly, the transactivation capacity of the GR was reduced in this patient, while transrepression (important for the immunosuppressive actions of GCs) was intact. The reduction in transactivation capacity may result in GC resistance at the negative feedback level in the pituitary and hypothalamus, and thereby causing a compensatory raise in endogenous cortisol levels. These relatively elevated GC levels could increase the immunosuppressive action of GCs, since the transrespression capacity seems to be normal *(24)*, which can explain the clinical picture of this posttransplantation patient.

Other patients with GC resistance due to a dysfunctioning GR signaling have been reported, in which genetic alterations of the GR have not been studied yet *(7, 31–33)*. Some additional mechanisms leading to GC resistance, which have been postulated, are as follows: increased expression of 90-kDa heat shock protein (hsp90), one of the chaperone proteins *(34)*, altered phosphorylation status, hormone-induced conformation changes of the GR and nuclear transformation *(35)* and thermolability of the GR *(7)*.

In contrast to GC resistance also hypersensitivity to endogenous cortisol has been reported, resulting in Cushing's syndrome despite hypocortisolemia *(36)* or normal cortisol levels *(37)*. Recently, a female patient was reported, who presented with symptoms of tissue-specific glucocorticoid hypersensitivity. Charmandari et al found a novel, heterozygous G to C substitution in exon 2 of the *GR* gene, yielding an aspartic acid to histidine substitution in the amino-terminal domain of the GRα *(38)*. In vitro studies showed that the mutant receptor GRα (D401H) improved the transcriptional activity of glucocorticoid-responsive genes, which may explain the enhanced GC sensitivity in some tissues of this patient.

UNEXPLAINED GLUCOCORTICOID RESISTANCE

As described in the previous paragraph several underlying molecular mechanisms of patients with GC resistance have been revealed. However, there are a substantial number of patients with GC resistance of unknown origin, showing no mutations in the *GR* gene. In the past, several patients were reported, who all demonstrated an insufficient suppression after 1 mg dexamethasone and hyperandrogenism, but no classical Cushingoid features and an intact diurnal cortisol rhythm *(39)* and thus meeting the criteria of GC resistance. Two of these patients also suffered from chronic fatigue, of which one improved after treatment with dexamethasone. Analysis of the coding regions of the *GR* gene revealed only in two patients the ER22/23EK (two linked single nucleotide mutations in exon 2) alteration, which is also present in the normal population (frequency 5–12%) and later appeared to be associated with a mild GC resistance in healthy individuals *(28, 40)*. The importance of the presence of the ER22/23EK in patients with generalized GC resistance is unclear. No other mutations of the *GR* gene were found in these patients.

Previously, 12 unrelated patients with generalized cortisol resistance, which was defined by nonsuppression after the administration of dexamethasone, were studied by Ruiz et al. *(17)*. DNA analysis revealed in four of these patients a previously reported polymorphism (N766N), consisting of an AAT to AAC change both coding for an asparagine, of which the clinical implications are not known at present. Although it is a silent polymorphism, a functional role cannot be ruled out yet. In two of these 12 GC resistant patients, mutations in the *GR* gene were observed (R477H and G679S, see also Table 1). In vitro assays showed that these mutations lead to an impaired receptor function. However, the exact molecular background of the other patients with clinical GC resistance remains to be elucidated at present.

Russcher et al reported nine patients with clinically abnormal GC sensitivity (8 GC resistance and one with GC hypersensitivity) *(24)*. For three of these patients mutations in the *GR* gene have been demonstrated to underlay the GC resistance *(15, 19, 20)*. In one patient the above mentioned ER22/23EK polymorphism *(39)* without other *GR* gene mutations was present, and in one patient two intronic mutations, leading to increased GRβ expression, were found. However, *GR* gene analysis of the other five patients yielded no mutations, although they clearly suffered from systemic GC resistance. Thus, the pathophysiology of their GC resistance remains to be revealed.

In a recent report, Drigo et al demonstrated a 16-year-old girl with Takayasu's arteritis *(34)*. Interestingly, this patient did not clinically or biochemically respond to longterm treatment with high dose GCs. In addition, she did not suffer from any adverse effects, suggesting generalized GC resistance. Further analysis showed a reduced number of GR on peripheral blood mononuclear leukocytes (PBMLs), while the affinity of the receptor was unchanged. Partial sequencing of the *GR* gene (exon 4 to 9α) did not yield any mutations. However, in PBMLs of this patient an increased expression of hsp90 was found. Hsp90 proteins are known to have an important function in the stabilization of the GR in a conformation, which makes the GR available for ligand binding *(41)*. Subsequently, alterations in these hsp proteins could theoretically lead to GC resistance *(42)*. The mRNA expression levels of hsp90 beta in cultured fibroblasts from GC resistant patients with and without GR defects were studied by Bronnegard et al. Interestingly, they found that the GR defects are related to increased hsp90 beta mRNA levels, but no increase was observed in hsp90 levels in the patients with an intact GR *(43)*.

OTHER FORMS OF GC RESISTANCE

Classical generalized GC resistance, as caused by *GR* gene mutations, is not the only form of resistance to GCs. GC resistance can be acquired, as occurs in some types of neoplasms; ectopic ACTH syndrome *(44)*, pituitary tumors (Nelson's syndrome) *(45)*, and hematological malignancies *(46, 47)*. In many other diseases also forms of GC resistance have been demonstrated, e.g. major depression *(48)*, asthma *(49, 50)*, rheumatoid arthritis *(51)*, inflammatory bowel disease *(52)*, autoimmune hepatitis *(53)*, AIDS *(54)*, and Cushing's disease *(55, 56)*. Additionally, in septic shock a transient state of GC resistance has been reported *(57)*. By administering RU486, a GR antagonist, or chemotherapeutic treatment of leukemic cell line, resulting in deletions of the GR gene, GC resistance can also iatrogenically be induced *(46, 58)*.

Theoretically, a subtle systemic resistance to endogenous GCs could predispose to any disease, which responds well to exogenously administered GCs. In this view, auto-immune diseases, e.g. rheumatoid arthritis, asthma and systemic lupus erythematosus, provide good possibilities to study this potential enhanced vulnerability. Resistance to the immunosuppressive effects of GCs, including endogenous cortisol, may enhance activity of the immune system. The response of 39 patients with lupus nephritis to GCs was studied by Jiang et al. They examined the function of the GR, and the molecular structure of the GR in PBML *(59)*. ACTH or GC levels and ligand affinity of GR did not differ between the lupus patients and controls. Interestingly, GR number on mononuclear cells of lupus patients was reduced compared to the controls. In eight of the 39 studied lupus nephritis patients a polymorphism in exon 9 of the GR was found. This variant consists of an adenine insertion at the 2439 base pair of the *GR* gene, resulting in an additional 20 amino acids being translated into the GR protein. This phase-shift mutation, may affect GR functioning. The polymorphism in exon 9 and the lower GR number may be related to a slight GC resistance, and thereby contribute to the pathophysiology in lupus nephritis.

In addition, in asthma, GC resistance is a well-known clinical problem *(49, 50)*. Unlike most cases with familial GC resistance syndrome GR gene mutations seem not to cause this steroid-resistence in asthma *(60)*. Several underlying mechanisms leading to steroid-resistant asthma have been postulated: e.g increased expression of the GRβ splice variant, which is supposed to exert a dominant-negative effect on the GRα *(61, 62)*, reduced affinity in inflammatory cells (such as T-lymphocytes) induced by certain cytokines (e.g. interleukin (IL)-2, IL-4, IL-13) yielding local GC resistance *(63, 64)*, and impaired nuclear localization *(65)*, which may be related to alterations in GR phosphorylation *(64)*. Another factor, which has been suggested to be involved in the development of central GC resistance during inflammation, is leukemia inhibitory factor (LIF) *(66)*. This is a pleiotropic cytokine, which is stimulated in peripheral and cerebral tissues during inflammatory or chronic autoimmune diseases, and is thereby a potent stimulator of the HPA-axis. Animal studies showed that LIF treatment markedly decreased GR mRNA levels in the murine hypothalamus and pituitary and decreased GR protein levels, suggesting that LIF maintains the HPA axis activation by decreasing GR expression and may thereby contribute to GC resistance.

MILD GLUCOCORTICOID RESISTANCE DUE TO POLYMORPHISMS IN THE GLUCOCORTICOID RECEPTOR GENE

Not only in patients, but also within the healthy, normal population variation in GC sensitivity has been demonstrated *(67, 68)*. Several single nucleotide polymorphisms in the GR gene have been found to be at least partially responsible for this variability in GC sensitivity *(69)*. The ER22/23EK polymorphism seems to cause a mild GC resistance and results in reduced GC effects in many organs and metabolic processes, yielding increased insulin sensitivity, lower total and LDL-cholesterol levels *(40, 70)*, smaller waist in females and greater height and muscle mass in males *(40, 70, 71)*. In elderly, ER22/23EK variant has been shown to be associated with lower C-reactive protein levels, an increased survival rate *(72)*, and unexpectedly, higher HbA1C levels *(71)*. In vitro experiments showed that the ER22/23EK polymorphism resulted in a reduction of transactivating capacity, while transrepressing capacity of the GR was unaltered *(28)*. Recently, the underlying molecular mechanism of this polymorphism has been reported *(73)*: an increased amount of the GR-A translational isoform is formed. This GR-A isoform is known to have a lower transcriptional activity compared to the shorter GR-B isoform *(74)*, which can explain the subtle GC resistance.

Another polymorphism has been reported in the 3' UTR of exon 9β, which is the terminal exon of the mRNA of the GRβ splice variant. This variant consists of an A to G nucleotide substitution. Several previous studies showed a dominant negative effect of the GRβ splice variant on GRα functioning *(75, 76)*. Because of the nucleotide substitution in exon 9β an "ATTTA" motif is changed into "GTTTA." In vitro this yielded more stable GRβ mRNA and in vivo possibly a relative GC resistance and increased risk of developing rheumatoid arthritis *(77)*. After suppression with a low dose of dexamethasone, cortisol concentrations were not different between individuals carrying the various 9β genotypes *(78)*. However, in vitro experiments demonstrated that the 9β genotype may have diminished transrepressional activity with normal transactivation *(79)*. In children with idiopathic nephrotic syndrome two GR haplotypes were reported to be related to GC resistance *(80)*. Interestingly, two other polymorphisms of the GR (N363S and *BclI*) were found to increase GC sensitivity and are associated in some populations, but not all, with an increased fatmass or body mass index and lower amount of lean mass (*69*, for review).

DIAGNOSIS OF GLUCOCORTICOID RESISTANCE

The main characteristics of the syndrome of glucocorticoid resistance are hypercortisolism accompanied by hypertension, hypokalemia, as signs of overproduction of mineralocorticoids, and in particular in females, also hyperandrogenism (acne, hirsutism, male pattern of baldness and menstrual irregularities, infertility). More importantly, GC resistant patients do not suffer from the classical Cushingoid effects, such as a moon face, abdominal obesity with red striae, hyperglycemia, myopathy etcetera, despite their elevated cortisol levels. The chronic fatigue has also been suggested to result from a relative GC deficiency because of insufficient compensation for certain target tissues *(7)*. Patients can also be asymptomatic *(1, 22)*. Figure 2 shows a practical scheme showing clinical and biochemical tests, which can be used for the diagnosis of GC resistance.

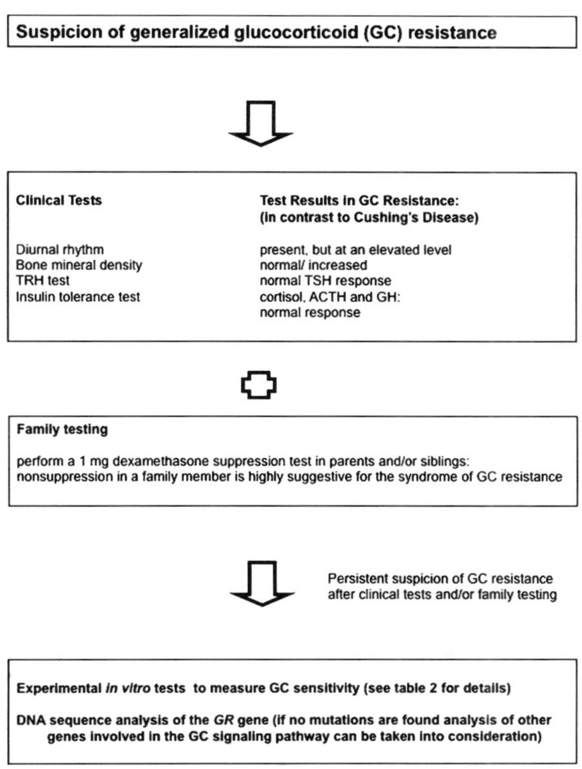

Fig. 2. Flow-chart of differential diagnostic considerations of suspected generalized GC resistance.

Typically, patients with GC resistance have elevated plasma ACTH and serum cortisol concentrations. In contrast to Cushing's syndrome, the diurnal rhythm, however, is maintained, although it is set to an elevated level *(15, 81, 82)*. After an overnight suppression test with 1 mg dexamethasone, cortisol levels are not adequately suppressed. No exact cut-off level is defined, however, above 70 nmol/l and even more above 140 nmol/l is suggestive for GC resistance. The urinary excretion of cortisol is increased. As a result of the compensatory elevated ACTH concentrations serum concentrations of adrenal androgens (dehydroepiandrosterone (DHEA), DHEA-S, and androstenedione) and of ACTH-dependent mineralocorticoids (cortisol, deoxycorticosterone, and corticosterone) are also increased. The adrenal glands are normal to slightly enlarged, which is aspecific.

To differentiate between GC resistance and Cushing's disease a helpful tool to monitor tissue effects of cortisol is measurement of bone mineral density (BMD). In patients with Cushing's disease BMD is decreased, but the BMD is normal or even increased in patients with GC resistance. This may be due to an absent deleterious effect of hypercortisolism together with in most instances, increased androgen production in the syndrome of GC resistance.

In the clinical and biochemical presentation of the disease considerable variability has been demonstrated. When the diagnosis is difficult based on the mentioned parameters indirect evidence for GC resistance can be obtained by a normal response of serum TSH to TRH administration and/or the demonstration of a normal response of growth hormone to an insulin induced hypoglycemia, which are invariably impaired in patients with Cushing's disease. Additional tests to confirm the diagnosis of GC resistance can be performed in an experimental setting, see Table 2 *(24)*.

Besides the various mentioned tests to diagnose hereditary GC resistance, a quick and easy manner to confirm the diagnosis could be performing dexamethasone suppression tests in family members.

TREATMENT OF GLUCOCORTICOID RESISTANCE

There is no standard therapy for patients suffering from GC resistance. The importance of treatment is that it should be individually directed to the signs and symptoms of the patient. In GC resistance, early morning ACTH levels can be suppressed by a low dose of dexamethasone taken around midnight.

Table 2
Experimental Laboratory Tests to Measure Indicators of GC Sensitivity

Method	*Measurements*
Analysis of GR characteristics	Number of GR per cell (n) and receptor affinity (dissociation constant (K_D)) *(2)*, coding sequence *(87)*, GR expression and mRNA splice variants (GR-α, GR-β, GR-P) by real-time quantitative PCR *(88)*
Evaluation of ex vivo GC sensitivity by measuring responses of target genes, which are sensitive to endogenous GCs	Measuring GC-induced leucine zipper and interleukin-2 *(89)*
Measuring the inhibition of mitogen stimulated proliferation	Phytohemagglutinin-stimulated incorporation of ^{3}H-thymidine or concanavalin A) by dexamethasone *(2, 68)*
Obtaining permanent cell lines (before starting treatment)	Transforming B lymphocytes with Ebstein-Barr virus. This test has recently been shown to be able to serve as a sensitive bio-assay, since the upregulation of the number of GR during culturing strongly correlates with GC sensitivity *(24, 90)*

GR glucocorticoid receptor; *GC* glucocorticoid

Hereby the ACTH-related activation of adrenal mineralocorticoid and androgen production is reduced. The most beneficial treatment seems to titrate to a dose of dexamethasone, which normalizes androgens, blood pressure and serum potassium. Once normalization of mineralocorticoids and androgens is reached the dexamethasone dose to maintain this suppression can be carefully titrated down. To taper the dose of dexamethasone over time is important to minimize the risks of an additive effect of dexamethasone and remaining endogenous cortisol production. To check potential effects of too high doses of dexamethasone in combination with the endogenous cortisol production, a yearly measurement of BMD is recommended. Treatment can be started with a dose of about 1 mg dexamethasone at night. This dose can be slowly decreased to 0.5 mg or even 0.25 mg/day. With respect to the treatment of hypertension, thiazide or loop diuretics should not be used because of their potassium-losing effects. To adequately control blood pressure, aldosterone antagonists are recommended, which have additional beneficial effects because of their potassium sparing and antiandrogenic effects.

REFERENCES

1. Charmandari E, Kino T, Chrousos GP. Familial/sporadic glucocorticoid resistance: clinical phenotype and molecular mechanisms. Ann N Y Acad Sci 2004;1024:168–181.
2. Lamberts SW, Koper JW, Biemond P, den Holder FH, de Jong FH. Cortisol receptor resistance: the variability of its clinical presentation and response to treatment. J Clin Endocrinol Metab 1992;74:313–321.
3. Chrousos GP, Gold PW. The concepts of stress and stress system disorders. Overview of physical and behavioral homeostasis. JAMA 1992;267:1244–1252.
4. Taylor AL, Fishman LM. Corticotropin-releasing hormone. N Engl J Med 1988;319:213–222.
5. Antoni FA. Hypothalamic control of adrenocorticotropin secretion: advances since the discovery of 41-residue corticotropin-releasing factor. Endocr Rev 1986;7:351–378.
6. Lundblad JR, Roberts JL. Regulation of proopiomelanocortin gene expression in pituitary. Endocr Rev 1988;9:135–158.
7. Bronnegard M, Werner S, Gustafsson JA. Primary cortisol resistance associated with a thermolabile glucocorticoid receptor in a patient with fatigue as the only symptom. J Clin Invest 1986;78:1270–1278.
8. Pratt WB, Toft DO. Steroid receptor interactions with heat shock protein and immunophilin chaperones. Endocr Rev 1997;18:306–360.
9. Toft DO. Recent advances in the study of hsp90 structure and mechanism of action. Trends Endocrinol Metab 1998;9:238–243.
10. Schaaf MJ, Cidlowski JA. Molecular determinants of glucocorticoid receptor mobility in living cells: the importance of ligand affinity. Mol Cell Biol 2003;23:1922–1934.
11. Diamond MI, Miner JN, Yoshinaga SK, Yamamoto KR. Transcription factor interactions: selectors of positive or negative regulation from a single DNA element. Science 1990;249:1266–1272.
12. Yang-Yen HF, Chambard JC, Sun YL, et al. Transcriptional interference between c-Jun and the glucocorticoid receptor: mutual inhibition of DNA binding due to direct protein-protein interaction. Cell 1990;62:1205–1215.
13. Yudt MR, Cidlowski JA. The glucocorticoid receptor: coding a diversity of proteins and responses through a single gene. Mol Endocrinol 2002;16:1719–1726.
14. Vingerhoeds AC, Thijssen JH, Schwarz F. Spontaneous hypercortisolism without Cushing's syndrome. J Clin Endocrinol Metab 1976;43:1128–1133.
15. Hurley DM, Accili D, Stratakis CA, et al. Point mutation causing a single amino acid substitution in the hormone binding domain of the glucocorticoid receptor in familial glucocorticoid resistance. J Clin Invest 1991;87:680–686.
16. Brufsky AM, Malchoff DM, Javier EC, Reardon G, Rowe D, Malchoff CD. A glucocorticoid receptor mutation in a subject with primary cortisol resistance. Trans Assoc Am Physicians 1990;103:53–63.
17. Ruiz M, Lind U, Gafvels M, et al. Characterization of two novel mutations in the glucocorticoid receptor gene in patients with primary cortisol resistance. Clin Endocrinol (Oxf) 2001;55:363–371.
18. Malchoff DM, Brufsky A, Reardon G, et al. A mutation of the glucocorticoid receptor in primary cortisol resistance. J Clin Invest 1993;91:1918–1925.
19. Karl M, Lamberts SW, Detera-Wadleigh SD, et al. Familial glucocorticoid resistance caused by a splice site deletion in the human glucocorticoid receptor gene. J Clin Endocrinol Metab 1993;76:683–689.
20. Karl M, Lamberts SW, Koper JW, et al. Cushing's disease preceded by generalized glucocorticoid resistance: clinical consequences of a novel, dominant-negative glucocorticoid receptor mutation. Proc Assoc Am Physicians 1996;108:296–307.

21. Mendonca BB, Leite MV, de Castro M, et al. Female pseudohermaphroditism caused by a novel homozygous missense mutation of the GR gene. J Clin Endocrinol Metab 2002;87:1805–1809.
22. Vottero A, Kino T, Combe H, Lecomte P, Chrousos GP. A novel, C-terminal dominant negative mutation of the GR causes familial glucocorticoid resistance through abnormal interactions with p160 steroid receptor coactivators. J Clin Endocrinol Metab 2002;87:2658–2667.
23. Charmandari E, Raji A, Kino T, et al. A novel point mutation in the ligand-binding domain (LBD) of the human glucocorticoid receptor (hGR) causing generalized glucocorticoid resistance: the importance of the C terminus of hGR LBD in conferring transactivational activity. J Clin Endocrinol Metab 2005;90:3696–3705.
24. Russcher H, Smit P, van Rossum EF, et al. Strategies for the characterization of disorders in cortisol sensitivity. J Clin Endocrinol Metab 2006;91:694–701.
25. Lamberts SW. Hereditary glucocorticoid resistance. Ann Endocrinol (Paris) 2001;62:164–167.
26. Charmandari E, Kino T, Ichijo T, Zachman K, Alatsatianos A, Chrousos GP. Functional characterization of the natural human glucocorticoid receptor (hGR) mutants hGRalphaR477H and hGRalphaG679S associated with generalized glucocorticoid resistance. J Clin Endocrinol Metab 2006;91:1535–1543.
27. de Lange P, Koper JW, Huizenga NA, et al. Differential hormone-dependent transcriptional activation and -repression by naturally occurring human glucocorticoid receptor variants. Mol Endocrinol 1997;11:1156–1164.
28. Russcher H, Smit P, van den Akker EL, et al. Two polymorphisms in the glucocorticoid receptor gene directly affect glucocorticoid-regulated gene expression. J Clin Endocrinol Metab 2005;90:5804–5810.
29. Leung DY, Hamid Q, Vottero A, et al. Association of glucocorticoid insensitivity with increased expression of glucocorticoid receptor beta. J Exp Med 1997;186:1567–1574.
30. de Lange P, Segeren CM, Koper JW, et al. Expression in hematological malignancies of a glucocorticoid receptor splice variant that augments glucocorticoid receptor-mediated effects in transfected cells. Cancer Res 2001;61:3937–3941.
31. Iida S, Gomi M, Moriwaki K, et al. Primary cortisol resistance accompanied by a reduction in glucocorticoid receptors in two members of the same family. J Clin Endocrinol Metab 1985;60:967–971.
32. Nawata H, Sekiya K, Higuchi K, Kato K, Ibayashi H. Decreased deoxyribonucleic acid binding of glucocorticoid-receptor complex in cultured skin fibroblasts from a patient with the glucocorticoid resistance syndrome. J Clin Endocrinol Metab 1987;65:219–226.
33. Vecsei P, Frank K, Haack D, et al. Primary glucocorticoid receptor defect with likely familial involvement. Cancer Res 1989;49:2220s-2221s.
34. Drigo I, Saccari A, Bacchin C, et al. Glucocorticoid resistance in a girl with Takayasu's arteritis. Ann Rheum Dis 2006;65:689–691.
35. Bamberger CM, Schulte HM, Chrousos GP. Molecular determinants of glucocorticoid receptor function and tissue sensitivity to glucocorticoids. Endocr Rev 1996;17:245–261.
36. Iida S, Nakamura Y, Fujii H, et al. A patient with hypocortisolism and Cushing's syndrome-like manifestations: cortisol hyperreactive syndrome. J Clin Endocrinol Metab 1990;70:729–737.
37. Newfield RS, Kalaitzoglou G, Licholai T, et al. Normocortisolemic Cushing's syndrome initially presenting with increased glucocorticoid receptor numbers. J Clin Endocrinol Metab 2000;85:14–21.
38. Charmandari E, Ichijo T, Jubiz W, et al. A novel point mutation in the amino terminal domain of the human glucocorticoid receptor (hGR) gene enhancing hGR-mediated gene expression. J Clin Endocrinol Metab 2008;93:4963–4968.
39. Huizenga NA, de Lange P, Koper JW, et al. Five patients with biochemical and/or clinical generalized glucocorticoid resistance without alterations in the glucocorticoid receptor gene. J Clin Endocrinol Metab 2000;85:2076–2081.
40. van Rossum EFC, Koper JW, Huizenga NA, et al. A polymorphism in the glucocorticoid receptor gene, which decreases sensitivity to glucocorticoids in vivo, is associated with low insulin and cholesterol levels. Diabetes 2002;51:3128–3134.
41. Pratt WB. The role of heat shock proteins in regulating the function, folding, and trafficking of the glucocorticoid receptor. J Biol Chem 1993;268:21455–21458.
42. Kang KI, Meng X, Devin-Leclerc J, et al. The molecular chaperone Hsp90 can negatively regulate the activity of a glucocorticosteroid-dependent promoter. Proc Natl Acad Sci U S A 1999;96:1439–1444.
43. Bronnegard M, Boos J, Marcus C, McGuire J, Werner S, Gustafsson JA. Expression of hsp90 beta messenger ribonucleic acid in patients with familial glucocorticoid resistance – correlation to receptor status. J Steroid Biochem Mol Biol 1995;52:345–349.
44. Gaitan D, DeBold CR, Turney MK, Zhou P, Orth DN, Kovacs WJ. Glucocorticoid receptor structure and function in an adrenocorticotropin-secreting small cell lung cancer. Mol Endocrinol 1995;9:1193–1201.
45. Karl M, Von Wichert G, Kempter E, et al. Nelson's syndrome associated with a somatic frame shift mutation in the glucocorticoid receptor gene. J Clin Endocrinol Metab 1996;81:124–129.

46. Palmer LA, Hukku B, Harmon JM. Human glucocorticoid receptor gene deletion following exposure to cancer chemotherapeutic drugs and chemical mutagens. Cancer Res 1992;52:6612–6618.
47. Hillmann AG, Ramdas J, Multanen K, Norman MR, Harmon JM. Glucocorticoid receptor gene mutations in leukemic cells acquired in vitro and in vivo. Cancer Res 2000;60:2056–2062.
48. Pariante CM. Glucocorticoid receptor function in vitro in patients with major depression. Stress 2004;7:209–219.
49. Sher E, Leung D, Surs W, Harbeck R, Nimmagadda S, Szefler S. Steroid resistant asthma: Cellular mechanisms contributing to inadequate response to glucocorticoid therapy. J Clin Invest 1995;93:33–39.
50. Ito K, Chung KF, Adcock IM. Update on glucocorticoid action and resistance. J Allergy Clin Immunol 2006;117:522–543.
51. Chikanza IC, Petrou P, Kingsley G, Chrousos G, Panayi GS. Defective hypothalamic response to immune and inflammatory stimuli in patients with rheumatoid arthritis. Arthritis Rheum 1992;35:1281–1288.
52. Munkholm P, Langholz E, Davidsen M, Binder V. Frequency of glucocorticoid resistance and dependency in Crohn's disease. Gut 1994;35:360–362.
53. Rai T, Ohira H, Tojo J, et al. Expression of human glucocorticoid receptor in lymphocytes of patients with autoimmune hepatitis. Hepatol Res 2004;29:148–152.
54. Norbiato G, Bevilacqua M, Vago T, et al. Cortisol resistance in acquired immunodeficiency syndrome. J Clin Endocrinol Metab 1992;74:608–613.
55. Lamberts SW. Glucocorticoid receptors and Cushing's disease. Mol Cell Endocrinol 2002;197:69–72.
56. Huizenga NA, De Herder WW, Koper JW, et al. Decreased ligand affinity rather than glucocorticoid receptor down-regulation in patients with endogenous Cushing's syndrome. Eur J Endocrinol 2000;142:472–476.
57. Molijn GJ, Spek JJ, van Uffelen JC, et al. Differential adaptation of glucocorticoid sensitivity of peripheral blood mononuclear leukocytes in patients with sepsis or septic shock. J Clin Endocrinol Metab 1995;80:1799–1803.
58. Lamberts SW, Koper JW, de Jong FH. The endocrine effects of long-term treatment with mifepristone (RU 486). J Clin Endocrinol Metab 1991;73:187–191.
59. Jiang T, Liu S, Tan M, et al. The phase-shift mutation in the glucocorticoid receptor gene: potential etiologic significance of neuroendocrine mechanisms in lupus nephritis. Clin Chim Acta 2001;313:113–117.
60. Lane SJ, Arm JP, Staynov DZ, Lee TH. Chemical mutational analysis of the human glucocorticoid receptor cDNA in glucocorticoid-resistant bronchial asthma. Am J Respir Cell Mol Biol 1994;11:42–48.
61. Sousa AR, Lane SJ, Cidlowski JA, Staynov DZ, Lee TH. Glucocorticoid resistance in asthma is associated with elevated in vivo expression of the glucocorticoid receptor beta-isoform. J Allergy Clin Immunol 2000;105:943–950.
62. Goleva E, Li LB, Eves PT, Strand MJ, Martin RJ, Leung DY. Increased glucocorticoid receptor beta alters steroid response in glucocorticoid-insensitive asthma. Am J Respir Crit Care Med 2006;173:607–616.
63. Leung DY, Spahn JD, Szefler SJ. Immunologic basis and management of steroid-resistant asthma. Allergy Asthma Proc 1999;20:9–14.
64. Irusen E, Matthews JG, Takahashi A, Barnes PJ, Chung KF, Adcock IM. p38 Mitogen-activated protein kinase-induced glucocorticoid receptor phosphorylation reduces its activity: role in steroid-insensitive asthma. J Allergy Clin Immunol 2002;109:649–657.
65. Matthews JG, Ito K, Barnes PJ, Adcock IM. Defective glucocorticoid receptor nuclear translocation and altered histone acetylation patterns in glucocorticoid-resistant patients. J Allergy Clin Immunol 2004;113:1100–1108.
66. Kariagina A, Zonis S, Afkhami M, Romanenko D, Chesnokova V. Leukemia inhibitory factor regulates glucocorticoid receptor expression in the hypothalamic-pituitary-adrenal axis. Am J Physiol Endocrinol Metab 2005;289: E857—E863.
67. Huizenga NA, Koper JW, de Lange P, et al. Interperson variability but intraperson stability of baseline plasma cortisol concentrations, and its relation to feedback sensitivity of the hypothalamo-pituitary-adrenal axis to a low dose of dexamethasone in elderly individuals. J Clin Endocrinol Metab 1998;83:47–54.
68. Chriguer RS, Elias LL, da Silva IM, Jr., Vieira JG, Moreira AC, de Castro M. Glucocorticoid sensitivity in young healthy individuals: in vitro and in vivo studies. J Clin Endocrinol Metab 2005;90:5978–5984.
69. van Rossum EFC, Lamberts SWJ. Polymorphisms in the glucocorticoid receptor gene and their associations with metabolic parameters and body composition. Recent Prog Horm Res 2004;59:333–357.
70. van Rossum EFC, Voorhoeve PG, te Velde SJ, et al. The ER22/23EK Polymorphism in the Glucocorticoid Receptor Gene is Associated with a Beneficial Body Composition and Muscle Strength in Young Adults. J Clin Endocrinol Metab 2004;89:4004–4009.
71. Kuningas M, Mooijaart SP, Slagboom PE, Westendorp RG, van Heemst D. Genetic variants in the glucocorticoid receptor gene (NR3C1) and cardiovascular disease risk. The Leiden 85-plus Study. Biogerontology 2006;7(4):231–238.
72. van Rossum EFC, Feelders RA, Van Den Beld AW, et al. Association of the ER22/23EK polymorphism in the glucocorticoid receptor gene with survival and C-reactive protein levels in elderly men. Am J Med 2004;117:158–162.

73. Russcher H, van Rossum EF, de Jong FH, Brinkmann AO, Lamberts SW, Koper JW. Increased expression of the glucocorticoid receptor-A translational isoform as a result of the ER22/23EK polymorphism. Mol Endocrinol 2005 19: 1687–1696.
74. Yudt MR, Cidlowski JA. Molecular identification and characterization of a and b forms of the glucocorticoid receptor. Mol Endocrinol 2001;15:1093–1103.
75. Bamberger CM, Bamberger AM, de Castro M, Chrousos GP. Glucocorticoid receptor beta, a potential endogenous inhibitor of glucocorticoid action in humans. J Clin Invest 1995;95:2435–2441.
76. Oakley RH, Sar M, Cidlowski JA. The human glucocorticoid receptor beta isoform. Expression, biochemical properties, and putative function. J Biol Chem 1996;271:9550–9559.
77. Derijk RH, Schaaf MJ, Turner G, et al. A human glucocorticoid receptor gene variant that increases the stability of the glucocorticoid receptor beta-isoform mRNA is associated with rheumatoid arthritis. J Rheumatol 2001;28:2383–2388.
78. Stevens A, Ray DW, Zeggini E, et al. Glucocorticoid sensitivity is determined by a specific glucocorticoid receptor haplotype. J Clin Endocrinol Metab 2004;89:892–897.
79. van den Akker EL, Russcher H, van Rossum EF, et al. Glucocorticoid receptor polymorphism affects transrepression but not transactivation. J Clin Endocrinol Metab 2006;91:2800–2803.
80. Ye JW, Ding J, Huang JP, et al. [Analysis on association of glucocorticoid receptor gene polymorphism with steroid-resistance in idiopathic nephrotic syndrome of children]. Zhonghua Er Ke Za Zhi 2003;41:661–665.
81. Chrousos GP, Vingerhoeds A, Brandon D, et al. Primary cortisol resistance in man. A glucocorticoid receptor-mediated disease. J Clin Invest 1982;69:1261–1269.
82. Lamberts SW, Poldermans D, Zweens M, de Jong FH. Familial cortisol resistance: differential diagnostic and therapeutic aspects. J Clin Endocrinol Metab 1986;63:1328–1333.
83. Kino T, Stauber RH, Resau JH, Pavlakis GN, Chrousos GP. Pathologic human GR mutant has a transdominant negative effect on the wild-type GR by inhibiting its translocation into the nucleus: importance of the ligand-binding domain for intracellular GR trafficking. J Clin Endocrinol Metab 2001;86:5600–5608.
84. Charmandari E, Kino T, Souvatzoglou E, Vottero A, Bhattacharyya N, Chrousos GP. Natural glucocorticoid receptor mutants causing generalized glucocorticoid resistance: molecular genotype, genetic transmission, and clinical phenotype. J Clin Endocrinol Metab 2004;89:1939–1949.
85. Raef H, Baitei EY, Zou M, Shi Y. Genotype-phenotype correlation in a family with primary cortisol resistance: possible modulating effect of the ER22/23EK polymorphism. Eur J Endocrinol 2008;158:577–582.
86. Charmandari E, Kino T, Ichijo T, et al. A novel point mutation in helix 11 of the ligand-binding domain of the human glucocorticoid receptor gene causing generalized glucocorticoid resistance. J Clin Endocrinol Metab 2007;92:3986–3990.
87. Koper JW, Stolk RP, de Lange P, et al. Lack of association between five polymorphisms in the human glucocorticoid receptor gene and glucocorticoid resistance. Hum Genet 1997;99:663–668.
88. ter Borg PC, Hagendorf A, van Buuren HR, Koper JW, Lamberts SW. A pilot study exploring the role of glucocorticoid receptor variants in primary biliary cirrhosis and primary sclerosing cholangitis. Neth J Med 2004;62:326–331.
89. Smit P, Russcher H, de Jong FH, Brinkmann AO, Lamberts SW, Koper JW. Differential regulation of synthetic glucocorticoids on gene expression levels of glucocorticoid-induced leucine zipper and interleukin-2. J Clin Endocrinol Metab 2005;90:2994–3000.
90. Tomita M, Brandon DD, Chrousos GP, et al. Glucocorticoid receptors in Epstein-Barr virus-transformed lymphocytes from patients with glucocorticoid resistance and a glucocorticoid-resistant New World primate species. J Clin Endocrinol Metab 1986;62:1145–1154.

20 Post-operative Replacement and Assessment of HPA Axis Recovery in Cushing's Syndrome

Sibylle Kohler, Niki Karavitaki, and John A. H. Wass

CONTENTS

SUMMARY

The management of patients following surgery for pituitary, adrenal or ectopic Cushing's syndrome is challenging, as adequate glucocorticoid replacement post-operatively is crucial to avoid hypoadrenalism. Following discharge from hospital, patients not only need to be seen regularly to assess for recurrence of Cushing's syndrome but also to identify patients with recovery of the HPA axis. This chapter aims to give an overview of current opinions on how to assess Cushing's patients following surgery and to offer guidelines on their treatment.

Key Words: Post-operative, Hypothalamo–pituitary–adrenal axis, ACTH axis, Cushing's syndrome, Cushing's disease, Relapse, Recovery

INTRODUCTION

The post-operative assessment and replacement of the hypothalamo–pituitary–adrenal axis following treatment of Cushing's syndrome is not well defined, as there are a number of views on how to ascertain whether a cure has been achieved. Furthermore, recurrence may occur months or years after apparently successful treatment of Cushing's syndrome, most commonly in cases of Cushing's disease. Assessment and treatment varies depending on the aetiology of Cushing's syndrome. Other pituitary hormones may also be affected by the glucocorticoid excess and require post-operative assessment, and health problems associated with Cushing's syndrome need close monitoring and therapy, including susceptibility to infections, cardiovascular complications such as hypertension and

From: *Contemporary Endocrinology: Cushing's Syndrome: Pathophysiology, Diagnosis and Treatment*
Edited by: M.D. Bronstein (ed.), DOI 10.1007/978-1-60327-449-4_20,

dyslipidaemia, low libido, impotence and menstrual disturbances *(1)*, anxiety, depression, mania and psychosis *(1, 2)*, osteopenia and osteoporosis, as well as impaired glucose tolerance and diabetes mellitus.

POST-OPERATIVE PITUITARY HORMONE REPLACEMENT

ACTH Axis

Cushing's disease

In order to assess whether post-operative cortisol replacement is necessary, the ACTH axis needs to be evaluated in each patient to determine whether pituitary surgery has been successful. However, there is no universally agreed threshold cortisol value to define cure after transsphenoidal surgery for Cushing's disease and no consensus regarding the timing of post-operative cortisol measurements *(3, 4)*. Common strategies are discussed below.

Definition of cure: Proposed definitions of cure include serum cortisol levels within the reference range *(5)*, a clinical appearance of remission combined with low serum and urinary cortisol levels *(6)* or suppression of cortisol on the low dose dexamethasone suppression test *(7)*. The most widely accepted view is that an undetectable post-operative serum cortisol (<50 nmol/L) is associated with the best long-term outcome and is the most valuable predictor of long-term cure *(8–13)*. The rationale for this derives from the fact that if removal of the adenoma is complete, lack of stimulation of the adrenal glands by ACTH leads to an undetectable serum cortisol because of the suppression of the hypothalamo–pituitary–adrenal axis [13].

Timing of post-operative cortisol measurements: The most widely accepted view is that basal serum cortisol should be measured between 8:00 *(12)* and 9:00 h *(9, 14)* 3–4 days after transsphenoidal surgery and at least 12 h after the last dose of hydrocortisone *(10, 13)*. Some authors suggest using cortisol values from the 6- to 12-week period following surgery, as these appear to offer better discrimination of continuing remission *(14, 15)*. Continued secretion of cortisol from hyperplastic adrenal tissue for at least 2 weeks after withdrawal of ACTH stimulation has been suggested as an explanation for the delayed decline in cortisol levels. It should be pointed out that these series were small and if cyclical cortisol secretion is excluded, it is difficult to reconcile the above findings with the majority of reports showing a gradual recovery of cortisol levels post-operatively over months or years *(13)*.

Hormone Replacement: Cushing's patients have an inadequate response to stress and therefore require glucocorticoids peri-operatively. Additionally, severe hypoadrenalism may develop in the early post-operative period due to the suppression of the normal pituitary corticotroph function by previous hypercortisolaemia *(16)*. Therefore, successfully treated Cushing's patients require physiologic glucocorticoid replacement with repeated subsequent assessments of their HPA axis, as the aim is to gradually reduce glucocorticoids as adrenal suppression recovers *(17)*. Hydrocortisone is suggested rather than dexamethasone, as the latter has a potent corticotroph suppressive effect and may hinder the subsequent HPA axis recovery *(3)*. Prednisolone also has a long half-life and leads to sustained ACTH suppression, making it less useful for replacement therapy *(10)*. As hydrocortisone cross-reacts with standard serum and urine assays of endogenous cortisol production, it must be discontinued for at least 12 h before measuring serum and urine cortisol levels *(3)*. Hydrocortisone should be dosed three times daily, as it has a half-life of 90–120 min, whereas dexamethasone can be administered once daily, as it has a much longer half-life (36–54 h) *(17)*. Hydrocortisone 20 mg is approximately equivalent to dexamethasone 0.75 mg and prednisolone 5 mg *(10)*. A possible dose regimen for the peri- and immediate post-operative period is hydrocortisone 20 mg orally or 100 mg intramuscularly with the induction of

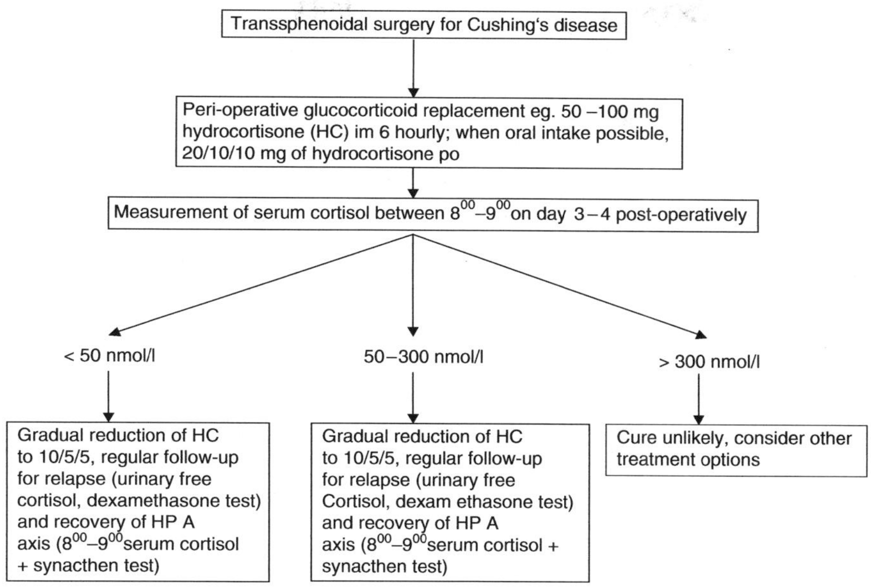

Fig. 1. Post-operative glucocorticoid replacement depending on post-operative serum cortisol levels.

anaesthesia followed by hydrocortisone 50–100 mg intramuscularly every 6 h after surgery *(10)*. As soon as the patient is able to eat and drink, intramuscular hydrocortisone is converted to oral hydrocortisone at a dose of 20 mg on waking, and 10 mg at lunchtime and at 17:00 h respectively (approximately double replacement). Depending on the basal morning cortisol levels measured 3–4 days after transsphenoidal surgery (see timing of post-operative cortisol measurements above) the hydrocortisone doses are adapted. If basal morning serum cortisol is undetectable (<50 nmol/L), hydrocortisone doses are gradually reduced to 10 mg on waking, 5 mg at lunchtime and 5 mg at 17:00 h (daily hydrocortisone doses are reduced by 2.5 mg every 1–2 weeks or as tolerated by the patient, as providing a glucocorticoid taper can alleviate symptoms of steroid withdrawal, including headache, fatigue, malaise or myalgia *(3)*) (Fig. 1).

If serum cortisol levels range between 50 and 300 nmol/L, hydrocortisone is reduced in the same way but the patient requires close monitoring for recurrence of hypercortisolism during the following months (see assessment for relapse of hypercortisolism below). Simultaneously, patients require regular monitoring for recovery of the HPA axis, making hydrocortisone replacement unnecessary (see assessment for recovery of HPA axis below). This is generally the case when 8:00–9:00 h serum cortisol levels rise above 400–450 nmol/L *(10, 17)*.

In a patient with a post-operative basal serum cortisol >300 nmol/L, no hydrocortisone replacement is required as surgical failure is likely and the patient requires further treatment *(10)*. The figure above illustrates the peri-operative management of patients with Cushing's disease.

Cushing's syndrome of adrenal origin

Adrenal tumours are responsible for 10–20% of cases of Cushing's syndrome in adults, adrenal adenoma for approximately 10%, adrenal carcinoma for approximately 8%, bilateral micronodular adrenal hyperplasia for 1% and bilateral macronodular hyperplasia for 1% *(10)*.

For adrenal adenomas unilateral adrenalectomy is curative, whereas bilateral micro- or macronodular adrenal hyperplasia is cured by bilateral adrenalectomy. In a patient with adrenal carcinoma, surgery is useful to debulk tumour mass, as up to 70% of patients have distant metastases at the time of diagnosis. Local recurrence during follow-up is common *(18)*. Post-operative basal serum cortisol levels are measured in the same way as for pituitary Cushing's syndrome, with a cortisol <50 nmol/L an indicator of cure.

Hormone replacement: Peri- and post-operative glucocorticoid cover is required for all patients with clinical or subclinical Cushing's syndrome attributed to adrenal tumours or hyperplasia *(10)*. Hydrocortisone is given as for pituitary surgery: 100 mg intramuscularly with induction of anaesthesia followed by hydrocortisone 50–100 mg intramuscularly every 6 h until the patient is eating and drinking and can take oral medication. Oral Hydrocortisone 20 mg is then given on waking with 10 mg at lunchtime and at 17:00 h. Hydrocortisone can be decreased to normal maintenance doses (10 mg on waking, 5 mg at lunchtime and 5 mg at 17:00 h) once the patient has recovered from surgery. Mineralocorticoid replacement is only required in patients who have undergone bilateral adrenalectomy, the recommended dose being 100 μg of fludrocortisone daily, which is adjusted according to blood electrolytes, postural blood pressure and renin measurements.

Ectopic Cushing's syndrome

The ectopic ACTH syndrome refers to excess ACTH production by a source outside of the pituitary, leading to signs of hypercortisolism; it accounts for approximately 12% of cases of Cushing's syndrome. The most common causes of this disorder are small cell lung carcinomas and carcinoid tumours particularly in the lungs, as well as islet cell tumours. Ectopic CRH secretion is very rare, and usually occurs in patients with fairly well differentiated pulmonary carcinoid tumours *(19)*. In a few patients, remission can be achieved by surgical excision of the tumour *(20–22)*. However, the tumour is not resectable at the time of diagnosis or has metastasized in the majority of patients, in which cases chemo- or radiotherapy may be helpful.

Hormone replacement: Patients with ectopic ACTH or CRH syndrome have an inadequate stress reponse and require glucocorticoid cover peri-operatively, as described for patients with Cushing's disease. Patients who have not had curative resection of the primary tumour require treatment with an adrenal enzyme inhibitor such as metyrapone, ketoconazole, etomidate or aminoglutethimide, which control hypercortisolism within a few days of commencement. The dose is adjusted to achieve normal 24-h urinary free cortisol excretion, or, alternatively, cortisol production is inhibited completely using enzyme inhibitors and replacement doses of glucocorticoids are given *(10)*. Medical adrenalectomy can also be achieved by giving mitotane. Octreotide, a long-acting somatostatin analogue, can reduce ectopic ACTH secretion rapidly. Uptake during radionucleotide scanning predicts a positive response to this drug and is a further treatment option.

Other Pituitary Hormones (FSH/LH, TSH, GH, ADH)

The vast majority of Cushing's syndrome is due to a pituitary ACTH-secreting corticotroph microadenoma, termed Cushing's disease. In these patients, an inherent risk of transsphenoidal pituitary surgery is the development of post-operative pituitary hormone deficiencies. The risk of hypopituitarism is correlated with the extent of pituitary resection *(8, 9, 23)*. Corticotroph adenomas can often be undetectable by radiological techniques and visual inspection and additionally, a subset of Cushing's disease is caused by diffuse corticotroph hyperplasia, which increases the complexity of surgery and makes post-operative hypopituitarism more likely *(8)*.

The following rates of pituitary hormone deficiency after transsphenoidal surgery have been reported: gonadotropins 3–48%, thyrotropin 13–45%, somatotropin 53–93% and antidiuretic hormone 0–46% *(3)*.

The integrity of the remaining pituitary function is usually assessed 4–6 weeks after transsphenoidal surgery *(10, 24)*. There is a risk of hypogonadism following extensive surgery *(8, 9, 23)*. In premenopausal women, the assessment of gonadal function is based on the menstrual history, as well as on the gonadotropin and the oestradiol levels. Replacement can be started at any time post-operatively in premenopausal women. A variety of options are available and the choice depends on the patient, their age and medical history *(25)*. In men, secondary hypogonadism is diagnosed by measuring morning testosterone and gonadotropin levels; in secondary hypogonadism the testosterone in low and the gonadotrophins are normal or low *(26)*. PSA is typically measured before commencing testosterone therapy, along with haemoglobin and a lipid profile. Testosterone can be administered transdermally as a patch or gel or by intramuscular injections, all of which are efficacious *(26, 27)*.

The thyroid axis can be assessed by measuring free T4 and TSH. In secondary hypothyroidism, the free T4 is low and the TSH low or normal. Levothyroxine is the treatment of choice, with a target free T4 level towards the upper end of normal *(28)*. The adequacy of treatment is assessed every 6–8 weeks by measuring free T4, the levothyroxine dose is adjusted until free T4 levels are within the target range.

Growth hormone (GH) deficiency is common in Cushing's disease, as hypercortisolaemia impairs GH secretion. Recovery of GH secretion is seen in a high proportion of patients following surgery for Cushing's disease, so that the definitive assessment of the GH secretory status should be postponed to 1–2 years after surgical cure of Cushing's disease *(29–31)*. The most definitive way to assess for GH deficiency involves provocative testing with an insulin tolerance test, which is the gold standard test. In the elderly, and in patients with cardiovascular disease or seizures, alternative tests such as the arginine or glucagon stimulation tests or the arginine in combination with GHRH test can be used *(10)*. In patients with three or more anterior pituitary hormone deficits, the chance of having GH deficiency is 95% and dynamic testing may not be required. If GH deficiency is found, growth hormone replacement is indicated.

Polyuria is not unusual in patients with Cushing's syndrome, and transient diabetes insipidus (DI) is more likely post-operatively in patients with Cushing's disease than after operations for other larger pituitary adenomas *(32)*. Evaluation for DI can be carried out when blood glucose, potassium and calcium levels are normal and appropriate steroid replacement has been commenced. Diabetes insipidus may occur due to the disruption of the hypothalamo–pituitary stalk or trauma to the posterior pituitary gland, thus temporarily impairing vasopressin secretion *(33)*. In most cases, vasopressin secretion recovers and diabetes insipidus lasts for just the first few days post-operatively, usually beginning within the first 48 h following surgery. Treatment is by giving vasopressin tablets or nasal spray.

Apart from a routine assessment of pituitary hormones following transsphenoidal surgery, patients' neurological status and visual function are assessed, including tests for visual acuity, extraocular movements and visual fields. Routine prophylactic peri-operative antibiotic coverage from induction of anaesthesia through to post-operative day 5 is undertaken by most centres *(10, 33)*, and the majority of studies suggest benefit from these *(34)*.

ASSESSMENT OF RECOVERY OF THE HPA AXIS AND FOLLOW-UP FOR RELAPSE

Cushing's Disease

Follow-up for relapse: Although post-operative hypoadrenalism is associated with a lower risk of relapse, several studies have shown return of hypercortisolism following a period of adrenal insufficiency *(7, 15, 35–37)*. The risk of relapse is estimated between 10 and 15%, as shown in a large European multicentre study by Bochicchio et al.; in this series, Cushing's disease relapsed in 12.7% of patients with undetectable serum cortisol levels in the post-operative period at a mean time of 39.3

months *(7)*. Similarly, Estrada et al. reported that 12% of patients with initially undetectable serum cortisol levels relapsed within 5 years *(37)*, and Pereira reported that 14% of patients with 2- and 12-week post-operative cortisol levels <50 nmol/L ultimately relapsed *(15)*. An explanation as to why some patients with undetectable post-operative cortisol levels do go on to relapse may be that the peri-operative steroid cover continues to cause negative feedback, despite the cessation of steroids for at least 24 h before measuring a 8:00 h cortisol. In addition, synthesis of ACTH may be arrested for days to weeks if glucocorticoids are administered, as these inhibit the transcription of ACTH in corticotroph cells within only 15 min of glucocorticoid exposure *(38)*. Another possible explanation for late relapse despite initial undetectable serum cortisol may be that the plasma ACTH concentration and therefore the serum cortisol concentration depend upon the number of adenomatous corticotroph cells remaining after pituitary surgery. The number of remaining cells may be too small to stimulate detectable cortisol secretion, but may be sufficient to eventually grow into a large enough adenoma to cause recurrent Cushing's disease *(39)*.

Patients who do not have undetectable post-operative serum cortisol levels but levels ranging from 50 to 300 nmol/L are at increased risk of relapse *(7, 15, 37, 40)*. In this population, the risk of relapse has been calculated to be approximately 77% after 5 years and 88% after 10 years using the Kaplan–Meier statistical method *(3)*. However, the risk is not absolute, as shown by Pereira et al. They followed 11 patients with a 9:00 h serum cortisol between 50 and 138 nmol/L and six patients with a cortisol level >138 nmol/L 2 weeks after surgery, all of which remained in remission during follow-up of 1–8 years *(15)*. Estrada et al. followed 17 patients with plasma cortisol levels of 306 ± 91 nmol/L post-operatively, 23% of which had not relapsed after 5 years and 12% of which had not relapsed after 10 years *(37)*. An explanation for long-term remission of Cushing's disease despite measurable post-operative cortisol levels may be that the remaining tumour cells undergo progressive necrosis during the first 3 months post-operatively.

As described above, clinical remission may be possible in patients despite measurable serum cortisol levels (50–300 nmol/L) post-operatively. These patients need careful assessment before a recommendation for repeat surgery or other treatment is made. In our opinion, decisions regarding further therapy should be based on 24-h urinary free cortisol levels and the response to low dose dexamethasone suppression *(3, 10, 12)*. Urinary free cortisol levels should remain within the reference range and low dose dexamethasone suppression lead to a complete suppression of cortisol <50 nmol/L. Because there is no absolutely reliable predictor of cure and long-term remission, all patients should undergo regular follow-up to detect relapse of Cushing's disease at least yearly for at least 10 years. Other biochemical tests for assessment of relapse include the corticotropin-releasing hormone stimulation test, metyrapone test or desmopressin test, although these tests do not seem to provide greater discrimination than 24-h urinary free cortisol measurements or the low dose dexamethasone test *(3, 12)* (Fig. 2).

Patients with persistent hypercortisolaemia (>300 nmol/L) following surgery are unlikely to have been cured and should be considered for re-exploration and/or radiotherapy *(10)*.

Factors associated with the risk of relapse of hypercortisolism: Various investigators have sought to define factors in patients that may be associated with the risk of relapse. Adenoma size seems to play a role, as surgical failure is more common with macroadenomas and extrasellar extension *(8, 41–43)*. However, not all studies suggest that there is a correlation between size and surgical success *(7, 44)*. If an adenoma is visualised on pre-operative imaging, some authors have found a higher chance of surgical success, with rates of 100% in patients with positive scans versus rates of 69% in patients with negative scans *(7, 8)*. However, other authors such as Invitti et al. and Yap et al. have not found significant differences in rates of surgical success *(7, 35, 45)*. Surgical failure has been reported to be more likely in patients who do not respond to corticotropin releasing hormone (CRH)

Fig. 2. Biochemical tests to assess the recovery of the HPA axis.

Tests to assess the recovery of the HPA axis
Morning serum cortisol (8.00–9.00)
Short synacthen test
Insulin tolerance test
Glucagon stimulation test
Corticotropin releasing hormone stimulation test
Metyrapone test

infusion with an ACTH and cortisol rise pre-operatively *(3, 7, 46)* and in patients with a paradoxical rise in cortisol after thyrotropin releasing hormone (TRH) or luteinizing hormone releasing hormone (LHRH) infusions *(3, 46)*. A decline in intraoperative ACTH levels did not prove to be a useful tool for predicting remission either *(47)*. When an adenoma was noted on post-operative histology, some series found higher remission rates of 75–78% vs 24–36% than when no adenoma was noted *(3, 6, 40)*. Other series found no correlation between positive histology for adenoma and likelihood of remission *(8, 12, 35, 37, 45)*.

Assessment for recovery of the HPA axis: Assessment of recovery of the HPA axis is recommended every 3–6 months during the first 2 years by measuring 8:00–9:00 h serum cortisol levels or the response to a short synacthen test after withholding hydrocortisone replacement for at least 24 h. Replacement therapy can be discontinued if a basal 8:00–9:00 h serum cortisol level above 400–450 nmol/L is obtained *(10, 17)* (although patients should be advised to start steroids if they feel unwell), or the cortisol level rises to >580 nmol/L at 30 min after ACTH stimulation *(10)*. It is however important to document the adequacy of the stress response once the patient has been weaned off glucocorticoid replacement therapy with an insulin tolerance test (ITT), especially when the response to ACTH stimulation is borderline *(10, 17)*. The normal response in an ITT is for cortisol to rise to >580 nmol/L, which demonstrates the ability to withstand stress without requiring glucocorticoid cover. Alternative tests to the ITT are the glucagon stimulation test, corticotropin-releasing hormone stimulation test or the metyrapone test.

Recovery of the HPA axis usually takes up to 1 year and occasionally up to 2 years. If the axis has not recovered after 2 years, recovery thereafter is unlikely. During the reduction of the post-operative glucocorticoid dosage, patients may experience symptoms suggestive of hypoadrenalism. The mechanism for this is not clear, but symptoms seem to be related to the re-adaptation of tissues to physiological glucocorticoid doses after prolonged exposure to supra-physiological levels *(24)*. It is useful to warn patients that such symptoms may occur. Severe symptoms can be relieved by temporarily increasing the dose of glucocorticoid replacement, but it should be reduced to a physiological level again gradually. Symptoms are transient and will clear eventually *(24)*.

Cushing's Syndrome of Adrenal Origin

Follow-up for relapse of hypercortisolism: As in Cushing's disease, 24-h urinary free cortisol measurements and low dose dexamethasone testing are used. Generally, surgery cures Cushing's syndrome in patients with adrenal adenoma or hyperplasia.

Patients with adrenal carcinoma should undergo regular staging with CT to detect progression and are treated with adjunctive oral mitotane *(48)*. Adrenostatic drugs such as metyrapone, ketoconazole, etomidate and aminoglutethimide, which inhibit P450 steroidogenic enzymes like 11β-hydroxylase and the side-chain cleavage enzyme, may additionally be needed to control hypercortisolism *(49)*.

Assessment for recovery of the HPA axis: It may take up to 2 years for the contralateral adrenal gland to recover fully after unilateral adrenalectomy. A first assessment for recovery can take place once 8:00–9:00 h cortisol levels rise to >50 nmol/L. A short synacthen test after the patient has discontinued hydrocortisone replacement for at least 24 h *(10)* can then be done and be repeated every 3–6 months until a normal result is achieved. To confirm an adequate stress response an insulin tolerance test should be obtained. If a patient has undergone bilateral adrenalectomy, lifelong glucocorticoid and mineralocorticoid replacement is necessary *(10)*.

Ectopic Cushing's Syndrome

Patients with ectopic Cushing's syndrome are evaluated for relapse using the same methods as described for Cushing's disease and adrenal Cushing's syndrome. Regular imaging studies are necessary to ensure the primary tumour does not progress. In some patients, the source of hypercortisolism cannot be identified, and these patients need regular reexamination with CT, MRI, radionucleotide scanning with octreotide, radiolabelled metaiodobenzylguanidine or PET *(10)*. The assessment of recovery of the HPA axis also follows the same algorithms as described for pituitary and adrenal Cushing's syndrome.

CONCLUSION

The management of patients undergoing surgical intervention for Cushing's syndrome is complex and includes the assessment and treatment of associated conditions, adequate glucocorticoid replacement peri-operatively, investigation as to whether cure has been achieved post-operatively and close observation to detect relapse of Cushing's syndrome and the recovery of the HPA axis. Various protocols exist, but as long as one is followed closely and none of the many aspects of the post-operative management of Cushing's syndrome are neglected, the final outcome can be optimized (Table 1).

Table 1
Assessment and Management of Associated Conditions in Patients with Cushing's Syndrome

Conditions associated with Cushing's syndrome	*Mechanism*	*Assessment*
Susceptibility to infectious disease	Immune suppression, enhanced viral replication	Clinical monitoring
Hypertension	Activation of renin/angiotensin system, mineralocorticoid effect	Regular blood pressure measurement
Dyslipidaemia	Insulin resistance	Lipid profile
Hypogonadotrophic hypogonadism	Suppression of gonadotropin secretion	Testosterone measurement, menstrual history
Depression, anxiety, mania	Glucocorticoid effect	Clinical monitoring
Osteopenia, -porosis	Increased bone resorption	Bone mineral density scan
Impaired glucose tolerance	Insulin resistance, increased glycogenolysis	Fasting glucose measurement

REFERENCES

1. Kelly WF. Psychiatric aspects of Cushing's syndrome. Q J Med 1996;89:543–551.
2. Loosen PT. Psychiatric manifestations of Cushing's syndrome. In: Blevins LS, ed. Cushing's syndrome. Boston: Kluwer Academic Publishers, 2002:45–64.
3. Utz A, Swearingen B, Biller B. Pituitary surgery and postoperative management in Cushing's disease. Endocrinol Metab Clin North Am 2005;34:459–478.
4. Arnaldi G, Angeli A, Atkinson AB, et al. Diagnosis and complications of Cushing's syndrome: a consensus statement. J Clin Endocrinol Metab 2003;88:5593–5602.
5. Mampalam TJ, Tyrell JB, Wilson CB. Transsphenoidal microsurgery for Cushing's disease. Ann Int Med 1988;109:487–493.
6. Invitti C, Giraldi FP, De Martin M, et al. Diagnosis and management of Cushing's syndrome: results of an Italian multi-centre study. J Clin Endocrinol Metab 1999;84:440–448.
7. Bochicchio D, Losa M, Buchfelder M, and the European Cushing's Disease Survey Study Group. Factors influencing the immediate and late outcome of Cushing's disease treated by transsphenoidal surgery: a retrospective study by the European Cushing's Disease Survey Group. J Clin Endocrinol Metab 1995;80:3114–3120.
8. Rees DA, Hanna FWF, Davies JS, Mills RG, Vafidis J, Scanlon MF. Long-term follow-up results of transsphenoidal surgery for Cushing's disease in a single center using strict criteria for remission. Clin Endocrinol 2002;56:541–553.
9. Trainer PJ, Lawrie HS, Verhelst J, Howlett TA, Lowe DG, Grossman AB, Savage MO, Afshar F, Besser GM. Transsphenoidal resection in Cushing's disease; undetectable serum cortisol as the definition of successful treatment. Clin Endocrinol 1993;38:73–78.
10. Turner HE, Wass JAH. Oxford Handbook of Endocrinology and Diabetes. Oxford, UK, Oxford University Press, 2006;785.
11. Burke CW, Adams CBT, Esiri MM, Morris M, Bevan JS. Transsphenoidal surgery for Cushing's disease: does what is removed determine the endocrine outcome? Clin Endocrinol 1990;33:525–537.
12. McCance DR, Gordon DS, Fannin TF, Hadden DR, Kennedy L, Sheridan B, Atkinson AB. Assessment of endocrine function after transsphenoidal surgery for Cushing's disease. Clin Endocrinol 1993;38:79–86.
13. McCance DR, Besser M, Atkinson AB. Assessment of cure after transsphenoidal surgery for Cushing's disease. Clin Endocrinol 1996;44:1–6.
14. Toms GC, McCarthy MI, Niven MJ, Orteu CH, King TT, Monson JP. Predicting relapse after transsphenoidal surgery for Cushing's disease. J Clin Endocrinol Metab 1993;76:291–294.
15. Pereira AM, van Aken MO, van Dulken H. Long-term predictive value of postsurgical cortisol concentrations for cure and risk of recurrence in Cushing's disease. J Clin Endocrinol Metab 2003;88:5858.
16. Fitzgerald PA, Arnold DC, Findling JW. Cushing's disease: transient secondary adrenal insufficiency after selective removal of pituitary microadenomas; evidence for a pituitary origin. J Clin Endocrinol Metab 1982;54:413–422.
17. Inder WJ, Hunt PJ. Glucocorticoid replacement in pituitary surgery: guidelines for perioperative assessment and management. J Clin Endocrinol Metab 2002;87:2745–2750.
18. Stojadinovic A, Ghossein RA, Hoos A, Nissan A, Marshall D, Dudas M, Cordon-Cardo C, Jacques DP, Brennan MF. Adrenocortical carcinoma: clinical, morphologic, and molecular characterization. J Clin Oncol 2002;20:941–950.
19. Orth DN. Corticotropin-releasing hormone in humans. Endocr Rev 1992;13:164.
20. Aniszewski JP, Young WF, Thompson GB. Cushing syndrome due to ectopic adrenocorticotropic hormone secretion. World J Surg 2001;25:934.
21. Ilias I, Torpy DJ, Pacak K. Cushing's syndrome due to ectopic corticotropin secretion: twenty years experience at the National Institute of Health. J Clin Endocrinol Metab 2005;90:4955.
22. Sidori AM, Kaltsas GA, Pozza C. The ectopic adrenocorticotropin syndrome: clinical features, diagnosis, management and long-term follow-up. J Clin Endocrinol Metab 2006;91:371.
23. Semple CG, Thomson JA, Teasdale GM. Transsphenoidal microsurgery for Cushing's disease. Clin Endocrinol 1984;21:621–629.
24. McKenna TJ. Perioperative Evaluation and Management. Cushing's syndrome. Boston, Kluwer Academic Publishers, 2002; 279–299.
25. Lamberts SW, De Herder WW, Van der Lely AJ. Pituitary insufficiency. Lancet 1998;352:127–134.
26. Bhasin S, Cunningham GR, Hayes FJ, et al. Testosterone therapy in adult men with androgen deficiency syndromes: an endocrine society clinical practice guideline. J Clin Endocrinol Metab 2006;91:1995–2010.
27. Bhasin S. Approach to the infertile man. J Clin Endocrinol Metab 2007;92:1995–2004.
28. Schneider HJ, Aimaretti G, Kreitschmann-Andermahr I, et al. Hypopituitarism. Lancet 2007;369:1461–1470.

29. Carroll PV, Monson JP, Grossman AB, Besser GM, Plowman PN, et al. Successful treatment of childhood-onset Cushing's disease is associated with persistent reduction in growth hormone secretion. Clin Endocrinol 2004;60: 169–174.
30. Hughes NR, Lisset CA, Shalet SM. Growth hormone status following treatment for Cushing's syndrome. Clin Endocrinol 1999;51:61–66.
31. Tzanela M, Karavitaki N, Stylianidou C, Tsagarakis S, Thalassinos NC. Assessment of GH reserve before and after successful treatment of adult patients with Cushing's syndrome. Clin Endocrinol 2004;60:309–314.
32. Nemergut E, Dumont A, Barry U, Laws E. Perioperative management of patients undergoing transsphenoidal pituitary surgery. Anesth Analg 2005;101:1170–1181.
33. Ausiello JC, Bruce JN, Freda P. Postoperative assessment of the patient after transsphenoidal pituitary surgery. Pituitary 2008;11(4):391–401.
34. Dumont AS, Nemergut EC, Jane JA, Jr, Laws ER, Jr. Postoperative care following pituitary surgery. J Intensive Care Med 2005;20:127–140.
35. Yap LB, Turner HE, Adams CB, Wass JAH. Undetectable postoperative cortisol does not always predict long-term remission in Cushing's disease: a single centre audit. Clin Endocrinol 2002;56:25–31.
36. Rollin GAFS, Ferreira NP, Junges M. Dynamics of serum cortisol levels after transsphenoidal surgery in a cohort of patients with Cushing's disease. J Clin Endocrinol Metab 2004;89:1131–1139.
37. Estrada J, Garcia-Uria JL, Lamas C. The complete normalisation of the adrenocortical function as the criterion of cure after transsphenoidal surgery for Cushing's disease. J Clin Endocrinol Metab 2001;86:5695–5699.
38. Eberwine JH, Roberts JL. Analysis of pro-opiomelanocortin gene structure and function. DNA 1983;2:1–8.
39. Salenave S, Gatta B, Pecheur S, et al. Pituitary magnetic resonance imaging findings do not influence surgical outcome in adrenocortitropin-secreting microadenomas. J Clin Endocrinol Metab 2004;89: 3371–3376.
40. Guilhaume B, Bertagna X, Thomsen M, Bricaire C, Vila-Porcile E. Transsphenoidal pituitary surgery for the treatment of Cushing's disease: results in 64 patients and long-term follow-up studies. J Clin Endocrinol Metab 1988;66:1056–1064.
41. Hammer GD, Tyrrell JB, Lamborn KR. Transsphenoidal microsurgery for Cushing's disease: initial outcome and long-term results. J Clin Endocrinol Metab 2004;89:6348–6357.
42. Blevins LSJ, Christy JH, Khajavi M. Outcomes of therapy for Cushing's disease due to adrenocorticotropin-secreting pituitary macroadenomas. J Clin Endocrinol Metab 1998;83:63–67.
43. Cannavo S, Almoto B, Dall'Asta C. Long-term results of treatment in patients with ACTH-secreting pituitary macroadenomas. Eur J Endocrinol 2003;149:195–200.
44. Chee GH, Mathias DB, James RA. Transsphenoidal pituitary surgery in Cushing's disease: can we predict outcome? Clin Endocrinol 2001;54:617–626.
45. Booth GL, Redelmeier DA, Grosman H. Improved diagnostic accuracy of inferior petrosal sinus sampling over imaging for localizing pituitary pathology in patients with Cushing's disease. J Clin Endocrinol Metab 1998;83:2291–2295.
46. Pieters GFFM, Hermus ARMM, Meijer E. Predictive factors for initial cure and relapse rate after pituitary surgery for Cushing's disease. J Clin Endocrinol Metab 1989;69:1122–1126.
47. Graham KE, Samuels MH, Raff H. Intraoperative adrenocorticotropin levels during transsphenoidal surgery for Cushing's disease do not predict cure. J Clin Endocrinol Metab 1997;82:1776.
48. Baudin E, Pellegriti G, Bonnay M, Penfornis A, Laplanche A, Vassal G, Schlumberger M. Impact of monitoring plasma 1,1-dichlorodiphenildichloroethane (o,p′DDD) levels on the treatment of patients with adrenocortical carcinoma. Cancer 2001;92:1385–1392.
49. Luton JP, Cerdas S, Billaud L, Thomas G, Guilhaume B, Bertagna X, Laudat MH, Louvel A, Chapuis Y, Blondeau P, Bonnin A, Bricaire H. Clinical features of adrenocortical carcinoma, prognostic factors, and the effect of mitotane therapy. N Engl J Med 1990;322:1195–1201.

21 Special Aspects of Cushing's Syndrome: Pregnancy

Dima Abdelmannan and David C. Aron

CONTENTS

SUMMARY

Cushing's syndrome (CS) is rare during pregnancy because it is associated with infertility in approximately 71% of female patients who have the disease. The diagnosis of CS is challenging in the nonpregnant state and even more so during pregnancy for several reasons. First, pregnant women without CS develop some features of Cushing's, such as hypertension, hyperglycemia, and striae. Second, the various yet normal functional alterations involving the hypothalamic-pituitary axis during pregnancy make it difficult to use the standard testing normal ranges that are used to diagnose Cushing's in nonpregnant states (e.g., low-dose dexamethasone suppression testing and assessment of 24-h urinary free cortisol and salivary cortisol). However, because hypercortisolism is associated with unfavorable maternal and fetal outcomes, it is important to have a high index of suspicion of the disease to prevent delay in diagnosis. In this chapter, we explore the different causes of CS during pregnancy, as well as the normal changes affecting the hypothalamic-pituitary-adrenal (HPA) axis and how to incorporate that information into the interpretation of biochemical testing data. We propose a general approach to treatment with both medical and surgical options, while keeping in mind the paramount importance of individualizing therapy.

Key Words: Cushing's syndrome, Pregnancy, Cortisol, ACTH, Hypothalamic-pituitary-adrenal axis

From: *Contemporary Endocrinology: Cushing's Syndrome: Pathophysiology, Diagnosis and Treatment*
Edited by: M.D. Bronstein (ed.), DOI 10.1007/978-1-60327-449-4_21,

INTRODUCTION

Despite the fact that Cushing's syndrome (CS) occurs most commonly in women of childbearing age, the coexistence of pregnancy and CS is rare. This rarity results from the infertility associated with suppression of gonadotropin secretion by elevated cortisol levels and androgens; oligomenorrhea or amenorrhea occurs in approximately 75% of women of reproductive age *(1)*. The first case report of pregnancy in a patient with CS (by Hunt and McConaghy) occurred 21 years after Harvey Cushing's classic 1932 description of the disorder. The number of reported cases now exceeds 100, but their relative rarity has meant that there are no large case series from a single institution *(2–4)*. In addition, despite the fact that pituitary-dependent CS is the most common etiology in women of childbearing age, cortisol-producing adrenal tumors account for a larger proportion of cases in pregnancy. The fact that hypercortisolism may be associated with unfavorable maternal and fetal outcomes obligates the clinician to have a high index of suspicion of the disease, despite its rarity and difficulties in diagnosis.

CLINICAL FEATURES

It is now well established that CS can present with the classic features or with far more subtlety *(1)*. However, most of the reported cases of CS during pregnancy describe the typical signs and symptoms, a fact that probably represents underdiagnosis. Some women have more than one term pregnancy or spontaneous abortion before hypercortisolism is recognized *(5)*. Because pregnancy itself can exhibit some of the clinical features of CS, e.g., hypertension, hyperglycemia, and striae, a high index of clinical suspicion must be maintained to prevent delay in diagnosis *(6, 7)*. In fact, CS is frequently diagnosed in mid pregnancy (12–26 weeks gestation), possibly because of the overlap of clinical features *(8)*.

The classical features of CS are well-known – central obesity, thin skin, easy bruisability, striae, hypertension, etc. The characteristic purple striae are depressed and wide (often 0.5–2.0 cm) in contrast to the pinkish-white striae seen in pregnant Caucasians. Striae are seen more commonly in younger patients with CS, the same individuals more likely to be pregnant. However, the striae of CS tend to occur in sites other than the abdominal wall (e.g., axilla, thighs, and breasts). Because many of these clinical features are similar to those that develop in pregnant women without CS, e.g., striae, hypertension, and gestational diabetes, it is important to consider which signs and symptoms have the greatest discriminatory value. As in nonpregnant patients, catabolic features such as bruising and proximal weakness may be the most useful signs, especially if they occur in a patient with hypertension and gestational diabetes *(6, 9)*.

BIOCHEMICAL AND IMAGING DIAGNOSIS

The evaluation of a patient for CS, although dependent upon clinical judgment, relies to a large extent on biochemical testing *(10)*. However, the biochemical diagnosis during pregnancy is further complicated by taking place in the context of the altered behavior of the hypothalamic-pituitary-adrenal axis during normal pregnancy. In diagnosis, we ask two basic questions: (*1*) does the patient have glucocorticoid excess? and (2) if so, what is the etiology?

Hypothalamus-Pituitary-Adrenal Axis in Pregnancy

In addition to the usual considerations when evaluating the hypothalamic-pituitary-adrenal axis, e.g., episodic secretion, circadian rhythm, negative feedback, total versus free cortisol in serum, and characteristics of the tests themselves, pregnancy presents special problems *(10, 11)*. In general, the hypothalamic-pituitary-adrenal axis in pregnancy is activated to achieve a state of physiologic hypercortisolism, without clinical manifestations *(8, 12–16)*. There is a two to threefold increase in hepatic production of cortisol binding globulin (CBG), an effect mediated by a progressive increase in estrogen. The highest levels are achieved during the latter part of pregnancy; the peak reached at about 6 months' gestation is maintained until delivery. This is associated with decreased clearance, but not increased production of cortisol. Since the plasma assays measure total plasma cortisol levels, the levels mainly represent the bound fraction and thus depend on cortisol-binding globulin levels. Therefore, total plasma cortisol levels are elevated. Carr et al. found AM levels (mean ± SEM) of 14.9 ± 3.4 μg/dl at 11 weeks of gestation and 35.2 ± 9.0 μg/dl at 26 weeks of gestation, remaining elevated until labor and delivery *(17)*. These levels overlap those found in CS. However, in contrast to CS, the normal diurnal variation of plasma cortisol is maintained *(18)*. Not only do total plasma cortisol levels increase during pregnancy, but plasma free cortisol levels also rise. Likewise, urinary free cortisol concentrations increase to levels that may overlap those observed in CS. Lindolm et al. reported the mean urine cortisol in pregnancy to be 127 μg/24 h (range 68–252) compared to a control group mean of 37 μg/24 h (range 11–83) *(21)*. These levels in pregnancy overlap those found in CS. Urinary excretion of 17-hydroxycorticosteroids remains normal. Because total plasma cortisol levels are higher as a result of increased binding of dexamethasone, suppressibility as judged by standard criteria may be impaired. In addition, dexamethasone suppressibility of plasma free cortisol levels decreases as pregnancy advances. Dexamethasone suppressibility of urine free cortisol also is impaired. ACTH levels have been reported to be higher, the same and lower in early pregnancy compared to nonpregnant control women, although normal diurnal variation was maintained. It is clear that as pregnancy progresses, plasma adrenocorticotropic hormone (ACTH) levels rise. Why this occurs in the setting of increased plasma free cortisol is not clear. Suggested causes placental synthesis of corticotropin-releasing hormone (CRH) and ACTH, pituitary desensitization to cortisol feedback, or enhanced pituitary responsiveness to CRH or other factors, e.g., vasopressin. There is also decreased suppression of the hypothalamic-pituitary-adrenal axis by exogenous glucocorticoids. This decreased suppression can persist for up to five weeks postpartum *(8)*. Diurnal rhythm, although preserved, tends to be blunted. These changes may relate to the higher CRH levels in pregnancy.

Plasma CRH levels rise during pregnancy, reaching very high levels at term, and abruptly fall after delivery *(19)*. The primary source of plasma CRH during pregnancy is the placental unit. In contrast to the usual negative feedback that cortisol has on hypothalamic CRH production, there is increased production in placental CRH in response to cortisol *(20)*. Placental CRH drives ACTH in a noncircadian fashion. The CRH has been proposed to be a biological clock that times labor and delivery and may also have effects on maturation of the fetal adrenal, fetal–placental unit circulation, and a paracrine effect on the placenta. A high affinity binding protein for placental CRH blunts the ACTH-releasing activity of CRH *(21)*. Several cases of development of CS during pregnancy and spontaneous remission following miscarriage or delivery have been reported *(22)*. Whether these cases result from overproduction of placental CRH is not clear. Table 1 illustrates the major differences in CS between pregnant and nonpregnant states.

Establishing the Diagnosis of Cushing's Syndrome in Pregnancy

The biochemical diagnosis of CS is challenging under the best of circumstances *(10, 23)*. During pregnancy, it is particularly difficult. All three of the most commonly used approaches to establishing the diagnosis of CS – low-dose dexamethasone suppression testing, assessment of 24-h urinary free cortisol, and midnight salivary cortisol – present difficulties in the pregnant patient. With the overnight

Table 1
Major Differences in Cushing's Syndrome (CS) Between Pregnant and Nonpregnant States

	Pregnancy	*Nonpregnancy state*
Prevalence	No incidence available but 120 cases in the literature	Incidence of endogenous CS has been estimated at 13 cases per million individuals
Presentation	Pregnant women without CS develop some features of CS, such as hyper tension, hyperglycemia, and striae, a high index of clinical suspicion must be maintained to prevent delay in diagnosis	
Etiology	Adrenal adenomas cause approximately 40–50% of CS in pregnancy while pituitary adenomas causes approximately 30% of the causes	AA causes 15% of CS cases in nonpregnant cases while up to 70% are caused by pituitary adenomas
Biochemical changes		
ACTH	Plasma ACTH increases as pregnancy progresses In Cushing's patients, ACTH levels were not suppressed in half of those with primary adrenal disorders, perhaps because of continued stimulation of the maternal hypothalamic-pituitary-adrenal axis by placental CRH	
Cortisol	Serum cortisol levels rise two to threefolds in pregnancy, but the diurnal variability is maintained. In cases of CS, the diurnal variation is lost	
Salivary cortisol	Salivary cortisol rise two to threefold during normal pregnancy	
Urinary free cortisol	Urinary free cortisol concentrations increase during pregnancy to levels that may overlap those observed in CS In cases of CS, the urinary free cortisol is not suppressed appropriately after dexamethasone	
CBG	Plasma CBG levels increase in pregnancy due to increase in estrogen levels leading to elevated cortisol levels	
Other factors	Placental degradation of cortisol appears to protect the fetus from glucocorticoid excess	

dexamethasone suppression test, the reliance on total plasma cortisol levels results in a high false positive rate in high estrogen states like pregnancy. A 24-h urine collection for free cortisol also has a high false positive rate in pregnancy. Urinary free cortisol, though normal in the first trimester, increases to as high as three times the normal upper limit during the second and third trimesters. Thus, levels consistent with CS in nonpregnant women are by no means diagnostic during pregnancy. Another factor that complicates interpretation is the fact that much of the literature on CS is relatively old and studies have relied on older assay methodologies. The sensitivities of low-dose dexamethasone suppression testing and urinary free cortisol are not 100% in nonpregnant individuals, but would be expected to be closer to 100% during pregnancy so that their use can be considered as reasonable screening tests during pregnancy; the price of high false positive rates may be worth paying because of the clinical implications of the disorder. A promising alternative is measurement of late night salivary cortisol.

Salivary cortisols rise two to threefold during pregnancy, a magnitude similar to the increase in total plasma cortisol. Scott et al. found that the mean (±1 SD) hourly salivary cortisol level was 5.0 ± 1.4, 7.2 ± 1.2, and 13.6 ± 3.6 nmol/l in normal nonpregnant women, early pregnancy, and late pregnancy, respectively *(24)*. These levels are still below those usually observed in CS. In 1992, Billaud et al. reported three cases of adrenal cortex cancer that were diagnosed during pregnancy and compared the levels of free salivary and urinary cortisol levels in those three patients with those or normal subjects at the same stage of a normal pregnancy and found it to be significantly higher (50, 34, and 95 pg/ml; compared with 8.6 ± 4 pg/ml) *(25)*. Moreover, in normal pregnancy diurnal rhythm is maintained. Studies have shown that patients with CS have midnight salivary cortisol levels that usually exceed 0.4 µg/dl (normal range of 0.1–0.2 µg/dl) *(26)*. Viardot et al. compared nighttime to daytime salivary cortisol levels in a trial to see if it has less variability than day time salivary cortisol *(26)*. Their group included normal individuals, obese and late pregnant patients as well as patients with CS. Although nighttime salivary cortisol was superior to urinary free cortisol, the higher level of salivary cortisol in pregnant patients reduced test specificity to 75%. Despite salivary cortisol's increasing use, and despite its reflecting the unbound cortisol in the serum, there are not yet well validated threshold values for diagnosis of CS in pregnancy. Notwithstanding these limitations, it is a promising approach. Other tests, e.g., CRH/low-dose dexamethasone suppression test have been proposed, but relatively few studies have been performed and the total number of patients studied is small *(27)*. Moreover, the ACTH and cortisol response to CRH administration is blunted in pregnancy *(28–30)*. This test also requires a very sensitive plasma cortisol assay that is accurate at low levels. Such assay performance may not be readily achieved in routine clinical laboratory practice.

Determining the Etiology of Cushing's Syndrome in Pregnancy

Once the diagnosis of CS is made, the next step is to determine the etiology. The various types of CS are shown in Table 1. About half of the cases of CS in pregnancy are caused by adrenal adenomas and only about one third are caused by pituitary tumors. This is different from CS in nonpregnant states where adrenal adenomas account for only 15% of cases while about 70% are caused by pituitary adenomas. In theory, this should facilitate differential diagnosis, but the hormonal changes of pregnancy complicate the matter. In contrast to nonpregnant individuals with cortisol producing adrenal tumors who have low ACTH levels, pregnant patients with such tumors may not have a suppressed ACTH. This lack of suppression most likely reflects the effects of placental CRH. If the pregnant patient does have a suppressed ACTH, the diagnosis of ACTH-independent disease is confirmed and imaging can be performed to localize the adrenal tumor (adenoma or carcinoma) or identify nodular adrenal hyperplasia. Although CT scanning would be contraindicated because of the ionizing radiation, and MRI (even without contrast material) relatively contraindicated because of potential risks especially during the period of organogenesis, ultrasound can be used. Ultrasound has reasonably good sensitivity for the adrenal tumors associated with CS. Sensitivity is a function of both tumor size and operator expertise. It is more operator dependent than CT or MRI *(31)*. Even in this circumstance when ACTH is suppressed, there are difficulties. First, a number of patients with ACTH-independent pregnancy-dependent CS who have been reported showed no radiologic evidence of adrenal tumors *(32)*. Second, several cases with "adrenal adenomas" who were not surgically treated during pregnancy underwent spontaneous remission postpartum *(33–35)*. This fact suggests the possibility that the adrenal "tumors" were, in fact, incidental. It is known that adrenal incidentalomas occur in ~ 2% of individuals and that this is a potential cause of false positive adrenal imaging *(36)*. It has been suggested that the expression of "illicit" LH and beta-human chorionic gonadotropin (HCG) receptors on the adrenal gland could account for adrenal CS that resolves after delivery as the placenta is removed and therefore beta-HCG production ceases *(37)*.

When the ACTH is not suppressed, high-dose dexamethasone suppression testing can be tried. If there is suppression of cortisol, then the likelihood of a cortisol-producing adrenal tumor is very low, but lack of suppression is not very informative. Both pituitary CS and ectopic ACTH syndrome may not suppress. The role of CRH testing in pregnancy is unclear; there has not been a systematic study and ovine CRH is classified by the U.S. Food and Drug Administration (FDA) as a category C drug to be used in pregnancy only when absolutely clinically indicated. However, the limited data suggest that the test can distinguish adrenal Cushing's from CS caused by ACTH-secreting tumors. Distinguishing between pituitary CS (Cushing's disease or CD) and the ectopic ACTH syndrome by means of CRH testing is more problematic. Of note, only a few cases of ectopic ACTH syndrome during pregnancy have been reported and whether the prevalence of this disorder is the same during pregnancy as in the nonpregnant state is unknown. Moreover, many ACTH-secreting tumors, both pituitary and ectopic, are small making them difficult to localize by imaging studies. The MRI is relatively contraindicated and because gadolinium contrast is an FDA category C drug, it is contraindicated. Noncontrasted MRIs have lower sensitivity for pituitary tumors than contrasted MRIs *(10, 38)*. It is also important to recognize that the pituitary gland increases in size during pregnancy. How this would affect the test sensitivity is not known. In addition, there is a prevalence of incidental pituitary lesions of approximately 10% of the population in the age group from 20 to 50 years will have incidental tumors of the pituitary demonstrable by MRI. Therefore, some patients with ectopic ACTH syndrome will have radiographic evidence of a pituitary lesion. Interestingly, among patients with pituitary CS, the prevalence of pituitary macroadenomas is much higher in pregnancy. Whether this is a function of publication bias or the effects of pregnancy on the pituitary is not clear *(13)*.

The best test to differentiate pituitary-dependent disease from the ectopic ACTH syndrome is inferior petrosal sinus sampling with assessment of the ACTH response to CRH *(11)*. There are several reports of this procedure being performed and the pregnancies were uneventful. However, notwithstanding the special attention that can be paid to minimizing fetal exposure to ionizing radiation, the potential deleterious effects of ionizing radiation is a serious limitation *(13, 39)*. That said, Nieman and her colleagues have suggested a prudent approach *(8, 13)*. They state that for pregnant women with CRH and dexamethasone test responses consistent with CD, and pituitary lesions larger than at least 6 mm, usually require no additional testing. Petrosal sinus sampling may be necessary in other cases and when done, should be done in a center with special expertise. They also note that the usual criteria to establish a pituitary/systemic gradient may not apply in the pregnant state *(8, 13)*. In summary, diagnosis and differential diagnosis remain problematic, particularly during pregnancy. Nieman and colleagues recommend a combination of urinary free cortisol (UFC) and assessment of midnight salivary cortisol for screening of CS in pregnancy. In patients with confirmed CS, a low ACTH should prompt imaging of the adrenals. However, in cases with borderline ACTH, a combination of the 8-mg dexamethasone suppression test and CRH stimulation testing is suggested to establish the presence of, and distinguish between, the ACTH-dependent forms. Inferior petrosal sinus sampling (IPSS) may be necessary in a portion of cases with discordant biochemical or imaging findings *(8, 13)*. However, there have been case reports of CRH-dependent CS; in this circumstance CRH, possibly produced in the placenta, can produce ACTH cell hyperplasia, complicating the diagnostic process further.

OUTCOMES OF CUSHING'S SYNDROME IN PREGNANCY

The etiology of the state of hypercortisolism, severity of illness, stage of pregnancy at the time of diagnosis, and the potential beneficial impact of therapy on maternal and fetal outcomes all enter into the decision-making process about therapy. The quality of the evidence on which the decisions are based is only fair; there are no randomized controlled trials and the condition's rarity makes it unlikely that there ever will be. Comparison of outcomes based on multiple case reports is fraught with hazard. Moreover, the choice of therapy and its timing must be individualized because prognostication is so difficult. For example, Chico et al. described six pregnancies in five patients with Cushing's disease – four had undergone transsphenoidal surgery, with improvement but no cure of their hypercortisolism; the other woman became pregnant during initial workup *(40)*. Although fetal outcomes were poor in three cases, a remarkably uneventful and uncomplicated outcome with no clinical progression of cushingoid symptoms was observed in two of the three pregnancies followed to term, despite significant increases in urinary free cortisol.

Maternal Morbidity

The adverse outcomes in pregnant women with CS relate to excessive glucocorticoid action. Maternal morbidity occurs in about 70% of cases, although maternal mortality is infrequent. The frequency of hypertension and gestational diabetes is much greater than during normal pregnancy. In addition, pre-eclampsia and eclampsia appear to occur more commonly. Other reported problems include infection, osteoporotic fracture, and congestive heart failure. For example, Kamiya et al. reported a diabetic patient who exhibited congestive heart failure as an initial symptom *(41)*. Echocardiography revealed a remarkable thickening of the left ventricle without asymmetric hypertrophy. After an adrenal adenoma was removed in the 28th week of pregnancy, the congestive heart failure and hyperglycemia dramatically improved. Only four months after delivery, the thickening of her left ventricle was normalized. Maternal death related to CS has been reported rarely.

The beneficial impact of treatment of Cushing's in the nonpregnant state is clear. Early studies showed very high mortality rates for untreated CS with the primary causes of death being cardiovascular in nature *(9, 42)*. More recent data indicate that the mortality of *treated* CS is much closer to age- and sex-adjusted expected mortality rates *(43)*. This is particularly true for adrenal adenomas. The issue of timing of treatment of CS in the pregnant patient remains somewhat uncertain. The data that treatment during pregnancy has a positive impact on maternal outcomes is modest. However, the data provide stronger support for treatment for the purpose improving fetal outcomes.

Fetal Outcomes

The risk to the fetus depends upon the effects of glucocorticoids on both the fetus directly and the maternal–placental unit. The fetus itself is relatively protected from glucocorticoids. Placenta and all fetal tissues rapidly inactivate cortisol to cortisone, and in contrast to adult tissues, there is little capacity of fetal tissues to convert cortisone to cortisol. This inability to convert cortisone to cortisol persists in the neonatal period *(44)*. Because ACTH does not cross the placental barrier and steroid hormones cross readily, the high maternal corticosteroid levels can suppress fetal ACTH secretion during the last trimester of gestation and result in adrenal insufficiency in the newborn. However, this complication appears to be uncommon *(13)*. Even a case of neonatal CS from antenatal betamethasone treatment has been reported, but this is very rare *(45)*. Fetal virilization is a potential effect of androgen-secreting adrenal tumors *(45, 46)*. Although one case of a fetal abnormality has been reported in a patient with CS, the epidemiologic data on pregnant women with asthma treated with glucocorticoids indicate no increased risk of congenital anomalies *(47)*.

Fetal mortality is about 25–40% and is made up of spontaneous abortion, stillbirth, and early neonatal death due to prematurity. The actual fetal loss rate is really higher because of underdiagnosis of CS. Preterm delivery rate may be as high as 50%. These complications are the likely result of the adverse effects on the placenta of the complications associated with hypercortisolemia, e.g., hypertension and hyperglycemia. Comparison of fetal outcomes suggests that treatment during pregnancy is beneficial. Lindsey and Niemann reviewed 136 pregnancies in which treatment outcomes were available. When no active treatment was given, there were 59 live births (76%) compared with 50 live births (89%) in women in whom treatment was instituted at a mean gestational age of 20 ± 1 weeks *(13)*. Most patients reviewed had undergone adrenalectomy for adrenal adenomas and the live birth rate after unilateral or bilateral adrenalectomy was approximately 87%. Of the 40 women with pituitary CS, most were treated medically; 20% underwent transsphenoidal surgery *(13)*. This review suggests that treatment during pregnancy is associated with better fetal outcomes. However, there are important limitations of the data, especially in terms of the question of the comparability of the groups who did and did not undergo surgery. Moreover, even successful elimination of the hypercortisolism may not avert the development of adverse outcomes.

MANAGEMENT OF CUSHING'S SYNDROME DURING PREGNANCY

Surgical Treatment

In the nonpregnant individual with CS, the treatment is relatively straightforward, assuming that the etiology has been accurately determined. For pituitary CS, transsphenoidal surgery for pituitary tumor removal has replaced bilateral adrenalectomy *(48–51)*. The former is associated with cure/remission rates of about 80–90% in the most experienced hands. Surgical morbidity and mortality are quite low. Transsphenoidal adenomectomy for Cushing's disease during pregnancy was first described in 1987 followed by several other reports *(52–56)*. The maternal outcomes in general have been good and the control of the hypercortisolism resulted in decreased insulin requirements and improved blood pressure control. Successfully treated cases required replacement therapy for secondary adrenal insufficiency as would be expected. However, preterm labor and fetal death have occurred many weeks after surgery. It is also important to note that there is a larger experience with transsphenoidal surgery during pregnancy for management of prolactinoma, indicating the safety of the procedure in good hands. Bilateral adrenalectomy was the treatment of choice in the 1960s for Cushing's disease and it still has a role, although a much more limited one *(57)*. This procedure has been performed during pregnancy and in general, the maternal outcomes have been good, although there are problems with wound healing and infection. These case reports mostly date from the 1960s. All patients are expected to receive lifelong glucocorticoid and mineralocorticoid replacement therapy. The role for bilateral adrenalectomy during pregnancy is extremely limited, but with the development of laparoscopic adrenalectomy, a major advance in surgical technique in terms of reduction in surgical morbidity and mortality, it does remain an option for patients who can be treated in no other way *(58, 59)*.

For adrenal tumors, unilateral adrenalectomy for adrenal adenoma has been performed safely even into the early third trimester, although most surgery was performed between 6 and 28 weeks of gestation. However, for both transsphenoidal surgery and laparoscopic adrenalectomy, there are significant learning curves and treatment should be obtained at experienced centers. Radiotherapy is primarily limited to an adjunctive role, primarily for patients whose pituitary tumor resection has been incomplete, although Anderson and Walters reported a case of Cushing's disease where the patient underwent irradiation of the sella at 24 weeks of gestation *(60)*. This pregnancy resulted in a term pregnancy without complications. There are limited data on gamma knife procedures during pregnancy. Medical therapy in the nonpregnant state is generally reserved for patients with persistent disease postoperatively and for those who are not good surgical candidates where it is given either as preparation or as a substitute for surgery *(61)*. Medical therapy may have a larger role in CS in pregnancy, especially of nonadrenal origin.

Medical Treatment

The use of medical treatment in CS associated with pregnancy has been done in relatively few cases. Medical treatment in pregnancy is usually avoided to minimize the potential for teratogenesis and induction of fetal adrenal insufficiency. In addition to those patients who conceived while on medical treatment, the rationales for use have included temporary treatment until delivery, preparation for surgery, and refusal of surgery. It has also been used when pregnancy-induced CS was suspected. The greatest experience with medical treatment during pregnancy involves metyrapone, an agent which inhibits 11β-hydroxylation leading to a reduction in cortisol levels *(61)*. Metyrapone also decreases placental aromatase enzyme activity. The total daily dosage has usually been 0.5–3.0 g with dosage adjustment based on plasma and 24-h urine cortisol levels and clinical status *(62–65)*. It is generally well tolerated. Blood pressure must be monitored carefully because of the potential of metyrapone to exacerbate hypertension and contribute to pre-eclampsia and there has been one report of fetal hypoadrenalism after metyrapone *(13)*. Metyrapone was used in two consecutive pregnancies in a patient with pregnancy-induced CS *(66)*. In both pregnancies, metyrapone therapy was initiated at 14 weeks of gestation, and titrated to a dose of 2.5–3.0 g/day. There were no reported neonatal congenital abnormalities, except for intrauterine growth retardation in the second pregnancy.

Although ketoconazole is usually the drug of choice for medical therapy for pituitary CS in nonpregnant individuals, its use in pregnancy has been more limited *(61)*. Ketoconazole inhibits several P450 enzymes involved in steroid hormone biosynthesis, e.g., the 17α-hydroxylase activity and cholesterol side-chain cleavage enzyme in the maternal and fetal adrenal gland. Ketoconazole also has effects on steroid metabolism in the placenta. These actions suggest the potential for causing interference in normal sex differentiation. However, in the case of an adrenal adenoma, ketoconazole was used at 600 mg/day between 32nd and 37th week of gestation; in another patient who had Cushing's disease, 600–1,000 mg/day was used between 7th and 37th week of gestation *(67, 68)*. In both cases, the female and male infants were noted to have intrauterine growth retardation at birth, but no congenital anomalies, adrenal insufficiency, or sexual differentiation problems. For example, Berwaerts et al. reported a 30-year-old female with pituitary-dependent Cushing's disease, who refused transsphenoidal surgery and was treated with ketoconazole and cabergoline *(68)*. After approximately three years of therapy, the patient herself decided, without the knowledge of her treating physician, to interrupt contraception. The patient became pregnant and ceased the intake of all medication (at approximately the third week of pregnancy). Because of the development of clinical CS, ketoconazole and cabergoline were restarted and continued uneventfully until the 37th week. Vaginal delivery was also passed uneventfully. The newborn male did not demonstrate any congenital malformations and was normally sexually developed. Nevertheless, because ketoconazole crosses the placenta (in animal models) and is teratogenic, its use during pregnancy should be discouraged.

Experience with other drugs is even more limited. Mitotane (*o,p′*-DDD), used primarily in the management of adrenal carcinoma, is an adrenolytic agent with cytotoxicity specific to the adrenal cortex, but has potential teratogenicity *(61)*. Gerl et al. reported the use of mitotane in a pregnant patient with Cushing's disease when transsphenoidal surgery and other drugs failed to control hypercortisolism; a patient with Cushing's disease who became pregnant while being treated with mitotane underwent a therapeutic abortion because of suspected embryotoxicity early in pregnancy *(69, 70)*. Aminoglutethimide which inhibits cholesterol side chain cleavage enzyme may result in virilization of female fetuses when used in pregnancy. Hanson et al. reported the use of aminoglutethimide until 21 weeks of gestation in a patient with Cushing's disease without any adverse effects *(71)*. This patient had bilateral adrenalectomy at 21 weeks of gestation and gave birth to a term baby girl without virilization. Cyproheptadine, a serotonin antagonist has been used in a few cases without consistent effects *(72, 73)*. There were no reported congenital abnormalities. There is a subset of cases with Cushing's disease with hyperprolactinemia that respond to dopamine agonists such as bromocriptine *(61)*. While the safety of certain dopamine agonists during pregnancy has been established in patients with prolactinoma, it is not a primary therapy for Cushing's disease. The glucocorticoid antagonist Mifepristone (RU 486) could have potential, at least late in pregnancy. Mifepristone has been used to treat nonpregnant patients with CS, but its primary use is as an abortifacient and there are no reports of its use to control hypercortisolism during pregnancy *(74, 75)*.

In summary, biases and data limitations notwithstanding, there are certain general statements that can be made. First, the maternal and fetal outcomes of untreated CS are poor. Second, surgical procedures specific for the pituitary and the adrenal can be performed safely in the hands of experts. Third, even medical therapy can be utilized with apparent safety, although the number of cases is small. However, the importance of individualizing treatment based on patient preferences, individual risks, and physician and team experience cannot be overemphasized. For patients with pituitary CS diagnosed in the first, second, or even early in the third trimester, transsphenoidal surgery would be the most appropriate approach. We would not recommend bilateral adrenalectomy; there have been too many cases of spontaneous resolution of CS following delivery. In these cases and if the diagnosis of Cushing's disease is made in the third trimester, especially late, medical treatment combined with early delivery is preferred. There will also be some milder cases in which the risks of treatment merit expectant management. For patients with adrenal tumors, especially adenomas, unilateral adrenalectomy is the most appropriate approach. In addition, as a general rule, cesarean delivery should be avoided because of the problems of wound healing in hypercortisolism.

CONCLUSION

The CS is primarily a disorder of women of childbearing age, but fortunately is rare during pregnancy. The diagnosis of CS is challenging in the nonpregnant state and even more so during pregnancy. Pregnant women without CS develop some features of CS, such as hypertension, hyperglycemia, and striae. Both of the tests most commonly to establish the diagnosis of CS (low-dose dexamethasone suppression testing and assessment of 24-h urinary free cortisol) present difficulties because of normal changes in the hypothalamic-pituitary axis during pregnancy. However, hypercortisolism is associated with unfavorable maternal and fetal outcomes. Thus, it is important to have a high index of suspicion of the disease to prevent delay in diagnosis. Once the diagnosis is made, we propose a general approach to treatment, but recognized the importance of individualizing therapy.

REFERENCES

1. Yanovski JA, Cutler GB, Jr. Glucocorticoid action and the clinical features of Cushing's syndrome. Endo Metab Clin NA 1994;23:487–510.
2. Atallah D, Atallah C, Saade C, Mansour F, Kesrouani A, Abboud J. Cushing's syndrome and pregnancy: a case report and review of the literature. Contracept Fertil Sex 1999;27:61–64.
3. Hunt AB, McConaghy WM. Pregnancy associated with diseases of the adrenal glands. Am J Obstet Gynecol 1953;66: 970–987.
4. Sheeler L. Cushing's syndrome and pregnancy. Endo Metab Clin NA 1994;23:619–627.
5. Aron DC, Schnall AM, Sheeler LR. Cushing's syndrome and pregnancy. Am J Obstet Gynecol 1990;162:244–252.
6. Keely E. Endocrine causes of hypertension in pregnancy—when to start looking for zebras. Semin Perinatol 1998;22: 471–484.
7. Kreisberg R. Clinical problem-solving. Half a loaf. N Engl J Med 1994;330:1295–1299.
8. Lindsay J, Nieman L. The hypothalamic-pituitary-adrenal axis in pregnancy: challenges in disease detection and treatment. Endocr Rev 2005;26:775–799.
9. Ross EJ, Linch DC. Cushing's syndrome—killing disease: discriminatory value of signs and symptoms aiding early diagnosis. Lancet 1982;2:646–649.
10. Findling J, Raff H. Cushing's syndrome: important issues in diagnosis and management. J Clin Endocrinol Metab 2009;91:3746–3753.
11. Aron DC. Diagnostic implications of adrenal physiology and clinical epidemiology for evaluation of glucocorticoid excess and deficiency. In: DeGroot LJ, Jameson JL, ed. Endocrinology. 4 ed., 2000.
12. Chrousos GP, Torpy DJ, Gold PW. Interactions between the hypothalamic-pituitary-adrenal axis and the female reproductive systems: clinical implications. Ann Int Med 1998;129:229–240.
13. Lindsay J, Jonklaas J, Oldfield E, et al. Cushing's syndrome during pregnancy: personal experience and review of the literature. J Clin Endocrinol Metab 2005;90:3077–3083.
14. Magiakou MA, Mastorakos H, Rabin D, et al. The maternal hypothalamic-pituitary-adrenal axis in third trimester human pregnancy. Clin Endocrinol (Oxf) 1996;44:419–428.
15. Magiakou MA, Mastorakos G, Webster E, Chrousos GP. The hypothalamic-pituitary-adrenal axis and the female reproductive system. Ann NY Acad Sci 1997;816:42–56.
16. Nolten WE, Lindheimer MD, Rveckert PA, et al. Diurnal patterns and regulation of cortisol secretion in pregnancy. J Clin Endocrinol Metab 1980;31:466–472.
17. Carr BR, Parker CR, Madden JD, et al. Maternal plasma adrenocorticotropin and cortisol relationships throughout human pregnancy. Am J Obstet Gynecol 1981;139:416–422.
18. Cousins L, Rigg L, Hollingsworth D, et al. Qualitative and quantitative assessment of the circadian rhythm of cortisol in pregnancy. Am J Obstet Gynecol 1983;145:411–416.
19. Campbell EA, Linton EA, Wolfe CD, Scraggs PR, Jones MT, Lowry PJ. Plasma corticotrophin-releasing hormone concentration during pregnancy and parturition. J Clin Endocrinol Metab 1987;64:1054–1059.
20. Robinson BG, Emanuel RL, Frim DM, Majzoub JA. Glucocorticoid stimulates expression of corticotropin-releasing hormone gene in human placenta. Proc Natl Acad Sci USA 1988;85:5244–5248.
21. Trainer PJ, Woods RJ, Korbonits M, et al. The pathophysiology of circulating corticotropin-releasing hormone-binding protein levels in the human. J Clin Endocrinol Metab 1998;83:1611–1614.
22. Aron DC, Schnall AM, Sheeler LR. Spontaneous resolution of Cushing's syndrome after pregnancy. Am J Obstet Gynecol 1990;162:472–474.
23. Nieman LK, Biller BM, Findling JW, et al. The diagnosis of Cushing's syndrome: an Endocrine Society Clinical Practice Guideline. J Clin Endocrinol Metab 2008;93:1526–1540.
24. Scott EM, McGarrigle HHG, Lachelin CL. The increase in plasma and saliva cortisol levels in pregnancy is not due to the increase in corticosteroid-binding globulin levels. J Clin Endocrinol Metab 1990;71:639–644.
25. Billaud L, Sanson ML, Guilhaume B, Bertagna X, Abecassis JP, Luton JP. Cushing syndrome during pregnancy. New diagnostic methods used in 3 cases of adrenal cortex carcinoma. Presse Med 1992;21:2041–2045.
26. Viardot A, Huber P, Puder J, et al. Reproducibility of nighttime salivary cortisol and its use in the diagnosis of hypercortisolism compared with urinary free cortisol and overnight dexamethasone suppression test. J Clin Endocrinol Metab 2005;90:5730–5736.
27. Yanovski JA, Cutler GB, Jr., Chrousos GP, Nieman LK. The dexamethasone-suppressed corticotropin-releasing hormone stimulation test differentiates mild Cushing's disease from normal physiology. J Clin Endocrinol Metab 1998;83:348–352.

28. Hernandez C, Simo R. Provocation test with corticotropin liberating hormone in pregnancy. Med Clin (Barc) 1996; 107:477.
29. Schulte HM, Weisner D, Allolio B. The corticotrophin releasing hormone test in late pregnancy: lack of adrenocorticotrophin and cortisol response. Clin Endocrinol 1990;33:99–106.
30. Schulte HM, Chrousos GP, Avgerinos P, et al. The corticotropin-releasing hormone stimulation test: a possible aid in the evaluation of patients with adrenal insufficiency. J Clin Endocrinol Metab 1984;58:1064–1067.
31. Resnek RM, Armstrong P. The adrenal gland. Clin Endocrinol 1994;40:561–576.
32. Close CF, Mann MC, Watts JF, Taylor KG. ACTH-independent Cushing's syndrome in pregnancy with spontaneous resolution after delivery: control of the hypercortisolism with metyrapone. Clin Endocrinol (Oxf) 1993;39:375–379.
33. Margulies PL, Imperato-McGinley J, Arthur A, Peterson RE. Remission of Cushing's syndrome during pregnancy. Int J Gynaecol Obstet 1983;21:77–83.
34. Parra A, Cruz-Krohn J. Intercurrent Cushing's syndrome and pregnancy. Am J Med 1966;40:961–966.
35. Verdugo C, Donoso J, Meza H, et al. Cushing's syndrome and pregnancy with spontaneous remission after delivery. Rev Med Chil 1982;110:564–569.
36. Chidiac RM, Aron DC. Incidentalomas: a disease of modern technology. Endo Metab Clin NA 1997;26:233–253.
37. Polli N, Giraldi F, Cavagnini F. Cushing's disease and pregnancy. Pituitary 2004;7:237–241.
38. Dwyer AJ, Frank JA, Doppman JL, et al. Pituitary adenomas in patients with Cushing's disease: initial experience with Gd-DTPA enhanced MR imaging. Radiology 1987;63:421.
39. Pinette MG, Pan YQ, Oppenheim D, Pinette SG, Blackstone J. Bilateral inferior petrosal sinus corticotropin sampling with corticotropin-releasing hormone stimulation in a pregnant patient with Cushing's syndrome. Am J Obstet Gynecol 1994;171:563–564.
40. Chico A, Manzanares JM, Halperin I, Martinez de Osaba MJ, Adelantado J, Webb SM. Cushing's disease and pregnancy: report of six cases. Eur J Obstet Gynecol Reprod Biol 1996;64:143–146.
41. Kamiya Y, Okada M, Yoneyama A, et al. Surgical successful treatment of Cushing's syndrome in a pregnant patient complicated with severe cardiac involvement. Endocr J 1998;45:499–504.
42. Welbourn RB, Montgomery DA, Kennedy TL. The natural history of treated Cushing's syndrome. Br J Surg 1971; 58:1–16.
43. Swearingen B, Biller BM, Barker FG II, et al. Long-term mortality after transsphenoidal surgery for Cushing's disease. Ann Int Med 1999;130:821–824.
44. Hillman DA, Giroud CJP. Plasma cortisone and cortisol levels at birth and during the neonatal period. J Clin Endocrinol Metab 1995;25:243–248.
45. Bradley BS, Kumar SP, Mehta PN, Ezhuthachan SG. Neonatal cushingoid syndrome resulting from serial courses of antenatal betamethasone. Obstet Gynecol 1994;83:869–872.
46. Miyata M, Nishihara M, Tokunaka S, Yachiku S. A maternal functioning adrenocortical adenoma causing fetal female pseudohermaphroditism. J Urol 1989;142:806–808.
47. Fitzsimons R, Greenberger PA, Patterson MD. Outcome of pregnancy in women requiring corticosteroids for severe asthma. J Allergy Clin Immunol 2009;78:349–353.
48. Biller BM, Grossman A, Stewart PM, et al. Treatment of adrenocorticotropin-dependent Cushing's syndrome: a consensus statement. J Clin Endocrinol Metab 2008;93:2454–2462.
49. Laws ER, Jr., Thapar K. Pituitary surgery. Endo Metab Clin NA 1999;28:119–132.
50. Swearingen B, Biller BM, Barker FG II, et al. Long-term mortality after transsphenoidal surgery for Cushing's disease. Ann Int Med 1999;130:821–824.
51. Tyrrell JB, Wilson CB. Cushing's disease: therapy of pituitary adenomas. Endo Metab Clin NA 1994;23:925–938.
52. Casson IF, Davis JC, Jeffreys RV, Silas JH, Williams J, Belchetz PE. Successful management of Cushing's disease during pregnancy by transsphenoidal adenectomy. Clin Endocrinol (Oxf) 1987;27:423–428.
53. Coyne TJ, Atkinson RL, Prins JB. Adrenocorticotropic hormone-secreting pituitary tumor associated with pregnancy: case report. Neurosurgery 1992;31:953–955.
54. Mellor A, Harvey RD, Pobereskin LH, Sneyd JR. Cushing's disease treated by trans-sphenoidal selective adenomectomy in mid-pregnancy. Br J Anaesth 1998;80:850–852.
55. Pinette MG, Pan YQ, Oppenheim D, Pinette SG, Blackstone J. Bilateral inferior petrosal sinus corticotropin sampling with corticotropin-releasing hormone stimulation in a pregnant patient with Cushing's syndrome. Am J Obstet Gynecol 1994;171:563–564.
56. Ross RJ, Chew SL, Perry L, Erskine K, Medbak S, Afshar F. Diagnosis and selective cure of Cushing's disease during pregnancy by transsphenoidal surgery. Eur J Endocrinol 1995;132:722–726.
57. O'Riordain DS, Farley DR, Young WFJ, Grant CS, van Heerden JA. Long-term outcome of bilateral adrenalectomy in patients with Cushing's syndrome. Surgery 1994;116:1088–1093.

58. Acosta E, Pantoja JP, Gamiino R, Rull JA, Herrera MF. Laparoscopic versus open adrenalectomy in Cushing's syndrome and disease. Surgery 1999;126:1111–1116.
59. Finkenstedt G, Gasser RW, Hofle G, et al. Pheochromocytoma and sub-clinical Cushing's syndrome during pregnancy: diagnosis, medical pre-treatment and cure by laparoscopic unilateral adrenalectomy. J Endocrinol Invest 1999;22:551–557.
60. Anderson KJ, Walters AW. Cushing's syndrome and pregnancy. Aust NZ J Obstet Gynaecol 1976;16:225–230.
61. Sonino N, Boscaro M. Medical therapy for Cushing's disease. Endo Metab Clin NA 1999;28:211–222.
62. Cabezon C, Bruno OD, Cohen M, Garcia S, Gutman RA. Twin pregnancy in a patient with Cushing's disease. Fertil Steril 1999;72:371–372.
63. Close CF, Mann MC, Watts JF, Taylor KG. ACTH-independent Cushing's syndrome in pregnancy with spontaneous resolution after delivery: control of the hypercortisolism with metyrapone. Clin Endocrinol (Oxf) 1993;39:375–379.
64. Connell JM, Cordiner J, Davies DL, Fraser R, Frier BM, McPherson SG. Pregnancy complicated by Cushing's syndrome: potential hazard of metyrapone therapy. Case report. Br J Obstet Gynaecol 1985;92:1192–1195.
65. Gormley MJ, Hadden DR, Kennedy TL, Montgomery DA, Murnaghan GA, Sheridan B. Cushing's syndrome in pregnancy—treatment with metyrapone. Clin Endocrinol (Oxf) 1982;16:283–293.
66. Wallace C, Toth E, Lewanczuk R, et al. Pregnancy-induced Cushing's syndrome in multiple pregnancies. J Clin Endocrinol Metab 1996;81:15–21.
67. Amado JA, Pesquera C, Gonzalez EM, Otero M, Freijanes J, Alvarez A. Successful treatment with ketoconazole of Cushing's syndrome in pregnancy. Postgrad Med J 1990;66:221–223.
68. Berwaerts J, Verhelst J, Mahler C, Abs R. Cushing's syndrome in pregnancy treated by ketoconazole: case report and review of the literature. Gynecol Endocrinol 1999;13:175–182.
69. Gerl H, Benecke R, Knappe G, Rohde W, Stahl F, Amendt P. Pregnancy and partus in Cushing's disease treated with o,p'-DDD. Acta endocrinol (Kbh) 1992;126(Suppl. 4):133.
70. Leiba S, Weinstein R, Shindel B, et al. The protracted effect of o,p'-DDD in Cushing's disease and its impact on adrenal morphogenesis of young human embryo. Ann Endocrinol (Paris) 1989;50:49–53.
71. Hanson TJ, Ballonoff LB, Northcutt RC. Amino-glutethimide and pregnancy. JAMA 1974;230:963–964.
72. Kasperlik-Zaluska A, Migdalska B, Hartwig W, et al. Two pregnancies in a woman with Cushing's syndrome treated with cyproheptadine. Case report. Br J Obstet Gynaecol 1980;87:1171–1173.
73. Khir AS, How J, Bewsher PD. Successful pregnancy after cyproheptadine treatment for Cushing's disease. Eur J Obstet Gynecol Reprod Biol 1982;13:343–347.
74. Kehlet H, Binder C. Value of an ACTH test in assessing hypothalamic-pituitary-adrenocortical function in glucocorticoid-treated patients. BMJ 1973;2:147–149.
75. Koide SS. Mifepristone. Auxiliary therapeutic use in cancer and related disorders. J Reprod Med 1998;43:551–560.

22 Special Aspects of Cushing's Syndrome: Childhood

Martin O. Savage, Farhad Afshar, Nicholas P. Plowman, Renuka P. Dias, Ashley B. Grossman, and Helen L. Storr

Contents

Summary

Cushing's syndrome (CS) is a rare pediatric problem on which few pediatric endocrinologists have extensive experience. Hence, close collaboration with an adult endocrinologist colleague is strongly recommended. This chapter reviews the main types of CS occurring in the pediatric age range. Results are presented from the authors'own experience of management of over 50 cases of pediatric CS during the last 25 years. These include McCune–Albright syndrome in infancy, adrenocortical tumors, primary nodular adrenal hyperplasia, ectopic ACTH syndrome, and Cushing's disease. The major clinical features are described, including linear growth and puberty, and diagnostic techniques are discussed. From a personal database of 38 cases of Cushing's disease (CD), the relative benefits of pituitary MR imaging versus bilateral inferior petrosal sinus sampling for ACTH are appraised. Therapeutic strategy is discussed for primary adrenal CS and pituitary-dependent CD. The results of transsphenoidal surgery and pituitary radiotherapy are described together with the challenge of optimizing postcure linear growth and body composition.

Key Words: Cushing's syndrome, Pediatrics, Cushing's disease, Pituitary surgery, Pituitary radiotherapy

From: *Contemporary Endocrinology: Cushing's Syndrome: Pathophysiology, Diagnosis and Treatment*
Edited by: M.D. Bronstein (ed.), DOI 10.1007/978-1-60327-449-4_22,

Pediatric Cushing's syndrome (CS) presents a diagnostic and therapeutic challenge. CS is a rare problem in pediatric endocrine practice, and most pediatric endocrinologists have limited experience in the diagnosis and treatment of these children. Consequently, pediatricians can benefit from close consultation with adult colleagues. This chapter describes the clinical assessment and presentation, diagnosis, treatment and therapeutic outcome of CS in childhood and adolescence. We present data from our personal series of 52 cases of pediatric CS, managed over the last 26 years. CS may occur throughout childhood and adolescence, but certain etiologies present more frequently at certain ages *(1)* (Fig. 1).

McCune–Albright Syndrome

CS in infancy is usually associated with McCune–Albright syndrome (MAS) caused by activating mutations of arginine 201 in the guanine nucleotide-binding protein (G protein) α-subunit *(2)*. In infancy, MAS, occurring predominantly in females, may present with CS, often with additional endocrine dysfunction such as hyperthyroidism and precocious puberty *(3)*. The CS is usually severe and potentially life-threatening, requiring bilateral adrenalectomy. Histological appearance shows nodular adrenocortical hyperplasia *(4)*.

Adrenocortical Tumors

Adrenocortical tumors (ACT) comprise 0.3–0.4% of neoplasms in children and are an important cause of pediatric CS *(5)*. Much has been learnt from experience in Southern Brazil, where the incidence is 3.4–4.2 per million children, i.e., 10–15 times higher than in other geographical areas *(6, 7)*. Adrenocortical carcinoma is also associated with Li–Fraumeni syndrome and germline point mutations of the p53 tumor suppressor gene *(TP53)* encoding an R337H amino acid substitution *(6)*. The genetics of adrenal tumors has recently been reviewed *(8)*. In the Brazilian series, ACT occurred most commonly under 4 years of age and was usually associated with virilization (56%) or mixed hormone secretion, including cortisol (29.2%), with pure cortisol-secreting ACT making up 5.5 and 3% of patients in two series *(7)*.

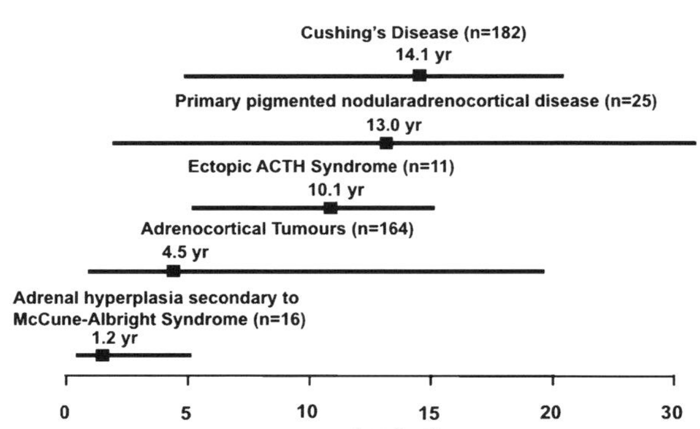

Fig. 1. Different etiologies of pediatric Cushing's syndrome from the literature (n = 398 cases) shown at ages of peak incidence (*boxes*) *(1)*.

Ectopic ACTH Syndrome

Ectopic ACTH syndrome (EAS) is extremely rare in children and adolescents *(1)*. However, pediatric EAS is well documented *(9)*. Carcinoid tumors predominate as cause of pediatric EAS, and most are bronchial or thymic, but renal oncocytic carcinoid, duodenal carcinoid, and clear-cell sarcoma also have been reported, as have neuroendocrine tumors of the pancreas and Wilms' tumor *(1)*.

Primary Nodular Adrenal Hyperplasia

Primary bilateral adrenocortical hyperplasia is a rare but important cause of pediatric CS *(10)*. Primary pigmented adrenocortical disease (PPNAD) is usually associated with the multiple endocrine neoplasia (MEN) syndrome designated as Carney complex. Carney complex (CNC; MIM 160980) *(11)* is an autosomal dominant syndrome characterized by lentigines, cardiac myxomas, endocrine, and nonendocrine tumors, and PPNAD is its most frequent presentation in children and young adults *(12)*.

PPNAD typically occurs in adolescence or early adulthood *(13)*. The adrenal pathology shows multiple, small, pigmented, adrenocortical nodules surrounded by cortical atrophy *(10)*. The hypercortisolemia of PPNAD may rarely be subclinical or cyclical, and it has been suggested that classical CS may be absent in childhood. In our series of seven cases, all patients displayed typical features of CS including hypertension and virilization *(13)*.

Cushing's Disease

Pediatric pituitary-dependent Cushing's disease (CD) caused by an ACTH-secreting corticotroph adenoma accounts for 75–80% of CS and is almost always caused by a pituitary microadenoma *(1, 14)*. We have seen only one macroadenoma in 37 pediatric cases. The commonest age of presentation of pediatric CD falls in adolescence (Fig. 1), and our youngest patient was aged 5.8 years.

In adults, CD has a female preponderance, but in 50 CD patients aged 6–30 years, we found a strong predominance of males in the prepubertal patients *(15)*. In our current series of 37 cases, aged from 5.8 to 17.8 years, there are 24 males and 13 females. Our report *(15)* was the first to describe this male predominance in young children; however, the large series from the NIH *(14)* shows the same phenomenon.

CLINICAL ASSESSMENT OF THE CHILD WITH SUSPECTED CUSHING'S SYNDROME

The recognition of features that can alert the clinician to the diagnosis of CS is of crucial importance. Most cases have a change in facial appearance consistent with CS. However, this is frequently not recognized by parents and pediatricians as being pathological, and the mean length of symptoms prior to diagnosis in our series was more than two years. All patients complained of weight gain. However, the young child can present with obesity and poor growth without the classical features of plethora, hirsutism, acne, and striae. Emotional lability and fatigue are also frequently present.

Linear Growth

Growth failure is common in all children with CS *(16)*, and short stature was present in half of our CD patients, and growth velocity, when available, was subnormal. Height SDS was almost always below the mean, and BMI SDS was consistently above it (Fig. 2). Comparison of height and BMI

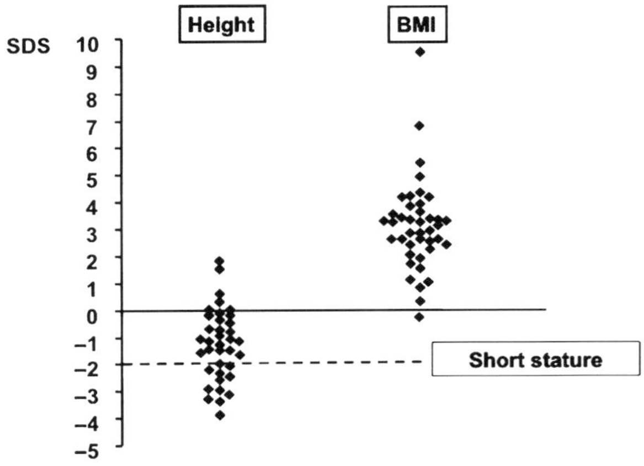

Fig. 2. Height and body mass index (BMI) SDS values in 42 pediatric patients with Cushing's syndrome; Cushing's disease (n = 35) primary nodular adrenal hyperplasia (n = 7). The *dotted line* indicates the SDS value below which patients are significantly shorter than average.

SDS values in 25 pediatric CD patients and 44 age-matched subjects with simple obesity showed a significant difference in the ratio of these two variables between the two groups *(17)*, height being increased in simple obesity and decreased in CD. Bone age (BA) at diagnosis in 17 CD patients was delayed by a mean of 2.0 "years" and the degree of delay correlated negatively with height SDS, duration of symptoms, and age at diagnosis *(18)*.

Puberty Development

There are few detailed reports of puberty in CD, although virilization with pseudo-precocious puberty is an important feature *(14)*. We analyzed clinical pubertal development in 27 CD patients and identified abnormal virilization in 12 *(19)*. In these patients, serum androstenedione, DHEAS, and testosterone SDS were higher than in subjects without abnormal virilization, and SHBG SDS values were lower (p= 0.006). Gonadotropin levels were suppressed.

INVESTIGATION OF CUSHING'S SYNDROME

Investigation protocols of CS have been extensively reviewed *(1, 20, 21)*. We will highlight aspects that we have found helpful during the management of 52 pediatric CS patients over the past 25 years. Investigations in children should be based on those performed in adults *(20, 21)*. The protocol consists initially of confirmation or exclusion of the diagnosis of CS followed by definition of etiology.

Confirmation or Exclusion of Cushing's Syndrome

We first perform three consecutive 24 h urine collections for urinary free cortisol (UFC). Three normal UFC levels have high specificity for exclusion of CS. If there is still uncertainty, we would admit the child for measurement of serum cortisol at three time points (09:00, 18:00 h, and midnight [sleeping]) to assess circadian rhythm. Midnight cortisol should be <50 nmol/L (1.8 μg/dL), although young children may reach their cortisol nadir earlier than midnight. Elevation of midnight sleeping serum cortisol has the greatest sensitivity of all tests for CS in children *(22)*. Precannulation is essential, so as not to wake the child.

We then perform a low-dose dexamethasone suppression test (LDDST), using 0.5 mg 6 hourly (at 09:00, 15:00, 21:00, and 03:00 h) for 48 h, unless the child weighs <40 kg, when we use the NIH-recommended dose of 30 μg/kg/day *(14)*. In the LDDST, blood is taken for serum cortisol at 0 and at 48 h, when it should be undetectable (<50 nmol/L). These tests, individually and in combination, have a high sensitivity for CS and an even higher specificity for the exclusion of this diagnosis.

Definition of the Etiology of Cushing's Syndrome

Having confirmed the presence of CS, ACTH-dependent or ACTH-independent disease needs to be established. Determination of 09:00 h plasma ACTH showed that all our patients with an ACT or nodular adrenal hyperplasia (*n*= 8) had undetectable ACTH *(13)*, which is a clear indication for adrenal MRI. Conversely, in all of our patients with CD, ACTH was detectable, ranging from 12 to 128 ng/L (NR 10–50 ng/L). The combination of elevated midnight cortisol and detectable 09:00 h ACTH confirms ACTH-dependent CS (Fig. 3).

We routinely perform a CRH test (1.0 μg/kg IV), usually before the LDDST, and in 27 CD patients serum cortisol increased by >20% (range 106–554%) *(23)*. Although it is arguable that the rarity of EAS in children does not justify the CRH test, we find that in children with CD, the response is always exuberant and an increased response contributes to this diagnosis. We have discontinued the high-dose dexamethasone suppression test (HDDST) because in 24 patients with CD, mean baseline serum cortisol values of 590.7 ± 168.8 nmol/L (21.4 ± 6.1 μg/dL) decreased to 337.4 ± 104.0 nmol/L (12.2 ± 3.8 μg/dL) at 48 h during LDDST, showing that cortisol suppression during LDDST strongly supports the diagnosis of CD *(24)*.

Biochemical Features in Nodular Adrenal Hyperplasia

In our series, all patients with PPNAD had typical primary adrenal CS with raised UFC levels, failure of cortisol to suppress on L and HDDST, undetectable plasma ACTH, and no cortisol response during a CRH test *(13, 23)*. In addition, a paradoxical increase of UFC and/or 17-hydroxy-corticosteroids is reported in the second phase of a HDDST, which can be diagnostic for PPNAD *(10)*.

Genetics of Nodular Adrenal Hyperplasia

PPNAD may occur in association with CNC, and linkage studies have suggested two predominant genetic loci. The 2p16 locus (CNC2) was identified first, but the gene responsible remains

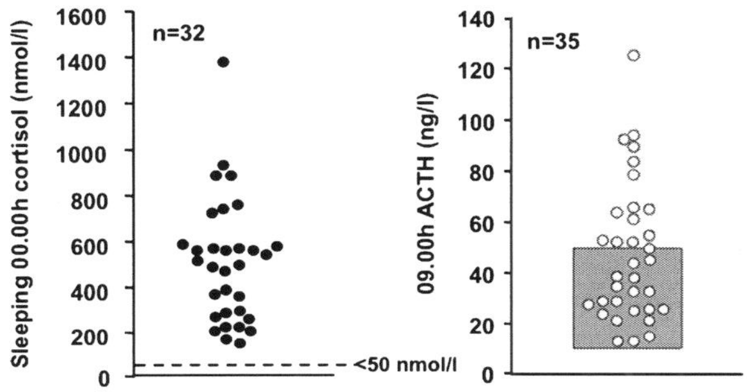

Fig. 3. Midnight serum cortisol and 09:00 h plasma ACTH values in children and adolescents with Cushing's disease. Note loss of circadian variation with elevation of midnight cortisol and detectable ACTH values. Normal ACTH range shown by the *gray box*.

unknown *(25)*. Recently, inactivating mutations of the regulatory subunit type 1-α of the protein kinase A (PRKAR1A) have been reported at the second genetic locus (17q22–24) *(11)*. Mutations are found most frequently in exons 4B, 2, and 6 of the PRKAR1A gene resulting in a premature stop codon *(26)*. The genetic features of CNC and PPNAD have recently been reviewed extensively *(27)*.

Adrenal Imaging

Adrenal imaging is an essential part of the investigation of primary adrenal CS. The differential diagnosis is between ACT and primary nodular adrenal hyperplasia. Most adrenal tumors are visible on MRI scan. In PPNAD, the adrenals are usually of normal size *(13)*. Although the adrenocortical nodules are small (often <6 mm), they may be visualized on CT or MR scanning. Unilateral or bilateral macronodules may be visible and can be quite large (10–30 mm) *(13)*.

Pituitary Imaging

Pituitary MR imaging is an important step towards the successful treatment of Cushing's disease by transsphenoidal surgery (TSS). Most pediatric ACTH-secreting pituitary tumors are microadenomas with diameters <5 mm *(28)*. These have a hypointense signal, which fails to enhance with gadolinium *(20)*. In the NIH series, approximately 50% of microadenomas were visible on pituitary MRI *(14)*. In our experience, pituitary imaging was relatively unhelpful, showing a normal appearance in over half of the patients, with a low predictive value of the position of the adenoma, as identified at surgery *(29)*. Details are shown in Table 1.

Bilateral Inferior Petrosal Sinus Sampling for ACTH

Bilateral inferior petrosal sinus sampling for ACTH (BIPSS) was developed mainly at the NIH and is now performed in pediatric patients *(14, 30)*. Owing to the rarity of EAS, the aim of BIPSS is primarily to demonstrate the site of ACTH secretion, i.e., either laterally or in the midline. The first pediatric data reported a predictive value of lateralization of 75–80% *(14)*. In our experience, ACTH sampling gave a better prediction of the site of the microadenoma than pituitary imaging *(29)*. Our most recent results are shown in Table 2.

BIPSS is a specialized technique and in our unit is performed by the same radiologist who studies adult patients on a regular basis. We generally do not use general anesthesia (GA) to avoid potential alteration of ACTH secretion. The youngest patient we studied without GA was aged 8.4 years, but we have recently performed BIPSS under GA in two patients aged 6.4 and 5.8 years. We have now performed BIPSS in 29 pediatric CD patients, without complications, and have shown lateralization

Table 1
Pediatric Cushing's Disease: Pituitary Imaging, Surgical Identification of Adenoma, and Cure by TSS

Total patients (n)	*Adenoma CT/MRI image (n)*	*Concordance of image with surgery (n)*	*Cure by TSS (n)*
37	19/36 (53%)	10/36 (28%)	24/37 (65%)

n number of patients, *MRI* magnetic resonance imaging, *CT* computed tomography imaging, *TSS* transsphenoidal selective adenomectomy

Table 2
BSIPSS Results, Surgical Identification of Adenoma, and Cure by TSS

Total patients (n)	*BSIPSS results* *Lateralization (n)*	*BSIPSS results* *Nonlateralization (n)*	*Concordance of BSIPSS result with surgery (n)*	*Cure by TSS (n)*
29	23 (79%)	6 (21%)	24 (83%)	22/29 (76%)

n number of patients, *BSIPSS* bilateral simultaneous inferior petrosal sinus sampling, *TSS* transsphenoidal selective adenomectomy

(interpetrosal sinus ACTH ratio of >1.4 after CRH) in 79% and nonlateralization (ISPG < 1.4) in 21% (Table 2). A more recent study from the NIH has described BIPSS in 94 pediatric patients and reported localization of ACTH secretion concurring with the site of the adenoma at surgery in 58% of cases, concluding that the technique was not essential in the pediatric investigation protocol *(31)*. The percentage of lateralization, however, increased to 70% (51/73) after exclusion of 18 centrally located and four bilateral lesions.

TREATMENT OF CUSHING'S SYNDROME

Treatment will be described for primary adrenal and then pituitary-dependent CS.

Primary Adrenal Lesions

First-line therapy for cortisol-secreting ACTs is surgical excision. Glucocorticoid replacement is required pre- and postoperatively due to suppression of the contralateral adrenal. The definitive treatment of PPNAD is open or laparoscopic bilateral adrenalectomy *(1, 13)*. This is not only to treat the CS but also to prevent the secondary complications of hypercortisolemia and the risk of development of adrenocortical neoplasia. We give metyrapone therapy to normalize cortisol levels preoperatively. After cure by surgery, patients will require long-term steroid replacement and lifelong endocrine follow-up with regular screening for features of CNC, especially if a *PRKAR1A* mutation is identified.

Cushing's Disease

Cushing's disease requires prompt and expert treatment, which should be curative. The approach to the treatment has evolved over the years. Initially, bilateral adrenalectomy was widely practiced, and though effective, the pituitary adenoma remained in situ, and there was a risk of Nelson's syndrome *(32)*. In the management of 37 cases, we have performed adrenalectomy twice when the patients were critically ill and unfit for pituitary surgery. In one of these patients, hypercortisolaemia could only be controlled by IV etomidate prior to adrenalectomy *(33)*.

Transsphenoidal Surgery

Transsphenoidal pituitary surgery (TSS) consisting of selective removal of the adenoma is now considered the first-line therapy for pediatric CD. TSS is considered a safe and effective procedure in children *(34, 35)*. Adult CD studies show variable surgical success rates depending on which definition of cure is adopted. Our adult endocrine unit has taken undetectable postoperative serum cortisol

(<50 nmol/L) as the criterion for cure. We use the same definition. Following cure by TSS in 24 patients, we have not seen recurrence of CD.

Selective microadenomectomy is technically very difficult in children. The microadenomas may be very small *(28)*, and an appreciable rate of failure, in terms of definite cure, exists even in the most experienced hands. We have recently analyzed our experience over the past 25 years and considered the factors which contributed to successful surgical therapy *(29)*. The overall cure rate in 37 pediatric patients treated by TSS from 1982 to 2008 was 65%, and in 29 patients with microadenomas who underwent preoperative BIPSS, the cure rate was 76% (Table 2). We, therefore, feel that the ability of BIPSS to identify the lateral or central position of the adenoma has contributed to an increased rate of surgical success. Other pediatric series report cure rates varying from 45 to 78% *(14, 34)*.

Successful TSS consists of removal of the microadenoma with retention of normal pituitary tissue, which is vital for the child's future development. Postoperative hypopituitarism is, therefore, a potential complication. An important potential hormone deficiency for future growth is that of growth hormone (GH) (see below).

Pituitary Radiotherapy

Pituitary radiotherapy (RT) has been a therapeutic option for pediatric CD for many years. Children with CD respond more rapidly than adults *(36)*. In our centre, external beam RT is used as second-line therapy, following unsuccessful TSS. Our practice is to make a decision to proceed to RT, usually within 2–4 weeks of TSS, when it is clear from cortisol levels that removal of the adenoma has been incomplete *(37)*. We deliver 45 Gy in 25 fractions over 35 days *(37)*. We have treated 13 patients during the past 26 years with a successful cure rate of 85%, which occurred at a mean interval of 0.8 years (range 0.3–2.9). Our analysis on long-term pituitary function in six patients showed that GH deficiency was frequent, but they may recover *(38)*. Gonadotropin secretion was generally preserved with normal or early puberty, and TSH and ACTH deficiency was minimal *(38)*.

POST-CURE GROWTH AND DEVELOPMENT

Most patients with CS have subnormal growth and short stature *(1, 13)*. A key article from the NIH described abnormalities of height and GH secretion in CD together with a rather pessimistic view of posttreatment catch-up growth and adult height *(39)*. We attribute poor catch-up growth to continuing GH deficiency, occurring either from TSS or from pituitary RT *(40)*. In CD, we test for GH deficiency 3 months after TSS or completion of RT. If GH therapy is demonstrated, then GH therapy is started possibly with a GnRH analogue. Catch-up growth usually occurs and adult height within range of target height is achieved in most patients *(41)*. Normal body composition is more difficult to achieve. Many patients remained obese, and BMI SDS was elevated ($p < 0.01$) at a mean interval of 3.9 years after cure in 14 patients *(41)*. In a long-term follow-up study, total body fat and the ratio of visceral to subcutaneous fat were abnormally high *(42)*.

CONCLUSIONS

In pediatric CS, early diagnosis remains a challenge due to the frequent lack of appreciation of the nature of the pathology by parents and general practitioners. Once suspected, investigation requires a formal protocol, and the choice and interpretation of tests is productively discussed with an adult endocrinologist. Cushing's disease presents the most difficult challenge in terms of investigation linked to effective therapy. Ideally, a centre combining pediatric and adult endocrinology, TSS, and pituitary RT would be optimal. The choice of neurosurgeon who is experienced in TSS in children is likely to significantly improve the chance of cure. Posttreatment management presents challenges for normalization of growth, puberty, and body composition.

REFERENCES

1. Storr HL, Chan LF, Grossman AB, Savage MO. Paediatric Cushing's syndrome: epidemiology, investigation and therapeutic advances. Trends Endocrinol Metab 2006;18:167–174.
2. Lumbroso S, Paris F, Sultan C. Activating Gsα mutations: analysis of 113 patients with signs of McCune-Albright syndrome – a European collaborative study. J Clin Endocrinol Metab 2004;89:2107–2113.
3. Kirk JM, Brain CE, Carson DJ, Hyde JC, Grant DB. Cushing's syndrome caused by nodular adrenal hyperplasia in children with McCune-Albright syndrome. J Pediatr 1999;134:789–792.
4. Boston BA, Mandel S, LaFranchi S, Bliziotes M. Activating mutation in the stimulatory guanine nucleotide-binding protein in an infant with Cushing's syndrome and nodular adrenal hyperplasia. J Clin Endocrinol Metab 1994;79:890–893.
5. Mayer SK, Oligny LL, Deal C, Yazbeck S, Gagné N, Blanchard H. Childhood adrenocortical tumors: case series and reevaluation of prognosis – a 24-year experience. J Pediatr Surg 1997;32:911–915.
6. Ribeiro RC, Sandrini F, Figueredo B, Zambetti GP, Michalkiewicz E, Lafferty AR, Lacerda L, Rabin M, Cadwell C, Sampaio G, Cat I, Stratakis CA, Sandrini R. An inherited p53 mutation that contributes in a tissue-specific manner to pediatric adrenal cortical carcinoma. Proc Natl Acad Sci USA 2001;98:9330–9335.
7. Michalkiewicz E, Sandrini R, Figueiredo B, Miranda EC, Caran E, Oliveira-Filho AG, Marques R, Pianovski MA, Lacerda L, Cristofani LM, Jenkins J, Rodriguez-Galindo C, Ribeiro RC. Clinical and outcome characteristics of children with adrenocortical tumours: a report from the International Pediatric Adrenocortical Tumour Registry. J Clin Oncol 2004;22:838–845.
8. Stratakis CA, Boikos SA. Genetics of adrenal tumors associated with Cushing's syndrome: a new classification for bilateral adrenal hyperplasias. Nat Clin Pract Endocrinol Metab 2007;11:748–757.
9. Ilias I, Torpy DJ, Pacak K, Mullen N, Wesley PA, Nieman LK. Cushing's syndrome due to ectopic corticotropin secretion: twenty years experience at the National Institutes of Health. J Clin Endocrinol Metab 2005;90:4955–4962.
10. Stratakis CA, Sarlis N, Kirschner LS, Carney JA, Doppman JL, Nieman LK, Chrousos GP, Papanicolaou DA. Paradoxical response to dexamethasone in the diagnosis of primary pigmented adrenocortical disease. Ann Intern Med 1999;131: 585–591.
11. Stratakis CA, Kirschner LS, Carney J. Clinical and molecular features of the Carney complex: diagnostic criteria and recommendations for patient evaluation. J Clin Endocrinol Metab 2001;86:4041–4046.
12. Gunther DF, Bourdeau I, Matyakhina L, Cassarino D, Kleiner DE, Griffin K, Courkoutsakis N, Abu-Asab M, Tsokos M, Keil M, Carney JA, Stratakis CA. Cyclical Cushing's syndrome presenting in infancy: an early form of primary pigmented nodular adrenocortical disease or a new entity? J Clin Endocrinol Metab 2004;89:373–382.
13. Storr HL, Mitchell H, Swords FM, Main KM, Hindmarsh PC, Betts PR, Shaw NJ, Johnston DI, Clark AJL, Reznek RH, Grossman AB, Savage MO, Clinical features, diagnosis, treatment and molecular studies in paediatric Cushing's syndrome due to primary nodular adrenocortical hyperplasia. Clin Endocrinol 2004;61:553–559
14. Magiakou MA, Mastorakos G, Oldfield EH, Gomes MT, Doppman JL, Cutler GB, Nieman LK, Chrousos GP. Cushing's syndrome in children and adolescents. Presentation, diagnosis and therapy. New Engl J Med 1994;331:629–636.
15. Storr HL, Isidori AM, Monson JP, Besser GM, Grossman AB, Savage MO. Pre-pubertal Cushing's is more common in males, but there is no increase in severity at diagnosis. J Clin Endocrinol Metab 2004;89:3818–3820.
16. Magiakou MA, Chrousos GP. Cushing's syndrome in children and adolescents: current diagnostic and therapeutic strategies. J Endocrinol Invest 2002;25:181–194.
17. Greening JE, Storr HL, Mckenzie SA, Davies KM, Martin L, Grossman AB, Savage MO. Linear growth and body mass index in paediatric patients with Cushing's disease or simple obesity. J Endocrinol Invest 2006;29:885–887.
18. Peters CJ, Ahmed ML, Storr HL, Davies KM, Martin LJ, Allgrove J, Grossman AB, Savage MO. Factors influencing skeletal maturation at diagnosis of paediatric Cushing's disease. Horm Res 2007;68:231–235.
19. Dupuis C, Storr HL, Perry LA, Ho JTF, Ahmed L, Ong KK, Dunger DB, Monson JP, Grossman AB, Besser GM, Savage MO. Abnormal puberty in paediatric Cushing's disease; relationships with adrenal androgens, sex hormone binding globulin and gonadotrophin concentrations. Clin Endocrinol 2007;66:838–843.
20. Newell-Price JP, Trainer P, Besser GM, Grossman AB. The diagnosis and differential diagnosis of Cushing's and pseudo-Cushing's syndrome. Endocrine Rev 1998;19:647–672.

21. Niemann LK, Biller BM, Findling JW, Newell-Price J, Savage MO, Stewart PM, Montori V. The diagnosis of Cushing's syndrome: an Endocrine Society clinical practice guideline. J Clin Endocrinol Metab 2008;93:1526–1540.
22. Batista DL, Riar J, Keil M, Stratakis CA. Diagnostic tests for children who are referred for the investigation of Cushing's syndrome. Pediatrics 2007;120:575–586.
23. Peters CJ, Storr HL, Grossman AB, Savage MO. The role of corticotrophin-releasing hormone in the diagnosis of Cushing's syndrome. Eur J Endocrinol 2006;155:S93–S98.
24. Dias RP, Storr HL, Perry LA, Isidori AM, Grossman AB, Savage MO. The discriminatory value of the low-dose dexamethasone suppression test in the investigation of paediatric Cushing' syndrome. Horm Res 2006;65:159–162.
25. Carney JA, Hruska LS, Beauchamp GD, Gordon, H. Dominant inheritance of the complex of myxomas, spotty skin pigmentation and endocrine over-reactivity. Mayo Clin Proc 1986;61:165–172.
26. Stratakis CA, Carney JA, Lin JP, Papnicolaou DA, Karl M, Kastner DL, Pras E, Chrousos GP. Carney complex a familial multiple neoplasia and lentiginosis syndrome. Analysis of 11 kindreds and linkage to the short arm of chromosome 11. J Clin Invest 1996;97:699–705.
27. Horvath A, Stratakis CA. Clinical and molecular genetics of acromegaly, MEN1, Carney complex, McCune-Albright syndrome, familial acromegaly and genetic defects in sporadic tumors. Rev Endocr Metab Disord 2008;9:1–11.
28. Fahlbusch R. Neurosurgical management of Cushing's disease in children. In: Savage MO, Bourguignon JP, Grossman AB, eds. Frontiers of Paediatr Neuroendocrinol.Oxford: Blackwell Scientific Publications, 1994:68–72.
29. Storr HL, Afshar F, Matson M, Sabin I, Savage KM, Evanson J, Plowman PN, Besser GM, Monson JP, Grossman AB, Savage MO. Factors influencing cure by transsphenoidal selective adenomectomy in paediatric Cushing's disease. Eur J Endocrinol 2005;152:825–833.
30. Lienhardt A, Grossman AB, Dacie JE, Evanson J, Huebner A, Afshar F, Plowman PN, Besser GM, Savage MO. Relative contributions of inferior petrosal sinus sampling and pituitary imaging in the investigation of children and adolescents with ACTH-dependent Cushing's syndrome. J Clin Endocrinol Metab 2001;86:5711–5714.
31. Batista D, Gennari M, Riar J, Chang R, Keil MF, Oldfield EH, Stratakis CA. An assessment of petrosal sinus sampling for localisation of pituitary microadenomas in children with Cushing disease. J Clin Endocrinol Metab 2006;91:221–224.
32. Hopwood NJ, Kenny FM. Incidence of Nelson's syndrome after adrenalectomy for Cushing's disease in children: results of a nationwide survey. Am J Dis Child 1977;131:1353–1356.
33. Greening JE, Brain CE, Perry LA, Mushtaq I, Sales Marques J, Grossman AB, Savage MO Efficient short-term control of hypercortisolaemia by low-dose etomidate in severe paediatric Cushing's syndrome. Horm Res 2005;64:140–143.
34. Kanter AS, Diallo AO, Jane JA Jr, Sheehan JP, Asthagiri AR, Oskouian RJ, Okonkwo DO, Sansur CA, Vance ML, Rogol AD, Laws ER Jr. Single-center experience with pediatric Cushing's disease. J Neurosurgery 2005;103(5 Suppl): 413–420.
35. Joshi SM, Hewitt RJ, Storr HL, Rezajooi K, Ellamushi H, Grossman AB, Savage MO, Afshar F. Cushing's disease in children and adolescents: 20 years of experience in a single neurosurgical centre. Neurosurgery 2005;57:281–285.
36. Jennings AS, Liddle GW, Orth DN. Results of treating childhood Cushing's disease with pituitary irradiation. New Eng J Med 1977;297:957–962.
37. Storr HL, Plowman PN, Carroll PV, Francois I, Krassas G, Afshar F, Besser GM, Grossman AB, Savage MO. Clinical and endocrine responses to pituitary radiotherapy in pediatric Cushing's disease. J Clin Endocrinol Metab 2003;88:34–37.
38. Chan LF, Perry LA, Besser GM, Grossman AB, Savage MO. Long-term anterior pituitary function in patients with paediatric Cushing's disease treated with pituitary radiotherapy. Eur J Endocrinol 2007;156:477–482.
39. Magiakou MA, Mastorakos G, Chrousos GP. Final stature in patients with endogenous Cushing's syndrome. J Clin Endocrinol Metab 1994;79:1082–1085.
40. Lebrethon M-C, Grossman AB, Afshar F, Plowman PN, Besser GM, Savage MO. Linear growth and final height after treatment of Cushing's disease in childhood. J Clin Endocrinol Metab 2000;85:3262–3265.
41. Davies JH, Storr HL, Davies K, Monson JP, Besser GM, Afshar F, Plowman PN, Grossman AB, Savage MO. Final adult height and body mass index after cure of paediatric Cushing's disease. Clin Endocrinol 2005;62:466–472.
42. Leong G, Abad V, Charmandari E, Reynolds JC, Hill S, Chrousos GP, Nieman LK. Effects of child- and adolescent-onset endogenous Cushing syndrome on bone mass, body composition and growth: a 7-year prospective study into young adulthood. J Bone Miner Res 2007;22:110–118.

23 Special Aspects of Cushing's Syndrome: Cyclic Cushing's Syndrome

Nora Albiger and Franco Mantero

CONTENTS

SUMMARY

Cyclic Cushing's syndrome (CS) involves rhythmic fluctuations in ACTH secretion resulting in a variation of adrenal steroid production. Generally accepted criterion for establishing the diagnosis of a truly cyclic condition includes at least three peaks and two troughs of cortisol production. In most cases, cyclic CS is caused by an ACTH-secreting pituitary adenoma, but it can also be due to an ectopic ACTH production, adrenal adenomas or nodular hyperplasias.

This condition should be strongly suspected in patients who present with signs and symptoms of CS but with normal or discrepant biochemical findings, patients with biochemical evidence for cortisol excess but low clinical suspicion of CS, and patients with the presence of conflicting patterns of cortisol response to dexamethasone or an anomalous response to medical treatment.

The diagnosis of cyclic CS is sometimes difficult and may require overlengthy periods of observation to be confirmed. The repeated use of urinary free cortisol measurements and midnight salivary cortisol test is recommended, if possible, making it coincide with clinical symptoms.

Given the variations in cortisol production, the response to medical treatment and surgery for cyclic CS needs to be interpreted with caution.

Key Words: Cyclic Cushing's syndrome periodic hormonogenesis, fluctuating cortisol values

From: *Contemporary Endocrinology: Cushing's Syndrome: Pathophysiology, Diagnosis and Treatment*
Edited by: M.D. Bronstein (ed.), DOI 10.1007/978-1-60327-449-4_23,

INTRODUCTION

Episodic cortisol secretion may be part of a complex clinical picture involving cyclic forms of Cushing's syndrome (CS) that can pose unusual diagnostic problems. Cyclic ACTH secretion may result in a more or less predictable rhythmic variation in adrenal cortisol production, alternating more or less regularly between high and normal levels, and following a clinical course with periodic symptoms of hypercortisolism.

Generally accepted criterion for establishing the diagnosis of a truly cyclic condition includes at least three peaks and two troughs of cortisol production, while any other cases are described as fluctuating or intermittent cortisol secretion *(1)*. Due to the long-term variation of the intercyclic period present in some patients, this criterion cannot be readily applied in all patients.

Although early publications already described fluctuating or intermittent cortisol secretion in patients with Cushing's syndrome *(2–5)*, cyclic Cushing's syndrome was described for the first time as a new and distinct entity in 1971. The case was a female patient with a very slow-growing carcinoid-type malignant bronchial adenoma causing hypercortisolism with cyclic changes in cortisol production and superior vena cava syndrome. The pattern of cortisol metabolite excretion over a 45-day period of study indicated a cortisol production phase lasting approximately 18 days. The authors chose the term "periodic hormonogenesis" to describe this phenomenon *(6)*.

The first series of patients with well-established cyclic Cushing's syndrome was described in 1985, suggesting that this condition was not so rare *(7)*: in this series, five out of nine patients fulfilled the criteria for cyclic Cushing's syndrome when sequential daily urine samples were studied to estimate their cortisol/creatinine ratio.

Cyclic Cushing's syndrome was subsequently described in another three cases whose cyclic condition was first diagnosed after transsphenoidal microsurgery for Cushing's disease. The condition was suspected because patients' signs and symptoms slowly settled and their endocrine results varied considerably *(8)*.

An attempt was made by Shapiro et al. *(9)* to classify patients with cyclic Cushing's syndrome. The clinical expression was correlated with the cortisol production pattern, distinguishing between regular or irregular cyclic hormonogenesis, but it is clear that not all patients can really be classified in this way, and it seems more appropriate to consider this condition as a single clinical entity.

Cyclic Cushing's syndrome is uncommon, but it is seen more often in children than in adults *(10–12)*, while the gender distribution remains much the same as in the classical forms of CS (i.e., it is more common among women) *(13)*.

Due to the frequent variations in cortisol secretion levels and the potentially cyclic or periodic hypercortisolism, hormone assessment is recommended on at least two, and preferably three, separate days when a diagnosis of Cushing's syndrome is suspected. The results of dynamic tests are easier to interpret during a sustained period of hypercortisolism, whereas they may prove difficult during cyclic episodes because paradoxical responses to dexamethasone may reflect an increasing or decreasing endogenous activity rather than the action of the agent administered *(14, 15)*. The physiopathology of this condition remains to be clarified, though several possible mechanisms have been proposed.

Normal cortisol secretion between cycles may complicate medical therapy because patients may show unexpected clinical and biochemical signs of hypocortisolism.

CAUSES AND POTENTIAL MECHANISMS IMPLICATED IN THE PHYSIOPATHOLOGY OF CYCLIC CUSHING'S SYNDROME

A cyclic behavior may be a feature of several forms of Cushing's syndrome (ACTH-dependent or -independent), but pituitary-dependent cause seem to be characterized by more frequent and more severe secretory episodes than ectopic or ACTH-independent forms *(16)*.

The most common causes of cyclic Cushing's syndrome are associated with ACTH-secreting pituitary adenomas *(9, 14, 15)*, but it has also been reported in association with ectopic ACTH secretion due to typical bronchial carcinoid *(17)*, atypical thymic carcinoid *(18)*, oncocytic carcinoid of the kidney *(19)*, gastric carcinoid *(20)*, pancreatic carcinoid *(21)*, malignant carcinoid tumor of the lung *(22)*, bronchial adenoma *(23)*, and pheochromocytoma *(24)*. Other causes, such as adrenal adenoma *(25)* and rare forms of the pigmented variant of micronodular adrenocortical hyperplasia (primary pigmented nodular adrenocortical disease, or PPNAD), also have a role in cyclic Cushing's syndrome *(10, 11, 26)*.

Data suggesting a hypothalamic origin of cyclic hypercortisolism emerge from a report on a patient with intermittent Cushing's syndrome following a cortisol hyperpulsatile pattern who had a sustained response to sodium valproate treatment. Sodium valproate is known to cause an increase in gamma amino-butyric acid (GABA), which in turn inhibits CRH secretion *(27)*. These data were not subsequently confirmed, however *(8)*.

It has also been suggested that rhythmic fluctuations in ACTH secretion may be at least partially due to a cyclic change in central dopaminergic tone because preoperative treatment with bromocriptine in a well-characterized patient with cyclic Cushing's syndrome was associated with a drop in cortisol levels *(28)*, although a prolonged trial was not performed.

Pituitary apoplexy can induce a remission of hypercortisolism *(29, 30)*, as described in a young woman who presented with a florid picture of Cushing's syndrome but with biochemical evidence of adrenal insufficiency *(31)*. MRI of the pituitary gland showed infarction of an ACTH-secreting macroadenoma. Over several years, the disease ran a fluctuating course characterized by periods of hypercortisolism alternating with adrenal insufficiency, and MRI showed changes in the pituitary adenoma due to repeated infarction episodes. Though it is difficult to explain why apoplexy of the adenoma can recur rhythmically, a careful follow-up of such patients is mandatory to establish the real course of their disease.

A serotoninergic influence may be involved in some way in the pathogenesis of cyclic Cushing's syndrome *(32)*, since urinary free cortisol (UFC) was strongly reduced in a patient with Cushing's disease and the cyclic secretion was contained by administering a serotonin antagonist. This hypothesis needs to be confirmed, however, because such a response might have been part of an intrinsic decrease in UFC in the case described.

There may be an unusual combination of Cushing's syndrome and corticosteroid-binding globulin (CBG) deficiency in patients with periodic ACTH and cortisol secretion presenting with high-plasma free cortisol levels and low CBG concentrations *(33)*.

Ectopic ACTH secretion may also be associated with cyclic Cushing's syndrome. The autocrine/paracrine modulatory effect of ghrelin on bronchial ACTH-secreting tumors has been suggested after a patient with a bronchial carcinoid reportedly, presented with cyclic hypercortisolism and an in vivo ACTH hyperresponsiveness to hexarelin that disappeared after the surgical removal of the tumor *(17)*.

Both types of ghrelin receptor (1a and 1b) were detected in the tumor, but not in the peritumoral lung tissue. Moreover, a cyclic pattern of hypercortisolism with a temporary drop in ACTH and cortisol levels during a lung infection occurring in a period of overt hypercortisolism was described in a patient with ectopic Cushing's syndrome *(34)*. It is well known that states of hypercortisolism may be complicated by opportunist infections *(35)*, and in cases of endogenous hypercortisolism, the likelihood of bacterial or opportunist infections is greatest in patients with particularly high ACTH and cortisol levels, as in ectopic ACTH secretion *(36)*. The mechanism behind the drop in cortisol levels during the infection may have to do with the action of inflammatory cytokines with antitumor properties, such as tumor necrosis factor (TNF) alpha *(37)*.

These mechanisms may help to explain a central effect causing rhythmic ACTH secretion, or they may at least explain the fluctuations seen in patients with ectopic ACTH secretion, but not the rhythms identified in adrenal cases.

A fluctuating daily cortisol production is generally seen in patients with food-dependent Cushing's syndrome and macronodular adrenal hyperplasia, though they do not follow a genuinely cyclic behavior. Fasting cortisol levels are low in these patients, increasing after food intake due to the aberrant expression of gastric inhibitory polypeptide (GIP) receptor on adrenocortical cells *(38)*. Transient ACTH-independent Cushing's syndrome has also been described during pregnancy in patients with mild bilateral adrenal hyperplasia *(39, 40)*. Hypercortisolism presented during pregnancy in these cases and regressed completely after delivery or spontaneous abortion. It may be that a mechanism associated with aberrant adrenal LH receptor expression lies behind the increase in cortisol production in such cases.

Cyclic Cushing's syndrome has been reported in a number of pediatric patients *(41, 42)*, most of them with ACTH-independent hypercortisolism due to micronodular adrenal hyperplasia *(10, 11, 26, 43–46)*. The best known variant of micronodular adrenal hyperplasia is called PPNAD. Familial and sporadic cases of PPNAD have been reported in association with germline-inactivating mutations of the *PRKAR1A* gene *(47–49)*. Moreover, PPNAD may be part of the Carney complex, an autosomal dominant multiple neoplasia syndrome, consisting of spotty skin pigmentation, myxomas, and other nonendocrine and endocrine tumors *(47, 48)*.

A new entity that has yet to be characterized has recently been proposed in the light of a description of a 3-year-old patient with cyclic Cushing's syndrome due to micronodular adrenal disease whose histology and genetic picture were not consistent with PPNAD, the Carney complex, or the McCune–Albright syndrome *(12)*.

CLINICAL PRESENTATION

Cyclic Cushing's syndrome must be suspected in patients with signs and symptoms of hypercortisolism but normal cortisol values, or patients with fluctuating cortisol values or conflicting patterns of cortisol response to dexamethasone or an anomalous response to medical treatment.

Clinically, cyclic Cushing's syndrome may present with one or many symptoms, depending on how long the disease has been active and the timing of the fluctuations, which can vary from a few days to several months, or even years *(6, 9)*. Clinical presentations can range from a single, outstanding symptom, such as recurrent edema or weight gain, to a complex clinical syndrome, but most patients present with at least two features characteristic of hypercortisolism, e.g., glucose intolerance, menstrual cycle disruptions, acne, hirsutism, or mood disorders *(13)*.

The cycles can also vary in duration, from a few hours to as long as 85 days *(9)*, sometimes with lengthy disease-free intervals *(34)*. Atkinson et al. *(7)* described a patient with cyclic CS due to a pituitary adenoma whose cortisol secretion followed two different rhythms, i.e., a 40-day period of cortisol excess was followed by 60–70 days of normal cortisol secretion; during the former period, cortisol secretion peaked every 3–6 days between troughs of normal cortisol levels.

A patient with four irregular, symptomatic cycles of hypercortisolism before ketoconazole therapy with a pituitary MRI revealing an empty sella has been described *(50)*. An empty sella is a neuroanatomical condition common in middle-aged, obese, multiparous females. It usually occurs with headache and visual disorders; most patients have a normal pituitary function, but Cushing's syndrome occurs in 2% of cases of primary empty sella *(51, 52)*.

DIAGNOSIS

The diagnosis of Cushing' syndrome is based on frontline screening tests that include measuring 24-hour UFC at least twice, a 1-mg overnight dexamethasone suppression test (DST), a longer low-dose DST, and a late-night salivary cortisol assay at least twice *(53)*.

The presence of cyclic hormonogenesis may further complicate the final diagnosis, and clinicians are often obliged to hospitalize patients several times before obtaining unequivocal biological evidence of cortisol excess, so accurate assessment and follow-up are needed in patients with consistently negative results suspected of having a cyclic disease. The repeated use of UFC and midnight salivary cortisol tests is recommended in these cases, if possible, making it coincide with clinical symptoms *(53)*.

Measuring salivary cortisol is an accurate method for assessing plasma free cortisol and a useful tool in the diagnosis of hypercortisolism *(54)*. There is also a strong correlation between free plasma and salivary cortisol concentrations *(55)*. Saliva sampling is simple, noninvasive, and can easily be done in an outpatient setting, or be used for long-distance follow-up purposes *(56, 57)*. It may also be a good tool for evaluating patients over a long period of time when an unpredictable pattern of urinary cortisol secretion makes it impossible to arrive at a final diagnosis *(58)*. Repeated midnight salivary cortisol sampling is, therefore, a highly effective option for patients with cyclic Cushing's syndrome.

DSTs are not recommended for the initial evaluation of patients with suspected cyclic hypercortisolism because cortisol response is strongly affected by the cyclic cortisol activity *(53)*. The DST should only be performed during a period of certain sustained hypercortisolism to avoid the risk of misdiagnosis because a DST performed when steroids are about to fall spontaneously might be erroneously interpreted as an adequate suppression.

A so-called paradoxical cortisol response to the DST has been reported by several authors *(11, 59, 60)*. For instance, Brown et al. *(14)* described a patient with CS due to a pituitary adenoma who had a paradoxical increase in cortisol after dexamethasone administration. The authors showed that plasma cortisol levels rose before the first dose of dexamethasone was administered, demonstrating a cyclic rise and fall in steroidogenesis. Theirs was the first accurate description of an apparently paradoxical response to dexamethasone being a purely fortuitous circumstance in a patient with a spontaneously rhythmic steroid production controlled by a mechanism not susceptible to the negative feedback action of steroids. This effect was demonstrated afterwards in a patient with hypercortisolism due to a pituitary adenoma in whom hypercortisolism alternated with a biochemical remission and a paradoxical cortisol response to dexamethasone, which was probably an expression of the periodic hormonogenesis *(15)*.

Paradoxical cortisol responses to DST have also been described in patients with micronodular adrenal hyperplasia *(11, 36, 59, 60)*. This phenomenon is reproducible in vitro and is associated with an increased expression of the glucocorticoid receptor in adrenal nodules *(61)*.

A more exhaustive study on these patients might well pinpoint a larger number of patients with cyclic Cushing's syndrome. Mullan et al. *(62)* suggest performing a continuous study for at least 28 days when a diagnosis of cyclic hypercortisolism is suspected, and when the patient's clinical condition allows.

When cyclic Cushing's syndrome is confirmed biochemically, further laboratory studies are needed to establish whether it is ACTH-dependent or -independent. Imaging needs are guided by biochemical assessments. MRI is the method of choice for Cushing's syndrome, but a pituitary adenoma is normally seen in no more than 36–78% of cases *(63, 64)*. Bilateral inferior petrosal sinus sampling is frequently required when it proves difficult to distinguish between pituitary and ectopic ACTH secretion. Specific biochemical testing for carcinoids or neuroendocrine tumors (NET) is warranted in cases of suspected ectopic ACTH production.

Scintigraphy with radionucleotide-labeled agonists for receptors commonly expressed by NET is used to seek occult ACTH-dependent disease, sometimes with disappointing results *(65)*.

Positron emission tomography (PET) has also been recommended for the diagnosis of NET. ^{18}F-FDG *(66)* identifies only highly metabolic undifferentiated tumors, so alternative radiotracers, such as whole-body (WB) PET with ^{11}C-5-hydroxytryptophan (5-HTP) *(67)*, ^{18}F-DOPA *(68)*, and ^{68}Gallium-peptides, especially ^{68}Ga-DOTA-peptides *(69, 70)*, have been used, with encouraging results.

In most cases, diagnosing ACTH-independent hypercortisolism is more straightforward because an adrenal lesion is usually detectable, but difficulties may arise not only in the differential diagnosis of adrenal adenomas and carcinomas but also with the rare forms of sporadic PPNAD in which patients may have a normal adrenal morphology *(60)*.

Difficulties in pinpointing the origin of cortisol excess may be accentuated by conditions that make it risky to attempt any invasive procedures.

We described a 67-year-old man with Cushing's syndrome who had severe mitral valve insufficiency and was at risk of bleeding due to a lack of high-molecular weight von Willebrand factor multimers, which was thought likely to be associated with the valve defect *(71)*. This patient's biochemical data suggested an ectopic origin of his ACTH secretion, but POMC levels were normal, and computed tomography scan and total body scintigraphy with^{111} In-pentreotide and PET images were negative. No inferior petrosal sinus catheterization could be used at initial diagnosis because of the abovementioned bleeding risk. Figure 1 shows the fluctuations in cortisol levels, the exaggerated response to ketoconazole probably due to spontaneous disease remission, and the cortisol response to surgical stress in a attempt to resolve the valve defect.

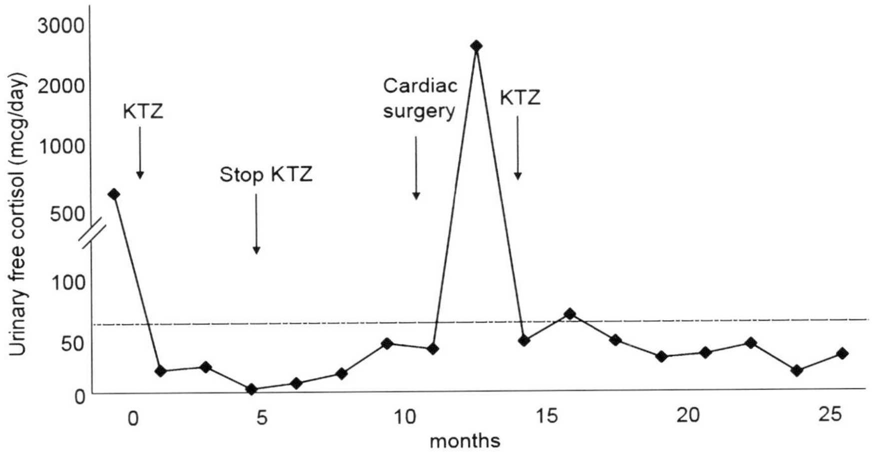

Fig. 1. Urinary free cortisol levels (UFC) in a patient with intermittent hypercortisolism. Ketoconazole (KTZ) was stopped due to hypocortisolism, probably due to spontaneous disease remission. (*dashed lines*) upper normal level of UFC.

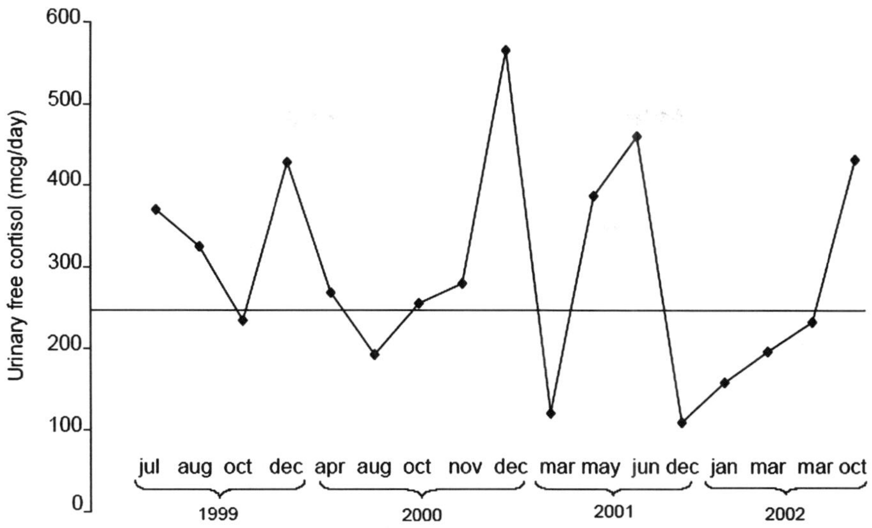

Fig. 2. Spontaneous urinary free cortisol (UFC) variations in a patient with ACTH-independent macronodular adrenal hyperplasia (AIMAH) during a 4-year follow-up (from 1999 to 2002). (*dashed lines*) upper normal level of UFC.

As in this case, the cause of Cushing's syndrome is often difficult to diagnose because there is currently no single, sufficiently accurate biochemical or imaging method available. Moreover, the association of cortisol excess with other diseases may complicate the final diagnosis, and the cyclic behavior of the condition may interfere with the response to medical treatment.

The evolution of UFC levels in a 71-year-old patient with ACTH-independent macronodular adrenal hyperplasia (AIMAH) causing cortisol excess is shown in Fig. 2. This patient had fluctuating cortisol levels during a 4-year follow-up. In patients with AIMAH, it may be useful to assess cortisol response to different exogenous stimuli to reveal any aberrant G-coupled receptor expression. Our patient had a cortisol response to food intake (94%), vasopressin (68%), and the postural test (37%), pointing to an aberrant receptor expression being involved in the cortisol production in this case. Abdominal CT showed bilateral macronodular adrenals (right: 30 mm; left: 55 mm). A I^{131}-norcholesterol scintiscan showed an asymmetric bilateral uptake, more prevalent on the left, and unilateral adrenalectomy of the largest gland was performed. After adrenalectomy, the patient had normal cortisol levels that persisted throughout a 66-month follow-up, ruling out any possibility of cortisol fluctuations. This case represents an unusual presentation of Cushing's syndrome in a patient with AIMAH and confirms that unilateral adrenalectomy of the largest gland may be a safe and effective treatment for selected patients with AIMAH, as demonstrated by our group in a larger series *(72)*.

THERAPY

When it comes to treatment, patients with cyclic Cushing's syndrome are no different from those with nonintermittent forms, but it is important to bear in mind that the former are quite likely to experience phases of relative adrenocortical insufficiency once medical therapy is begun, so an accurate follow-up is needed during their treatment to avoid this complication.

In addition, the risk of variations in steroidogenesis and the possibility of hypocortisolic episodes in patients with cyclic Cushing's syndrome may make the results of drug studies and surgery misleading, so they must be considered with caution.

The treatment of Cushing's syndrome is discussed in depth in another chapter, so only the main points are briefly summarized here.

Selective surgical resection of ACTH or cortisol-producing tumors is the optimal treatment for all forms of Cushing's syndrome. While adrenalectomy in patients with adrenal adenomas and the excision of an identified ectopic ACTH-secreting tumor may result in a high percentage of success, pituitary neurosurgery of an ACTH-secreting pituitary adenoma present a biochemical remission in 70–80% of cases, and a significant number of recurrences are seen during long-term follow-up, the rate ranging between 9 and 23% *(73, 74)*. Moreover, an accurate follow-up for several years is mandatory for patients with Cushing's disease treated by transsphenoidal surgery to avoid confusing real remission with a hitherto unrecognized cyclic hormonogenesis, particularly in patients whose symptoms, signs, and endocrine findings tend to vary *(7, 75, 76)*. Pituitary radiation and/or bilateral adrenalectomy are reserved for patients with Cushing's disease failing to respond to surgery. Medical treatment can be used before surgery in patients with overt CS and also in patients awaiting the response to pituitary radiation. Although significant advances have been made in the medical management of Cushing's syndrome, the challenge is still to find drugs capable of acting on the etiology of the different forms of the disease. Most of the available drugs can correct hypercortisolism, but they have little impact on tumor growth.

The identification of ectopic or abnormal hormone receptors in adrenal cortisol-secreting nodular hyperplasias has suggested new opportunities for the use of specific pharmacological therapies *(77–80)*.

CONCLUSION

Cyclic Cushing's syndrome poses unusual diagnostic problems. Clinicians and endocrinologists should be aware of the possibility of a cyclic cortisol production, and the syndrome should be suspected in patients with symptoms or signs of hypercortisolism, but normal cortisol levels, or fluctuating cortisol values, or an anomalous response to dexamethasone. Cyclic Cushing's syndrome may have both ACTH-dependent and -independent causes. Between cycles, patients may have a normal pituitary function, so UFC and salivary cortisol measurements are recommended in the initial diagnosis. Dynamic test findings are best interpreted if the tests are conducted during a sustained period of hypercortisolism.

Given the possible variations in steroidogenesis, the clinical and biochemical response to medical treatment and the outcome of drug studies and surgery for cyclic Cushing's syndrome need to be interpreted with caution.

REFERENCES

1. Mullan KR, Atkinson AB, Sheridan B. Cyclical Cushing's syndrome: an update. Curr Opin Endocrinol Diabetes Obes 2007;14:317–322.
2. Bassoe HH, Emberland R, Stoa KF. Fluctuating steroid excretion in Cushing's syndrome. Acta Endocrinol 1958;28:163–168.
3. Brooks RV, Jeffcoate SL, London DR, Prunty FT, Smith PM. Intermittent Cushing's syndrome with anomalous response to dexamethasone. J Endocrinol 1966;36:53–61.
4. Zondek H, Zondek GW, Leszynsky HE. Fluctuability of steroid excretion. Acta Endocrinol 1957;26:91–95.
5. Birke G, Diczfalusky E. Fluctuation in the excretion of adrenocortical steroids in a case of Cushing's syndrome. J Clin Endocrinol Metab 1956;16:286–290
6. Bailey RE. Periodic hormonogenesis – a new phenomenon. Periodicity in function of a hormone-producing tumor in man. J Clin Endocrinol Metab 1971;32:317–327.

7. Atkinson AB, Kennedy AL, Carson DJ, Hadden DR, Weaver JA, Sheridan B. Five cases of cyclical Cushing's syndrome. Br Med J (Clin Res Ed) 1985;291:1453–1457.
8. Atkinson AB, McCance DR, Kennedy L, Sheridan B. Cyclical Cushing's syndrome first diagnosed after pituitary surgery: a trap for the unwary. Clin Endocrinol (Oxf) 1992;36:297–299.
9. Shapiro MS, Shenkman L. Variable hormonogenesis in Cushing's syndrome. Q J Med 1991;79:351–363.
10. Gomez Muguruza MT, Chrousos GP. Periodic Cushing syndrome in a short boy: usefulness of the ovine corticotrophin releasing hormone test. J Pediatr 1989;115:270–273.
11. Carson DJ, Sloan JM, Cleland J, Russell CF, Atkinson AB, Sheridan B. Cyclical Cushing's syndrome presenting as short stature in a boy with recurrent atrial myxomas and freckled skin pigmentation. Clin Endocrinol (Oxf) 1988;28:173–180.
12. Gunther DF, Bourdeau I, Matyakhina L, Cassarino D, Kleiner DE, Griffin K, Courkoutsakis N, Abu-Asab M, Tsokos M, Keil M, Carney JA, Stratakis CA. Cyclical Cushing syndrome presenting in infancy: an early form of primary pigmented nodular adrenocortical disease, or a new entity? J Clin Endocrinol Metab 2004;89:3173–3182.
13. Meinardi JR, Wolffenbuttel BH, Dullaart RP. Cyclic Cushing's syndrome: a clinical challenge. Eur J Endocrinol 2007;157:245–254.
14. Brown RD, Van Loon GR, Orth DN, Liddle GW. Cushing's disease with periodic hormonogenesis: one explanation for paradoxical response to dexamethasone. J Clin Endocrinol Metab 1973;36:445–451.
15. Liberman B, Wajchenberg BL, Tambascia MA, Mesquita CH. Periodic remission in Cushing's disease with paradoxical dexamethasone response: an expression of periodic hormonogenesis. J Clin Endocrinol Metab 1976;43:913–918.
16. Sederberg-Olsen P, Binder C, Kehlet H, Neville AM, Nielsen LM. Episodic variation in plasma corticosteroids in subjects with Cushing's syndrome of differing etiology. J Clin Endocrinol Metab 1973;36:906–910.
17. Arnaldi G, Mancini T, Kola B, Appolloni G, Freddi S, Concettoni C, Bearzi I, Masini A, Boscaro M, Mantero F. Cyclical Cushing's syndrome in a patient with a bronchial neuroendocrine tumor (typical carcinoid) expressing ghrelin and growth hormone secretagogue receptors. J Clin Endocrinol Metab 2003;88:5834–5840.
18. Meinardi JR, van den Berg G, Wolffenbuttel BH, Kema IP, Dullaart RP. Cyclical Cushing's syndrome due to an atypical thymic carcinoid. Neth J Med 2006;64:23–27.
19. Hannah J, Lippe B, Lai-Goldman M, Bhuta S. Oncocytic carcinoid of the kidney associated with periodic Cushing's syndrome. Cancer 1988;61:2136–2140.
20. Hirata Y, Sakamoto N, Yamamoto H, Matsukura S, Imura H, Okada S. Gastric carcinoid with ectopic production of ACTH and beta-MSH. Cancer 1976;37:377–385.
21. Van Coevorden A, Laurent E, Rickaert F, van Reeth O, Van Cauter E, Mockel J. Cushing's syndrome with intermittent ectopic ACTH production. J Endocrinol Invest 1990;13:317–326.
22. Chajek T, Romanoff H. Cushing syndrome with cyclical edema and periodic secretion of corticosteroids. Arch Intern Med 1976;136:441–443.
23. Shapiro MS, Gutman A, Bruderman I, Myers B, Griffel WB. Cushing's syndrome associated with a bronchial adenoma. Possible periodic hormonogenesis. Isr J Med Sci 1975;11:919–914.
24. Terzolo M, Ali A, Pia A, Bollito E, Reimondo G, Paccotti P, Scardapane R, Angeli A. Cyclic Cushing's syndrome due to ectopic ACTH secretion by an adrenal pheochromocytoma. J Endocrinol Invest 1994;17:869–874.
25. Blau N, Miller WE, Miller ER Jr, Cervi-Skinner SJ. Spontaneous remission of Cushing's syndrome in a patient with an adrenal adenoma. J Clin Endocrinol Metab 1975;40:659–663.
26. Oelkers W, Bahr V, Hensen J, Pickartz H. Primary adrenocortical micronodular adenomatosis causing Cushing's syndrome. Effects of ketoconazole on steroid production and *in vitro* performance of adrenal cells. Acta Endocrinol (Copenh) 1986;113:370–377.
27. Beckers A, Stevenaert A, Pirens G, Flandroy P, Sulon J, Hennen G. Cyclical Cushing's disease and its successful control under sodium valproate. J Endocrinol Invest 1990;13:923–929.
28. Watanobe H, Aoki R, Takebe K, Nakazono M, Kudo M. In vivo and in vitro studies in a patient with cyclical Cushing's disease showing some responsiveness to bromocriptine. Horm Res 1991;36:227–234.
29. Dickstein G, Spindel A, Shechner C, Adawi F, Gutman H. Spontaneous remission in Cushing's disease. Arch Intern Med 1991;151:185–189.
30. Pignatta AB, Días AG, Gómez RM, Bruno OD. Spontaneous remission of Cushing's disease after disappearance of a microadenoma attached to the pituitary stalk. Pituitary 2004;7:45–49.
31. Alarifi A, Alzahrani AS, Salam SA, Ahmed M, Kanaan I. Repeated remissions of Cushing's disease due to recurrent infarctions of an ACTH-producing pituitary macroadenoma. Pituitary 2005;8:81–87.
32. Jordan RM, Ramos-Gabatin A, Kendall JW, Gaudette D, Walls RC. Dynamics of adrenocorticotropin (ACTH) secretion in cyclic Cushing's syndrome: evidence for more than one abnormal ACTH biorhythm. J Clin Endocrinol Metab 1982;55:531–537.

33. Watanobe H, Nigawara T, Nasushita R, Sasaki S, Takebe K. A case of cyclical Cushing's disease associated with corticosteroid-binding globulin deficiency: A rare pitfall in the diagnosis of Cushing's disease. Eur J Endocrinol 1995;133:317–319.
34. Peri A, Bemporad D, Parenti G, Luciani P, Serio M, Mannelli M. Cushing's syndrome due to intermittent ectopic ACTH production showing a temporary remission during a pulmonary infection. Eur J Endocrinol 2001;145:605–611
35. Aucott JN. Glucocorticoids and infection. Endocrinol Metab Clin North Am 1994;23:655–670.
36. Sarlis NJ, Chanock S, Nieman L. Cortisolemic indices predict severe infections in Cushing syndrome due to ectopic production of adrenocorticotropin. J Clin Endocrinol Metab 2000;85:42–47.
37. Wallach D, Boldin M, Varfolomeev E, Beyaert R, Vandenabeele P, Fiers W. Cell death induction by receptors of the TNF family: towards a molecular understanding. FEBS Lett 1997;410:96–106.
38. Lacroix A, Bolté E, Tremblay J, Dupré J, Poitras P, Fournier H, Garon J, Garrel D, Bayard F, Taillefer R. Gastric inhibitory polypeptide-dependent cortisol hypersecretion a new cause of Cushing's syndrome. N Engl J Med 1992;327:974–980.
39. Wallace C, Toth EL, Lewanczuk RZ, Siminoski K. Pregnancy-induced Cushing's syndrome in multiple pregnancies. J Clin Endocrinol Metab 1996;81:15–21.
40. Close CF, Mann MC, Watts JF, Taylor KG. ACTH-independent Cushing's syndrome in pregnancy with spontaneous resolution after delivery: control of the hypercortisolism with metyrapone. Clin Endocrinol (Oxf) 1993;39:375–379.
41. Levin ME The development of bilateral adenomatous adrenal hyperplasia in a case of Cushing's syndrome of eighteen years' duration. Am J Med 1966;40:318–324.
42. Robyn JA, Koch CA, Montalto J, Yong A, Warne GL, Batch JA. Cushing's syndrome in childhood and adolescence. J Paediatr Child Health 1997;33:522–527.
43. Sarlis NJ, Chrousos GP, Doppman JL, Carney JA, Stratakis CA. Primary pigmented nodular adrenocortical disease: reevaluation of a patient with Carney complex 27 years after unilateral adrenalectomy. J Clin Endocrinol Metab 1997;82:1274–1278.
44. Mellinger RC, Smith RW Jr. Studies of the adrenal hyperfunction in 2 patients with atypical Cushing's syndrome. J Clin Endocrinol Metab 1956;16:350–366.
45. Demoor P, Roels H, Delaere K, Crabbe EJ. Unusual case of adrenocortical hyperfunction. J Clin Endocrinol Metab 1965; 25:612–620.
46. Brooks RV, Jeffcoate SL, London DR, Prunty FT, Smith PM. Intermittent Cushing's syndrome with anomalous response to dexamethasone. J Endocrinol 1966;36:53–61.
47. Stratakis CA, Kirschner LS, Carney JA. Clinical and molecular features of the Carney complex: diagnostic criteria and recommendations for patient evaluation. J Clin Endocrinol Metab 2001;86:4041–4046.
48. Stratakis CA. Mutations of the gene encoding the protein kinase A type 1-alpha regulatory subunit (*PRKAR1A*) in patients with the "complex of spotty skin pigmentation, myxomas, endocrine overactivity, and schwannomas" (Carney complex). Ann NY Acad Sci 2002;968:3–21.
49. Groussin L, Jullian E, Perlemoine K, Louvel A, Leheup B, Luton JP, Bertagna X, Bertherat J. Mutations of the *PRKAR1A* gene in Cushing's syndrome due to sporadic primary pigmented nodular adrenocortical disease. J Clin Endocrinol Metab 2002;87:4324–4329.
50. Calvo-Romero JM, Morales-Pérez F, Díaz Pérez J. Cyclic Cushing's disease associated with primary empty sella. Eur J Int Med 2000;1:168–170.
51. Gallardo E, Schächter D, Cáceres E, Becker P, Colin E, Martinez C, Henríquez C. The empty sella: results of treatment in 76 successive cases and high frequency of endocrine and neurological disturbances. Clin Endocrinol (Oxf) 1992;37:529–533.
52. Manavela MP, Goodall CM, Katz SB, Moncet D, Bruno OD. The association of Cushing's disease and primary empty sella turcica. Pituitary 2001;4:145–151.
53. Nieman LK, Biller BM, Findling JW, Newell-Price J, Savage MO, Stewart PM, Montori VM. The diagnosis of Cushing's syndrome: an Endocrine Society Clinical Practice Guideline. J Clin Endocrinol Metab 2008;93:1526–1540.
54. Yaneva M, Mosnier-Pudar H, Dugué MA, Grabar S, Fulla Y, Bertagna X. Midnight salivary cortisol for the initial diagnosis of Cushing's syndrome of various causes. J Clin Endocrinol Metab 2004;89:3345–3351.
55. Vining RF, McGinley RA, Maksvytis JJ, Ho KY. Salivary cortisol – a better measure of adrenal cortical function than serum cortisol. Ann Clin Biochem 1983;20:329–335.
56. Nunes ML, Vattaut S, Corcuff JB, Rault A, Loiseau H, Gatta B, Valli N, Letenneur L, Tabarin A. Late-night salivary cortisol for diagnosis of overt and subclinical Cushing's syndrome in hospitalized and ambulatory patients. J Clin Endocrinol Metab 2009;94:456–462.
57. Mosnier-Pudar H, Thomopoulos P, Bertagna X, Fournier C, Guiban D, Luton JP. Long-distance and long-term follow-up of a patient with intermittent Cushing's disease by salivary cortisol measurements. Eur J Endocrinol 1995;133:313–316.

58. Hermus AR, Pieters GF, Borm GF, Verhofstad AA, Smals AG, Benraad TJ, Kloppenborg PW. Unpredictable hypersecretion of cortisol in Cushing's disease: detection by daily salivary cortisol measurements. Acta Endocrinol (Copenh) 1993;128:428–432.
59. Silverman SR, Marnell RT, Sholiton LJ, Werk EE Jr. Failure of dexamethasone suppression test to indicate bilateral adrenocortical hyperplasia in Cushing's syndrome. J Clin Endocrinol Metab 1963;23:167–172.
60. Stratakis CA, Sarlis N, Kirschner LS, Carney JA, Doppman JL, Nieman LK, Chrousos GP, Papanicolaou DA. Paradoxical response to dexamethasone in the diagnosis of primary pigmented nodular adrenocortical disease. Ann Intern Med 1999;131:585–591.
61. Bourdeau I, Lacroix A, Schurch W, Caron P, Antakly T, Stratakis CA. Primary pigmented nodular adrenocortical disease: paradoxical responses of cortisol secretion to dexamethasone occur in vitro and are associated with increased expression of the glucocorticoid receptor. J Clin Endocrinol Metab 2003;88:3931–3937.
62. Mullan KR, Atkinson AB, Sheridan B. Cyclical Cushing's syndrome: an update. Curr Opin Endocrinol Diabetes Obes 2007;14:317–322.
63. Invitti C, Pecori Giraldi F, De Martin M, Cavagnini F. Diagnosis and management of Cushing's syndrome: results of an Italian multicentre study. Study Group of the Italian Society of Endocrinology on the Pathophysiology of the Hypothalamic–Pituitary–Adrenal Axis. J Clin Endocrinol Metab 1999;84:440–448.
64. Tabarin A, Laurent F, Catargi B, Olivier-Puel F, Lescene R, Berge J, Galli FS, Drouillard J, Roger P, Guerin J. Comparative evaluation of conventional and dynamic magnetic resonance imaging of the pituitary gland for the diagnosis of Cushing's disease. Clin Endocrinol (Oxf) 1998;3:285–286.
65. Granberg D, Sundin A, Janson ET, Oberg K, Skogseid B, Westlin JE. Octreoscan in patients with bronchial carcinoid tumours. Clin Endocrinol (Oxf) 2003;59:793–799.
66. Eriksson B, Bergstrom M, Sundin A, Juhlin C, Orlefors H, Oberg K, Langstrom B. The role of PET in localization of neuroendocrine and adrenocortical tumors, Ann NY Acad Sci 2002;970:159–169.
67. Orlefors H, Sundin A, Garske U, Juhlin C, Oberg K, Skogseid B, Langstrom B, Bergstrom M, Eriksson B. Whole-Body ^{11}C-5-Hydroxytryptophan positron emission tomography as a universal imaging technique for neuroendocrine tumors: comparison with somatostatin receptor scintigraphy and computed tomography. J Clin Endocrinol Metab 2005;90:3392–3400.
68. Nanni C, Fanti S, Rubello D. ^{18}F-DOPA PET and PET/CT. J Nucl Med 2007;48:1577–1579.
69. Gabriel M, Decristoforo C, Kendler D, Dobrozemsky G, Heute D, Uprimny C, Kovacs P, Von Guggenberg E, Bale R, Virgolin IJ. ^{68}Ga-DOTA-Tyr3-octreotide PET in neuroendocrine tumors: comparison with somatostatin receptor scintigraphy and CT. J Nucl Med 2007;48:508–518.
70. Buchmann I, Henze M, Engelbrecht S. Comparison of $^{(68)}$Ga-DOTATOC PET and $^{(111)}$In-DTPAOC (Octreoscan) SPECT in patients with neuroendocrine tumours. Eur J Nucl Med Mol Imaging 2007;34:1617–1626.
71. Mantero F, Scaroni CM, Albiger NM. Cyclic Cushing's syndrome: an overview. Pituitary 2004;7:203–207.
72. Iacobone M, Albiger N, Scaroni C, Mantero F, Fassina A, Viel G, Frego M, Favia G. The role of unilateral adrenalectomy in ACTH-independent macronodular adrenal hyperplasia (AIMAH). World J Surg 2008;32:882–889.
73. Barbetta L, Dall'Asta C, Tomei G, Locatelli M, Giovanelli M, Ambrosi B. Assessment of cure and recurrence after pituitary surgery for Cushing's disease. Acta Neurochirurgia (Wien) 2001; 143:477–481.
74. Rees DA, Hanna FW, Davies JS, Mills RG, Vafidis J, Scanlon MF. Long-term follow-up results of transsphenoidal surgery for Cushing's disease in a single center using strict criteria for remission. Clin Endocrinol 2002;56:541–551.
75. McCance DR, Gordon DS, Fannin TF, Hadden DR, Kennedy L, Sheridan B, Atkinson AB. Assessment of endocrine function after transsphenoidal surgery for Cushing's disease. Clin Endocrinol 1993;38:79–86.
76. Streeten DH, Anderson GH Jr, Dalakos T, Joachimpillai AD. Intermittent hypercortisolism: a disorder strikingly prevalent after hypophysial surgical procedures. Endocr Pract 1997;3:123–129.
77. Lacroix A, Hamet P, Boutin JM. Leuprolide acetate therapy in luteinizing hormone-dependent Cushing's syndrome. N Engl J Med 1999;341:1577–1581.
78. Reznik Y, Allali-Zerah V, Chayvialle JA, Leroyer R, Leymarie P, Travert G, Lebrethon MC, Budi I, Balliere AM, Mahoudeau J. Food-dependent Cushing's syndrome mediated by aberrant adrenal sensitivity to gastric inhibitory polypeptide. N Engl J Med 1992;327:981–986.
79. Lebrethon MC, Avallet O, Reznik Y, Archambeaud F, Combes J, Usdin TB, Narboni G, Mahoudeau J, Saez JM. Food-dependent Cushing's syndrome: characterization and functional role of gastric inhibitory polypeptide receptor in the adrenals of three patients. J Clin Endocrinol Metab 1998;83:4514–4519.
80. Albiger NM, Occhi G, Mariniello B, Iacobone M, Favia G, Fassina A, Faggian D, Mantero F, Scaroni C. Food-dependent Cushing's syndrome: from molecular characterization to therapeutical results. Eur J Endocrinol 2007;157:771–778.

Index